PROGRESS IN OBSTETRICS AND GYNAECOLOGY

PROGRESS IN OBSTETRICS AND GYNAECOLOGY

Contents of Volume 7

PROGRESS IN OBSTETRICS AND GYNAECOLOGY
Volume Eight

EDITED BY

JOHN STUDD MD FRCOG

Consultant Obstetrician and Gynaecologist
King's College Hospital and Dulwich Hospital;
King's College Hospital Medical School, London

CHURCHILL LIVINGSTONE
EDINBURGH LONDON MELBOURNE AND NEW YORK 1990

CHURCHILL LIVINGSTONE
Medical Division of Longman Group UK Limited

Distributed in the United States of America by
Churchill Livingstone Inc., 1560 Broadway, New York,
N.Y. 10036, and by associated companies, branches and
representatives throughout the world.

First published 1990

ISBN 0-443-04170-9

ISSN 0261-0140

British Library Cataloguing in Publication Data
Progress in obstetrics and gynaecology.
   1. Gynaecology—Periodicals   2. Obstetrics
  —Periodicals
   618.05   RG1

**Library of Congress Cataloging in Publication
Data**
Progress in obstetrics and gynaecology.
   Includes indexes.
   1. Obstetrics—Collected works.   2. Gynecology—
Collected works.   1. Studd, John [DNLM:
1. Gynecology—Periodicals.   2. Obstetrics—
Periodicals.   W1 PR675PJ
RG39.P73   618   81-21699

Printed in Great Britain at The Bath Press, Avon

Preface

On reflection the most significant event in obstetrics and gynaecology during the last decade was not assisted conception, or the improvement in pre-natal diagnosis, or the advances in gynaecological endocrinology but the beginning of the HIV epidemic. It is a sobering thought that at the time of the first volume of *Progress in Obstetrics and Gynaecology* (or if you need a more substantial historical event, the inauguration of Ronald Reagan as President of the USA), AIDS had not been described. Now it is certain that the male disease of the 1980s will become equally a disease of women and children in the 1990s.

Even now more than 10% of notified new cases of HIV infection in the United Kingdom are women, many unaware that they (or their consorts!) were in a high risk group. The majority of sero-positive adults currently picked up by the Blood Transfusion Service are women because the high risk men have been screened out by the preliminary questionnaire.

Worldwide, AIDS is most commonly a heterosexual disease passed on by vaginal intercourse. No doubt promiscuity is important and vulvo-vaginal ulceration is a factor in African epidemiology but the rules of the disease in Africa, where even WHO have stopped worrying about over-population, are unlikely to be very different in Europe. Africa is merely 10 or so years ahead of us.

It has to be said that our specialty is fundamentally concerned, even pre-occupied, with sexual intercourse and procreation yet we have made little comment on the control and treatment of the disease in gynaecological patients or in mothers and babies. The high risk woman for HIV infection is simply somebody who has had unprotected vaginal intercourse. These women are hardly a rarity in our clinics but how many are screened for HIV? Whether we operate for cervical pathology, pelvic inflammatory disease, infertility or even deliver babies we are in a danger area for HIV but virtually none of us screen antenatal or pre-operative patients. Why not? It is unlikely that knowledge of sero-positivity will decrease the incidence of needlestick injuries for the surgeon with its less than 0.5% risk of infection but the patient herself needs to know.

Contemporary ethical standards, albeit a most flexible measure of propriety, would condemn screening without informed consent and two important chapters in *Volume 8* outline these arguments and the manner in which counselling can be undertaken in our clinics. It is a matter of some shame that we still have no idea of the incidence of HIV infection in an antenatal population and even the planned national anonymous antenatal screening programme allows patients to opt out. These may be those at highest risk. It is hard to justify the vast expense of this planned and predictable misinformation.

Apart from the need for epidemiological information the individual patient has the right to know her HIV status for many reasons. There are now many advances which have improved the prognosis of AIDS and it is better for the patient and her baby to be under the care of a specialist when the HIV infection turns into the clinical illness. In this way opportunistic infections will be dealt with promptly. As 25% of babies born to HIV positive mothers will be infected it is also desirable that women are able to make an informed decision about pregnancy before the event. The patient may also wish to change her lifestyle and inform appropriate persons about the infection. Perhaps the most important reason for the asymptomatic woman to know her status is the clear evidence that anti-viral drugs such as AZT delay the onset of AIDS in HIV positive adults.

As gynaecologists we can have some pride that we have so often been at the forefront of important medical and social issues. We led and the others followed. No other specialty reports their failures as a confidential triennial report. No other specialty took on the practice of contraceptive and abortion reform. We have even attempted the near impossible task of educating physicians and psychiatrists about the devastating effects of oestrogen deficiency. The examples are too numerous to go on but in our responsibility to women who may unknowingly be infected by HIV we have been in a deep sleep!

London, UK   J.S.
1990

Contributors

Hossam Ibrahim Abdalla MB ChB MRCOG
Director, Fertility and Endocrine Centre, Lister Hospital, London, UK

Sabaratnam Arulkumaran DCH FRCS(E) MRCOG
Senior Lecturer and Consultant, Department of Obstetrics and Gynaecology, The National
University Hospital, Singapore

Rod Baber MB BS BPharm MRCOG FRACOG
Visiting Obstetrician and Gynaecologist, The Royal North Shore Hospital of Sydney, St
Leonards, New South Wales, Australia

Carol M. Black MD FRCP
Consultant Rheumatologist, Rheumatology Unit, Royal Free Hospital, London, UK

Robert Bor DPhil CPsychol AFBPsS
District AIDS Counsellor, Principal Clinical Psychologist and Family Therapist, Royal Free
Hospital, London, UK

Mark Brincat PhD MRCOG
Senior Registrar, St George's Hospital Medical School, London, UK

Linda Cardozo MD MRCOG
Consultant Obstetrician and Gynaecologist, King's College Hospital, London, UK

Jonathan Carter MBBS DipRACOG FRACOG
Senior Registrar, King George V Hospital, and Royal Prince Alfred Hospital, Camperdown,
New South Wales, Australia

K. K. Chan FRCS FRCOG
Consultant Gynaecologist, The Birmingham and Midland Hospital for Women, Birmingham,
UK

James C. Dornan MD MRCOG
Senior Lecturer and Consultant, Queen's University, Belfast, Northern Ireland, UK

John Guillebaud MA FRCS(E) FRCOG
Medical Director, Margaret Pyke Centre for Study and Training in Family Planning,
London, UK

Kevin P. Hanretty MB ChB MRCOG
Lecturer and Honorary Senior Registrar, The Queen Mother's Hospital, Glasgow, UK

Ingemar Ingemarsson MD
Associate Professor, Department of Obstetrics and Gynaecology, University of Lund, Sweden

Margaret Anne Johnson MD MRCP
Consultant Physician, Royal Free Hospital, London, UK

Nicholas Johnson BMedSci BM BS MRCOG FRCS
Lecturer in Obstetrics and Gynaecology, St James's Hospital, Leeds, UK

Richard H. J. Kerr-Wilson FRCS(Ed) MRCOG
Consultant Obstetrician and Gynaecologist, St Paul's Hospital, Cheltenham, UK

Richard J. Lilford MRCOG MRCP PhD
Professor, and Head, Department of Obstetrics and Gynaecology, St James's University Hospital, Leeds, UK

Salvatore Lupoli MD
Research Fellow, Department of Rheumatology, Royal Free Hospital, London, UK

I. Z. MacKenzie MA MD FRCOG
Clinical Reader in Obstetrics and Gynaecology, University of Oxford; Honorary Consultant, Nuffield Department of Obstetrics and Gynaecology, John Radcliffe Hospital, Oxford, UK

Peter McParland MRCOG MRCPI
Senior Registrar, Hammersmith Hospital, London, UK

Adam L. Magos MB BS BSc MD MRCOG
Clinical Lecturer and Honorary Senior Registrar, Nuffield Department of Obstetrics and Gynaecology, University of Oxford, John Radcliffe Hospital, Oxford, UK

Riva Miller BA(Soc Science) Institute of Family Therapy
Senior Social Worker, AIDS Counselling Co-ordinator and Honorary Senior Lecturer, Royal Free Hospital, London, UK

L. M. Mynors-Wallis MA MRCP MRCPsych
Registrar, The Maudsley Hospital, London, UK

Robert Norman BSc MD FRCOG FCOG(SA) MRCPath
Senior Lecturer in Obstetrics and Gynaecology, University of Adelaide, Queen Elizabeth Hospital, Woodville, South Australia

C. W. E. Redman MD FRCS(Ed) MRCOG
Lecturer, University Department of Obstetrics and Gynaecology, Dudley Road Hospital, Birmingham, UK

Wendy D. Savage BA MB BCh FRCOG
Senior Lecturer in Obstetrics and Gynaecology, Joint Department of General Practice and Primary Care, St Bartholomew's Hospital and The London Hospital Medical College; Honorary Consultant, The London Hospital, London, UK

D. A. J. Sim MB MRCOG
Registrar, Department of Obstetrics and Gynaecology, Queen's University, Belfast, Northern Ireland, UK

Peter Stewart MA BM BCh MRCOG
Consultant Obstetrician and Gynaecologist, Department of Obstetrics and Gynaecology, Northern General Hospital, Sheffield, UK

John Studd MD FRCOG
Consultant Obstetrician and Gynaecologist, King's College Hospital, and Dulwich Hospital, London, UK

Chris Sutton MA MB BCh FRCOG
Consultant Obstetrician and Gynaecologist, Royal Surrey County Hospital, Guildford, UK

Yunus Tayob MA MB MRCOG
Lecturer, Academic Department of Obstetrics and Gynaecology, Royal Free Hospital, London, UK

Janet Treasure PhD MRCP MRCPsych
Senior Lecturer, Institute of Psychiatry, Denmark Hill, London, UK

Z. Van Der Spuy MB ChB PhD MRCOG
Senior Lecturer and Head of the Gynaecological Endocrine Laboratory and Service, Department of Obstetrics and Gynaecology, Observatory, Cape, South Africa

Eboo Versi MA DPhil MB BChir MRCOG
Senior Registrar, Department of Obstetrics and Gynaecology, The London Hospital, London, UK

Judith B. Weaver MD FRCS FRCOG
Consultant Obstetrician, Birmingham Maternity Hospital, Birmingham, UK

Alison Webster BSc MB BS MRCPath
Lecturer in Virology, Royal Free Hospital School of Medicine, London, UK

Martin J. Whittle MD FRCOG FRCP (Glasg.)
Consultant Obstetrician and Perinatologist, The Queen Mother's Hospital, Glasgow, UK

Contents

PART THREE: GYNAECOLOGY

PART ONE

General

1. Women in obstetrics and gynaecology

Wendy Savage

Since the first woman to qualify in medicine in England in 1865, Elizabeth Garrett Anderson, faced opposition from many doctors and medical students, who refused to be taught with her (Manton 1965), the position of women has improved. When the NHS was introduced in 1948 there was no difference in pay and conditions of service, although it has taken another 40 years for it to be accepted that a widower's pension should be paid to men whose doctor wives predeceased them, whilst a widow's pension has been paid from the outset.

However, women are under-represented at the top of the profession, as consultants, GP principals, BMA negotiators, top medical civil servants and on the councils of the Royal Colleges who have the power to change training requirements and speak on behalf of the profession. They are less likely to hold merit awards (Bruggen & Bourne 1982) and more likely than men to hold non-career posts, such as in the community health services, despite the fact that studies of women graduates have shown that women have been more intellectually successful as students and have gained more post-graduate qualifications (Ward 1981, Aird & Silver 1971). Whilst this might be due to the woman's own choice of putting her family before her career, many women who have reached the top of the hospital hierarchy have experienced discrimination because of their sex (Allen 1988, RCOG Working Party 1987). Comments such as 'Poor dears, they are at the mercy of their biology' are still made by senior surgeons when asked why so few women reach the top in this specialty (personal communication 1981, 1988). Lorber (1984) describes how the system of patronage favours young men compared with women.

As a consequence of this male-dominated power structure (no different from other professions or other institutions in this country, i.e. there are only 6% of MPs who are women in the current parliament), the way that obstetrics and gynaecology is organized is based on the way that men operate and the way men think is best for their female clientele. As Dora Russell said: 'I've seen more clearly why men are more conventional than women. Because, simply, the conventions suit them and are made for them' (Russell 1980).

The training programme does not take into account the likelihood that

3

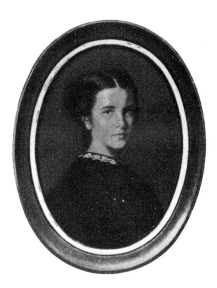

Fig. 1.1   Elizabeth Garrett Anderson LSA, portrait by Laura Herford in 1866. This was painted soon after her qualification. She was 29–30 years old. Courtesy of the Elizabeth Garrett Anderson Hospital for Women, London.

women will want to have children at the optimal biological time, i.e. between 20 and 35, and the demands of this programme have increased with changes in practice to make it almost intolerable to both sexes (Frazer 1987). In my view it is unrealistic to expect young doctors to continue working 80 or 100 hours a week when the country as a whole is moving towards a 35-hour week, and neither will younger consultants be prepared to work in this way. In Sweden, and more recently in New Zealand, junior doctors have negotiated a 40-hour week, and the present campaign in the UK (January 1989) looks more likely to succeed than the repeated attempts over the last 15 years which have merely resulted in a statement of intent by the DHSS to abolish one in two rotas—without the necessary funding or changes in the career structure to achieve this.

Isobel Allen's recent study, funded by the DHSS, of three cohorts of doctors showed that the youngest of these were the most likely to wish that they had never taken up medicine as a career, and over 40% of both men and women expressed this dissatisfaction (Allen 1988).

WOMEN IN OBSTETRICS AND GYNAECOLOGY TODAY

At the present time 12% of consultant posts in England and Wales in obstetrics and gynaecology are held by women, a proportion that has not increased over 25 years. During this time the proportion of women qualifying as doctors has risen from 25% to 45%, and the percentage of all women in consultant posts who are obstetricians and gynaecologists has fallen (Lefford 1986) despite the fact that of a number (3.3%) of those choosing this specialty, the proportion of women has risen from 40.6% in 1974–1980 to 48.9% in 1984 (Ellin & Parkhouse 1986). So why have they not reached their goal?

Despite reassuring statements made by health ministers in parliament (Hansard 1986), the situation is unlikely to change rapidly in the next decade unless radical action is taken by the profession now. In the first 6 months of 1988, 12 new consultants were appointed, only one of whom was a woman. Of consultants appointed between 1980 and 1985, only 12.5% were women and of honorary posts only 6.3% (DHSS 1987).

Almost 45% of SHOs are women (many SHOs of both sexes plan to do general practice), but as the seniority of the post increases, so does the proportion of women fall. 30% of registrars are female (although if overseas doctors are excluded the proportion of women rises to 40%) (Hansard 1986).

The grade which is the gateway to consultant status is that of senior registrar, and of these posts 76% were held by men in 1986. 21.3% of senior registrar appointments between 1980 and 1985 were given to women (DHSS 1987).

The average age at appointment to a consultant post is 37, and most consultants remain in the post to which they were appointed for their entire working life. This does have some advantages, particularly in providing stability in these days of constant managerial turmoil, but there are considerable disadvantages as well, making the system inflexible and difficult to change. For women who marry prior to their consultant appointment and especially if they marry another doctor, it can be very limiting. As far as planning is concerned, fluctuations in the needs of the population because of immigration or an increase in old or young women in the local population are difficult to deal with.

By contrast, in the USA doctors become specialists at a younger age and there is considerable job mobility after this. Despite a slower influx of women into medicine in the first half of this century compared with the UK, the effect of the women's movement in the 1960s has been to rapidly increase the proportion of women entering medicine and in the last decade those choosing obstetrics/gynaecology. Between 1976 and 1985 the proportion of women residents in this speciality rose from 14.6% to 38.8%, with 42.4% of first-year residents being women in 1985 (Hayashi & McIntyre-Seltman 1987).

To obtain a post in a teaching hospital an extra qualification is usually needed; the FRCS is now less favoured and an MD is increasingly acceptable, and a prerequisite for academic posts (Studd 1983).

The aims and objectives of the present system are not defined and it is assumed that the traditional type of post, combining obstetrics and gynaecology, with the conventional male occupant—active, busy and usually involved in private practice—is the only way that the service can be provided. For a woman planning to enter the specialty and for a sensitive man, the available role models are hard to emulate, and the demanding hours and lack of sleep, combined with the lack of job satisfaction entailed by the way that the work is organized, may lead to dissatisfaction with the training programme.

On both sides of the Atlantic, the years of training are physically demanding, and because of the nature of the job, require much on-call work living in the hospital. In the UK, in contrast to the shorter USA residency programme, there are frequent job moves and both sexes perceive the programme as disruptive of normal social and family life (RCOG 1987).

Women in particular, who wish to have children at the time they have learnt and seen from their daily work experience is most likely to be trouble free, may feel that the career demands are incompatible with achieving this aim. Many consultant obstetricians and managers are not positive about job-sharing or part-time training posts. The PM(79)3 Senior Registrar scheme is byzantine in its complexity—worthy of the most recondite of our civil servants—the woman's application is not certain to succeed, and takes an enormous amount of the applicant's time to organize. Very few women have succeeded in obtaining these posts in obstetrics and gynaecology: currently there are nine in training, and three of five gained manpower approval this year (but no funds as yet) out of 253 posts across the specialities. Criticism of part-time training in medicine has been voiced by some doctors (Burke & Black 1983).

In addition, women as patients are increasingly expressing their concern with the quality of the service offered to them, and more are asking to be seen by a gynaecologist of their own sex. In the USA this is accepted, and almost half of those on residency programmes are now women. In a presidential address in 1987 to the American Gynecological and Obstetrical Society, the positive aspects of their contribution was stressed (Hayashi & McIntyre-Seltman 1987).

The British response to what was seen as 'the problem' of the increasing number of women medical graduates was to set up a working party to look at the role of women doctors in obstetrics and gynaecology (the only college committee in which there was a majority of women). This group decided to do a survey of medical students and of doctors who had taken part 1 or 2 of the MRCOG examination, some of whom were now consultants. Significantly, the RCOG did not commission an outside body such as the Institute for Social Studies into Medical Care, with the necessary experience and expertise to do a survey efficiently. When the two hardworking gynaecologists who had conducted the survey presented their results to council, it took almost 2 years for the lengthy report to be reduced to a 16-page booklet for circulation to the Members and Fellows.

The RCOG Working Party thought that a ratio of one woman in four gynaecologists would enable women seeking care to have a choice of a woman gynaecologist, rather than the one in eight that it has been for the past 25 years. The idea that this might not be sufficient to cope with the demand was not mooted in the report, but even equal proportions may not be sufficient if women really could exercise choice (WNC 1984).

The council's recommendations to improve the situation were that the DHSS should increase the number of part-time training posts for women.

They apparently accepted without any question that many women did not aspire to the role of consultant and welcomed the new staff grade proposed in 'Achieving a Balance'. These attitudes were similar to those expressed in their report on 'Manpower in Obstetrics and Gynaecology' some years before, where the idea of a subconsultant grade was welcomed for posts such as medical gynaecology and ultrasound, thought to be suitable posts for women by the all-male committee.

This report was rejected by the Medical Women's Federation, who also expressed their disappointment at the 1987 council memorandum. It seems unlikely that, with the changing roles and expectations of women in society, large numbers of women now planning to do obstetrics and gynaecology will accept subconsultant posts.

The dissatisfaction expressed by 20% of those practising obstetrics and gynaecology, both male and female, and the 37% drop-out rate after the MRCOG were noted, but the clear message that the demands of the specialty were disruptive of family and personal life were not addressed. The president in his preface to the report did note that part-time consultant posts were needed but did not stress that men and women had similar wishes, with a minority—just over a fifth—wishing to work full time and 29% of men and 25% of women wanting to work 1–6 sessions. Those sampled had obtained part 2 MRCOG between 1969 and 1984, but the response rate was less than ideal, and it would have been better to re-circulate the sample during the 2-year period and improve the response rate, rather than to present the findings and dismiss the results as inadequate, as I have heard done by some council members.

This may appear to be a trivial point, but the response of a dominant group to change is usually to resist this. The history of the working party set up to look at the *role* of women in obstetrics and gynaecology is an example of how institutions maintain the status quo.

WOMEN FELLOWS OF THE RCOG

Dame Louise McIlroy, Professor of Obstetrics and Gynaecology at the Royal Free Hospital, was a founder Fellow of the Royal College of Obstetricians and Gynaecologists in 1929, and co-opted on to the first council. She had worked as a surgeon in France during World War I, for which she received the 'croix de guerre', and she also served in Serbia, Salonika and Constantinople.

Between 1929 and 1969, only 18 women were elected to the Fellowship, just over 5% of all Fellows. The first woman professor in Scotland, and five who founded medical schools in India, were honoured for their work, but despite the availability of domestic help, only one fellow was listed as being married with children.

The first woman to be elected rather than co-opted to the council was Mrs Hilda Lloyd in 1939, and she became the first (and up until now, only) woman president of the RCOG, in 1949. William Fletcher Shaw recorded the ambivalence felt by some at this 'revolutionary' appointment, but concluded that she was 'as effective a president as any' (Thompson 1988).

Now about 20% of Fellows in the London area, and less than 15% in Scotland and the rest of England and Wales, are women and they are under-represented as chairs of college committees and on council. Women appear to be willing to serve on committees, examine and sit on council but rarely seem to reach the positions of power. Without doing a study it is difficult to know why this is so, or why it seems that with increasing numbers in the profession, fewer reach the important positions in the college which influence policy and training.

There is now one woman amongst the 23 College Regional Advisors, but the suggestion that each region should have a woman, who has succeeded in combining the roles of consultant with marriage and motherhood, to advise women seeking careers advice was not welcomed by council—including some of the female members!

There is an equivalent female version of the Gynaecological Travellers Club but this has not been a successful pressure group for women trainees or women as patients.

WOMEN IN ACADEMIC OBSTETRICS AND GYNAECOLOGY

One wonders why women such as Coralie Rendle-Short, Una Lister and Jill Everett, who have held chairs and run departments competently in Uganda, Nigeria and Papua New Guinea respectively, did not obtain such a position in the UK. At present there is no female Professor of Obstetrics and Gynaecology in this country or Australia, New Zealand or the USA, and only one in the Scandinavian countries.

The proportion of women consultants at senior lecturer grade is similar to that for NHS consultants, but over a third of schools do not have a woman as teacher and role model for students, in the academic unit. I have the impression that there is a tendency for women academics to become the person who looks after the students and the teaching. Whilst respectable research is done by many women, only the late Anne Anderson stands out in my mind as an exceptional scientist over the last 20 years in the UK. However, I do not believe that this is the reason for the lack of women heading academic departments, as there are a number of professors who have not been noted for academic excellence in our specialty.

Is it, as Charles Douglas said at the RSM some years ago, that 'women are too sensible to want to be professors', or is it because women do not fit into the system designed by men? Do they opt out of the game or are they never really seen as players?

In the present university climate, where government funding is decreasing, academic posts are being lost, tenure is under threat and funds for research are increasingly hard to obtain, the honorary consultant contract and probationary 3-year appointment offered to many senior lecturers does not look attractive to trainees of either sex. However, if you can choose your post and your professor, the opportunities to influence teaching and modify the curriculum are exciting. Research may also change attitudes and practice as well as being intellectually fulfilling.

In the USA in 1986, 19.2% of obstetricians and gynaecologists who were faculty members were women compared with only 8% women amongst those who were board-certified, so this seems a more popular option for women there (Pearse et al 1987).

WOMEN AS CONSULTANTS IN OBSTETRICS AND GYNAECOLOGY

There is no research in this country which addresses the issue of the effect of the gender of the gynaecologist on their practice or the type of service provided. Some women have survived the training programme and adjusted to the system by becoming 'honorary men', and the expectation of the woman client or patient that her complaints will be understood and dealt with more sympathetically by a woman doctor is not always fulfilled.

However, Frey in Sweden surveyed male and female doctors and found differences in their attitudes towards patients which would support this idea, and Walton, who studied medical students during their psychiatry attachment, found the female students to be more conscientious, more caring, better at speaking to patients (and interestingly more likely to question their teachers). A study that I undertook at the London Hospital in 1978–1979 showed that, even as early as the second clinical year, male students responded in a negatively stereotyped way towards women as patients and as fellow students. The women students were more likely to respond positively to statements about birth and women's choice than the men after the obstetrics and gynaecology course.

Anecdotally, women's hospitals staffed by women doctors, such as the South London Hospital for Women and the Elizabeth Garrett Anderson Hospital, are said to have had a more relaxed atmosphere which women and trainees like. It is a pity that there has never been a study to ascertain the differences between this kind of women-directed care and the standard male-directed care. Not only would it have been scientifically interesting but it would also have enabled the battle to retain this choice for women to be fought on the basis of objective rather than hearsay evidence. However, whether this would have kept the hospitals open as designed is debatable.

Women obstetricians and gynaecologists have been said to be more sympathetic, more conservative surgeons, and less likely to intervene in obstetric cases than men, but again, hard data are lacking in the UK. In the USA, one survey has shown that women residents were more likely than men to support abortion and contraception for teenagers, and be interested in health education for women (Margolis et al 1983), and another of practising obstetricians and gynaecologists showed that women were more likely to support abortion in certain circumstances than men (ACOG Poll 1985). Weisman et al (1987) found that, in a survey of 1420 recently qualified specialists, women were more likely to provide abortion services and less likely to perform amniocenteses or some types of infertility services. Dominighetti et al (1985) reported a lesser rate of hysterectomy amongst Swiss women gynaecologists compared with their male colleagues.

The woman gynaecologist who made an indelible impression on me as a trainee obstetrician and gynaecologist was Miss Kathleen Robinson. Her ability to remember details of patients she had not seen for months, her quiet compassion and energy, and the way she treated the women as equal partners in the consultation was very different from the style of my male undergraduate teachers. It was not until many years later when I was examining with her that I realized how many feminist ideas I had learnt from her—she never let students get away with a chauvinistic or patronizing remark, but she made her point without raising her voice, or being unjust or unkind.

As a woman gynaecologist I get referrals from GPs of women who do not want to see a man, and some of these women would rather die than be examined by a member of the opposite sex. Hard as one may find this to imagine, these women do exist, and many more would prefer to see a woman for gynaecological complaints. In a survey of 600 women in Tower Hamlets who were asked about their knowledge and experience of cervical screening, 64.4% admitted to being embarrassed during the procedure, and the older women, most at risk, were most likely to feel embarrassment (87%) (Schwartz et al 1989). A quarter gave 'ability to see a woman doctor' as their first suggestion as to how to increase the rate of uptake of screening.

Some women gynaecologists will not see women who request to see a woman doctor as they fear that they will find their practice overloaded with neurotic patients, but I find the same incidence of psychological symptoms as in women without this preference.

CAREER OPTIONS IN OBSTETRICS AND GYNAECOLOGY

The majority of consultant posts combine obstetrics and gynaecology in the traditional way, but with the specialization suggested by the RCOG into fetal medicine, oncology, reproductive medicine and gynaecological urology, a few posts have been created in which the consultant concentrates on labour ward or gynaecological surgery.

In the next decade one would expect to see more of these specialized posts with consultant status as, for example, the general physician and surgeon are being replaced by cardiologists, gastroenterologists, neurologists, haematologists or rectal, breast and endocrine surgeons. In radiology there are specialists in ultrasound or neuro-radiology, so one should not expect that an expert in ultrasound or medical gynaecology would be employed as a clinical assistant rather than as a consultant within the specialty of obstetrics and gynaecology.

One would hope that there would be more flexibility, so that some consultant posts are for a 5- or 7-year period. Then, during different times in a woman's life—or indeed a man's when family commitments are heavy—a less arduous post in terms of hours and time on call could be selected, and later, a different permanent post selected.

WELL WOMEN'S SERVICES/COMMUNITY GYNAECOLOGY

In Tower Hamlets we created a post from existing family planning and abortion sessions as Director of Well Women's Services. This woman has had clinical and administrative responsibility for the Day Care Abortion Service, the contraceptive services (including psychosexual services) and cervical screening for the district. This post was at Senior Clinical Medical Officer grade with honorary consultant status. In future such posts (and one was recently advertised in City and Hackney as Community Gynaecologist) should be at consultant grade. Ideally there should be one such post in each district to co-ordinate these services for women and, as has happened in our district, to set up menopause and post-abortion counselling clinics if necessary. Collaboration with the schools about sex and health education and information about young people's services is another important part of the job, as is liaison with the health promotion services. Responsibility for sterilization services might also be part of this post, and both in- and out-patient operating sessions would be necessary.

ULTRASOUND

In some districts there is a consultant in ultrasound who is responsible for organizing these services and providing some of the scanning for anomalies, gynaecological work or amniocentesis. The person may be trained in radiology or obstetrics and gynaecology, and if in the latter may take on fetoscopy or genetic counselling or combine the work with obstetric sessions. This type of job may well appeal to women if it is accepted as of consultant status and is not a clinical assistant post of secondary status to combined posts.

MEDICAL GYNAECOLOGY

The same proviso applies. Some women have clinical assistant posts in infertility clinics or menopause clinics, but there is no reason why a full-time or sessional consultant post dealing with the wide range of procedures associated with modern infertility treatment and/or menopausal problems should not be a consultant one.

COLPOSCOPY

With the growth of this method of assessing abnormal cytology, there is, in some districts, enough work to create a full-time post for a consultant in colposcopy, who might also be the person responsible for the cervical screening in the district. She would liaise with the nearest gynaecological oncologist, be responsible for counselling women with abnormal smears and might have one or two in-patient operating sessions in gynaecology.

PRIVATE PRACTICE

There is a great demand for women gynaecologists in the private sector, and even without an NHS appointment, women can succeed. They tend to specialize in fertility control, colposcopy and medical gynaecology or psychosexual work. Private obstetrics is less widely practised but there is at least one woman practising successfully in partnership with a man and associated with a hospital in which active birth is encouraged.

OBSTETRIC POSTS

These tend to be centred on labour ward, and the specialty of perinatologist, in which the doctor is both obstetrician and neonatologist, as happens in some places across the Atlantic, has not been accepted here despite the attractions of such a combination of skills. Community obstetrics, in which the doctor works with GPs and midwives in the community and cares for women in hospital as necessary, is a new concept, although clinical assistant posts in antenatal care are quite common.

TRAINING

The present training programme is too long, entails much job mobility, and is insufficiently planned and co-ordinated. In this country 12–15 years after graduation is spent before a doctor becomes a consultant in obstetrics and gynaecology. In the USA, the residency programme is 4 years and then a year is spent in practice as board-certified during which time records are kept, and if oral examination on this practice is satisfactory the doctor is board-registered and free to practise. There is further training for specialization of 2–3 years for those wishing to work in teaching hospitals, but the majority of specialists are in practice by the time they are aged 30 years. The residency programme is in one place, and whilst arduous, averaging a working week of 80 hours with only 6 weeks holiday in one year, has a more carefully worked out programme of tuition and experience than in the British system based on apprenticeship.

PREGNANCY DURING TRAINING

Women may decide to become pregnant during their training programme, and Sayres et al (1986) looked at the incidence of this in Boston. They found that few women gave up their training, and that on average the women worked up to term and took only 5 weeks maternity leave. They suggested that programme directors should expect some pregnancies and plan for these, and thought that more generous maternity leave should be available. Grunebaum et al (1987) sent questionnaires to 1024 board-certified obstetricians and analysed the outcomes of 454 pregnancies which had occurred before, during and after obstetric residency training. They found that the mean birth weight of infants born to primiparous women was lower during and after residency than before, and that the rate of low birth weight and IUGR was increased in infants of all women born during residency, although the rate of pre-term delivery was unchanged. They discussed methods of reducing the workload of the pregnant resident and concluded that 'further exploration of the question of what to do when pregnancy occurs during residency and how to protect the fetus needs to be undertaken'.

In this country, leave from 28 weeks gestation until 6 weeks post delivery is allowed, but this causes problems for the department which does not receive extra money to pay for a locum and increases the stress on the woman who may feel she is letting the team down and who may continue to work (as I did myself) until in labour. Questions about pregnancy and plans for this are considered discriminatory under the Equal Opportunities Act, but guesses about a woman's intentions may weigh against her at interview, and not infrequently women are asked questions about their contraception and plans for a family in spite of the law. The regulations about maternity leave and pay are complicated and many NHS employers seem reluctant to give the woman her entitlement, another factor which may inhibit a woman from continuing with her chosen career.

PART-TIME TRAINING

This can be arranged with the approval of the RCOG and the agreement of sympathetic consultants and managers. Job-shares have been managed in a few places, notably Edinburgh and Newcastle, at Senior Registrar level. Criticisms by male chauvinists about part-time consultants being of little use can easily be countered by reference to the part-time NHS/private practice consultant. The RCOG Working Party study found that only a quarter of both sexes wanted to work full time as consultants, and about a fifth wanted to work between one and six sessions. If medical training was an ordinary 40-hour week, full-time post women could manage that and a family, but it is the fact that trainess spend so many years doing 60–80 hour weeks that makes part-time training necessary for some women.

THE FUTURE

Women should join together and, if practicable, recruit men to lobby the RCOG to change the training programme. Representatives from Women In Gynaecology and Obstetrics (WIGO) met with the president of the college and several officers in September, 1988, but so far our request for a working party to look at the training programme has not been granted.

The training programmes should be shortened to 5 or 6 years and should take place in one or two hospitals which are close together. One year would be spent doing an elective, as at present, in a related discipline and the part 2 MRCOG would be taken at the end of year 2 or 3. The training would be more systematic, with more time for tuition, reading and analysing the literature in a formal way.

There would be much less service work, particularly of an unsupervised nature. The log books being used by trainees at present could be used to move in this direction.

A prescribed amount of time would be spent or experience would be gained in the various sub-specialties. Some people would take out time after year 1 or 2 in order to do an MD, and those wishing to become teaching hospital consultants would do further training after accreditation. This would seem to fit in with the Plan for Action document produced by the DHSS as part of its 'Achieving a Balance' package.

This scheme would require more consultants, but in my view the present anxiety about litigation would best be solved by having more consultants responsible for fewer patients and doing more work themselves. If differential subscriptions are going to become the norm, it seems inevitable that consultant salaries will become less standard and related to hours of work and time spent on-call.

Women should expect to hold half the training and obtain half the new consultant posts in obstetrics and gynaecology by the year 2000, but this will not happen unless we act now. When one reads of the quiet determination of Elizabeth Garrett Anderson to become a doctor, and how she practised obstetrics and gynaecology in the face of personal abuse and outright opposition over 100 years ago, surely now that women make up 45% of medical graduates we can work together to change the training programme so that women patients will have the choices that they want, and women doctors will achieve their career aims and fulfil their potential.

The attitudes expressed in 1861 when the Middlesex Hospital medical students decided that Elizabeth Garrett was a threat to them (she had just obtained a certificate of honour in each subject)—that mingling of the sexes in the same class 'was a dangerous innovation likely to lead to results of an unpleasant character' (Manton)—betrays an ambivalent attitude towards women that exists up until today (Savage 1986). Women can contribute much to obstetrics and gynaecology—so let's do it.

REFERENCES

ACOG Poll 1985 Ob-Gyns' support for abortion unchanged since 1971. Family Planning Perspectives 17: 275–277

Aird L A, Silver P J S 1971 Women doctors from the Middlesex Hospital Medical School 1947–1967. British Journal of Medical Education 5: 132–141

Allen 1988a Any room at the top. Policy Studies Institute, London

Allen 1988b Doctors and their careers. Policy Studies Institute, London

Bruggen P, Bourne S 1982 The distinction awards system in England and Wales 1980. British Medical Journal 294: 1577–1580

Burke C W, Black N A 1983 Part-Time Senior Registrars, Registrars and Senior House Officers in General Medicine and its Specialties: A Report to The Royal College of Physicians. British Medical Journal 287: 1040–1044

DHSS 1986 Hospital medical staffing: achieving a balance. HMSO, London

DHSS 1987 Hospital medical staffing: plan for action. HMSO, London

DHSS Medical Manpower Division 1987 Medical and dental staffing prospects in the NHS in England and Wales in 1986. Health Trends 19: 1–7

Domenighetti G, Luraschi P, Marazzi A 1985 Hysterectomy and sex of the gynaecologist (letter). New England Journal of Medicine 313: 1482

Ellin D J, Parkhouse D F, Parkhouse J 1986 Career preferences of doctors qualifying in the NHS in England & Wales. Health Trends 18: 59–62

Frazer M 1987 Personal view. British Medical Journal 294: 570

Frey Helen 1980 Swedish men and women doctors compared. Medical Education 14: 145–153

Grunebaum A, Minkoff H, Blake D 1987 Pregnancy among obstetricians: a comparison of births before, during and after residency. American Journal of Obstetrics and Gynecology 157: 79–83

Hayashi T, McIntyre-Seltman K 1987 The role of gender in an obstetrics and gynecology residency programme. American Journal of Obstetrics and Gynecology 156: 769–777

Lefford F 1987 Women doctors: a quarter century track record. Lancet i: 1254–1256

Lorber J 1984 Women physicians. Careers, status and power (monograph). Tavistock Publications, London

Manton J O 1965 Elizabeth Garrett Anderson. Butler & Tanner, Frome

Margolis A J, Greenwood S, Heilbron D 1983 Survey of men and women residents entering United States obstetrics and gynaecology programs in 1981. American Journal of Obstetrics and Gynecology 146: 541–545

Pearse W, Fielden J, Sherline D 1987 Obstetric–Gynecologic Academic Manpower, 1986. Obstetrics and Gynecology 70: 403–405

Royal College of Obstetricians and Gynaecologists 1987 Memorandum of council on the role of women doctors in obstetrics and gynaecology. RCOG, London

Russell D 1980 The tamarisk tree, vol 2. Virago, London

Savage W, Tate P 1983 Medical students' attitudes to women: a sex-linked variable? Medical Education 17: 159–164

Savage W 1986 A savage enquiry: who controls childbirth? Virago, London

Sayres M, Wyshak G, Denterlein et al 1986 Pregnancy during residency. New England Journal of Medicine 314: 418–423

Schwartz M, Savage W, George J, Emohare L 1989 Community medicine. Cervical cytology: a failure of health education and medical organisation? (in press)

Studd J 1983 Obstetricians, gynaecologists & the FRCS. British Journal of Obstetrics and Gynaecology 90: 785–786

Thompson V 1988 Unpublished paper given at WIGO careers meeting (13.2.88). Royal Society of Medicine, London

Walton H J 1968 Sex differences in the ability and outlook of senior medical students. British Journal of Medical Education 2: 156–162

Ward A 1981 Careers of medical women (monograph). Medical Care Research Unit, Sheffield University

Weisman C, Nathanson C, Teitelbaum M, Chase G, King T 1987 Delivery of fertility control services by male and female obstetrician-gynaecologists. American Journal of Obstetrics and Gynecology 156: 464–469

Whitney R 1986 Hansard 13/3/86 col 1282. Women doctors (obstetrics and gynaecology). HMSO, London

Women's National Commission 1984 Women and the health service (monograph). The Cabinet Office, London SW1

2. Counselling for HIV screening in women

Riva Miller   Robert Bor

INTRODUCTION

This chapter sets out to describe an approach to counselling about AIDS in antenatal care. The HIV antibody test became available in 1985 and the issue of HIV testing in antenatal clinics followed from this (Hudson & Sharp 1988). Counselling has increasingly been recognized as an important aspect of the care of those with HIV infection, or those who have associated worries (Tedder 1988). Counselling is not a new task for staff in the antenatal clinic. On the contrary, genetic and infertility counselling and health education are inextricably linked to clinical care. Nor is screening a new task. Routine antenatal care involves screening for many conditions in both the mother and fetus. Using the approach to AIDS counselling described here it should be possible to integrate it into routine counselling of other issues. In this way it will not ultimately produce unwarranted stress for staff nor separate AIDS issues from comprehensive antenatal care (Bor et al 1988).

In the United Kingdom, the Department of Health and Social Security has issued guidelines stressing the importance of counselling in relation to testing for the HIV antibody. The World Health Organization also recognizes the role of counselling and health education in the prevention of transmission of HIV and the support of those infected, in all countries of the world.

The study of HIV in antenatal care can yield information about the incidence of the heterosexual spread of HIV; the effect on the mother's health of HIV and pregnancy, and subsequent pregnancies; the incidence of perinatal transmission and the health of the child; and the risks of HIV transmission associated with breast feeding (Novick & Rubinstein 1987).

Doctors may find that some mothers increasingly expect to be offered an HIV antibody test, if not at least to be counselled about AIDS when they first attend the antenatal clinic (Bradbeer 1989). Counselling has to be adapted to new information and to the evolving natural history of HIV infection. Ideally, AIDS should form an integral part of the discussion about other health-related issues with women. However, as the issues that emerge may be complicated and time consuming, there is a place for referral to specialist AIDS counsellors, in the same way as is already done for genetic counselling. In some cases, counselling may reveal other worries, such as in those who are frequently referred to as the 'worried well' (Bor et al 1989). Counselling is the remit of consultants, junior doctors, nurses, midwives, health visitors and general practitioners who have shared care.

The ideas and approach outlined are based on counselling in a clinical setting. AIDS counselling should be linked to clinical care, as, in addition to the many social, psychological, ethical and legal aspects, AIDS is a life-threatening illness (Miller & Bor 1988). There have been many views about HIV screening in antenatal clinics. A gap which remains in the literature is a procedure about *how* to counsel and *what* might be said about AIDS, in a clinical interview. Counselling is important because it will influence patients' decisions as to whether or not HIV antibody testing can be carried out.

In this chapter we will describe reasons for counselling, approaches to HIV screening in antenatal care, and examples of selected clinical cases.

WHY COUNSEL?

Counselling is important for those with AIDS/HIV infection and associated concerns because:

— There is no cure.
— AIDS is at present almost always fatal.
— HIV is infectious.
— Those most at risk are young and of childbearing age.
— HIV may be transmitted in-utero to the fetus.
— Information must be made available in a way which enables people to make informed decisions.
— There is often conflicting information.
— There are fears arising from uncertainty and incomplete knowledge.
— Co-ordination of care is needed because of the many medical specialities that might be involved in clinical and other care.
— If people are prepared for problems through counselling, some may be prevented, or their impact may be reduced.

At the beginning of the HIV epidemic there was little that could be offered in the way of medical treatment. Now, in 1989, those who are known to be anti-HIV positive can be offered clinical surveillance. This allows for early diagnosis and treatment of opportunistic infections which may improve survival and quality of life. Prophylactic treatment for specific infections is increasingly relevant in clinical care (Pinching 1988). The use of antiviral therapy for those who are anti-HIV positive and asymptomatic is currently being evaluated in clinical trials in the United Kingdom. Thus testing for HIV is becoming more relevant, with the emphasis increasingly on HIV infection in its asymptomatic phase.

DIFFERENT APPROACHES TO HIV SCREENING AND IMPLICATIONS FOR COUNSELLING

There are several approaches to HIV screening for women (Mills 1988):

1. *Anonymous testing.* Samples would be taken from all women and tested anonymously. Similar information could be obtained by screening neonatal cord blood or from samples taken for Guthrie testing. These results would only yield demographic and epidemiological data. The advantage of anonymous testing is that it would provide information to help develop services for those who are infected. It may also be the first necessary step in the introduction of more acceptable and routine HIV testing for women in antenatal care. The disadvantages of anonymous testing are that there is a very limited role for individual AIDS counselling, and it may be unwise clinically not to be able to identify and counsel a pregnant woman whose prognosis and that of her baby is poor (Johnson 1989).

2. *Routine HIV antibody testing with the option to 'opt out'.* All women would be counselled and tested unless they specifically request not to be. This is similar to scanning for fetal abnormalities. Those declining may be offered the option of being tested anonymously for the purposes of epidemiological data. The disadvantages of this approach are that all women, even those at very low risk, would need to be counselled, which may be time consuming in busy clinics. In addition, some people at higher risk might decline testing. The results may not be very useful for epidemiological purposes. The advantage of routine testing with consent is that it would be a way of screening and discussing HIV with all women attending the antenatal clinic.

3. *Women request the test ('opt in').* Under these circumstances women would be counselled and tested if they so wished, which is similar to screening and testing for Down's syndrome. It is important that requests for testing be accompanied by efforts to alert women to the availability and reasons for HIV antibody testing. This can be achieved by the distribution of leaflets in general practitioners' surgeries, antenatal and family planning clinics, and health centres. The advantages of this strategy are that counselling and testing would focus on those wishing to be tested. The main drawback is that some women who might be 'at risk' would not necessarily ask for the test, either because they do not want to know, or because they lack knowledge about it.

4. *Testing of 'high risk' women.* Women at high risk for HIV would be counselled and offered the test after taking a detailed medical and sexual history. This could be supplemented by questionnaires and leaflets. One advantage is that those admitting to a risk for HIV can be appropriately counselled. There are several disadvantages to this

approach. Some women may be unaware that their activities are risky. Others may not wish to disclose their risk. In addition, the person taking the history may not always have the necessary skills or knowledge to assess the nature and degree of risk.

5. *No testing in antenatal clinics.* HIV testing would only be carried out at alternative clinics, such as in genito-urinary medicine clinics and at special counselling and testing sites. The most important disadvantage of not testing at all in the antenatal clinic is that the counselling will not be linked to antenatal care facilities and thus may not always be able to offer the optimum information and support to pregnant women.

It seems inevitable that HIV screening will be eventually incorporated into the routine care of pregnant women. Counselling is essential to ensure adequate preparation for undergoing or declining the test. Where pre-test counselling for screening for fetal abnormalities has been neglected, the result has been a lack of information about such tests (Marteau et al 1988, Marteau et al, in press) and high levels of anxiety (Marteau et al 1988). If counselling and screening are not carefully implemented, similar consequences are likely, with a further possibility that some women may keep away from medical care and antenatal clinics. The epidemic, as far as heterosexual and perinatal transmission is concerned, will not be as effectively studied or controlled.

IMPLICATIONS OF AIDS FOR ANTENATAL CARE

The unique and specific issues about HIV infection in antenatal care are as follows:

— At present most women are *assumed* to be at low risk.
— HIV has a long latency and many patients will not have symptoms of infection.
— HIV is transmitted from male to female, and from female to male.
— HIV is transmitted through sexual activities (including anal and vaginal intercourse), and through blood products.
— HIV can be transmitted perinatally: in utero, in partum and post partum.
— HIV-infected women provide important information about heterosexual transmission.
— When women are found to be HIV antibody positive, their children and sexual partners must be considered for testing and clinical monitoring.
— Termination of pregnancy and fostering and adoption may have to be discussed in some cases. The babies of HIV-infected mothers should themselves be tested and followed up by paediatricians.

— There is practically no information about the effects of antiviral therapy on pregnant women and the fetus.
— Pre-test counselling and testing of women may help in preventing transmission of HIV to neonates and sexual partners.
— The timing of the HIV antibody test is important. There are fewer options for the obstetrician and mother if a positive result is found late in the course of pregnancy.
— Counselling about AIDS may 'rekindle' thoughts about past relationships, and this may be upsetting.
— Victims of rape and sexual abuse may also have to be counselled and tested for HIV.
— AIDS is co-terminus with death. Counselling about the test inevitably touches on fears of death.
— Counselling, or the offer of counselling, about AIDS may frighten some women, whilst others may regard such a discussion as insulting.
— There are infection control issues because of a high possibility of contact with infected blood and body fluids.
— Counselling for AIDS takes time, which is limited in busy antenatal clinics.
— There are still fears that insurance companies may place restrictions on women who are routinely counselled and tested in these settings. However, in general, *routine* screening with a negative result should not now affect insurance.

GUIDELINES FOR AIDS COUNSELLING

At its most basic, counselling is a conversation which includes the giving of information. A first step in AIDS counselling in the antenatal clinic is to talk about the HIV antibody test. The skills needed to do this are very similar to those already used to introduce other tests into antenatal clinics, such as maternal-serum alpha-fetoprotein screening to test for spina bifida and Down's syndrome. The interviews are time-limited and for this reason should be focused. In order to do this it can be helpful for staff in busy clinics to be guided by some basic principles: to follow a structure for the interview, as well as a protocol for HIV screening.

The most important principles of AIDS counselling are:

Assumptions should not be made about a patient's level of knowledge or risk about HIV. Making assumptions inhibits free discussion. The counselling conversation is best facilitated by a non-judgemental stance.

Complete reassurance cannot be given. There is, as yet, insufficient information to offer reassurance to women about the effect of HIV on their health and that of their baby.

The session should be focused in order to use the time available effectively. If the session is not focused, the patient may leave feeling more concerned and anxious. Unscheduled phone calls and visits from the patient may follow. Staff may then feel that they have failed in their task. This leads to lack of confidence, frustration, and what may be termed 'burn out'.

The structure of the interview

1. The first step is to *open the discussion and introduce the subject of HIV*:

   'We talk to all expectant mothers who attend this clinic about HIV and AIDS. Have you ever talked to anyone before about this?'

2. It is important to *establish the woman's view of her risk for HIV*:

   'Do you think that you have been at risk for HIV?'
   'Do you know how HIV is passed on?'
   'Do you know how it is *not* passed on?'
   'What exactly makes you think that you are at risk for HIV?'
   'What do you mean by having sex? Do you mean touching, kissing, penetrative anal or vaginal intercourse? Can you explain what you mean?'
   'Which of these activities do you think are most risky?'

3. *Giving information is essential in counselling, but the patient's knowledge about AIDS should first be checked.* An opportunity for patients to explain in their own words what they understand about AIDS is one way to begin to correct misinformation.

   'What do you understand about the risks associated with oral sex?'
   'What precautions are you taking to protect your sexual partner?'

4. *Discussion about the HIV antibody test takes place early in the interview*:

   'We offer all mothers the opportunity to have the HIV antibody test.'
   'Have you ever thought of having this test before?'
   'Can you tell me what you know about the test?'

   The window period between the risk for HIV and the appearance of antibodies must be taken into consideration:

   'When do you think was the last risk you had for HIV?'
   'Would you consider being tested again in a few weeks?'

   Some advantages and disadvantages of having the test should be discussed. The following is a *checklist*:
   ### Advantages
   a) Knowledge of a result can assist decision making.
   b) Symptoms of infection can be identified and treated early.
   c) Further transmission can be prevented with knowledge of a result.
   d) Knowledge of a result can reduce stress.
   ### Disadvantages
   a) Knowledge of a result can lead to difficulties in relationships.
   b) Social stigma can follow from knowledge and informing others of a result. Keeping secrets can be stressful.

    c) Life insurance and mortgage possibilities may be affected by HIV testing.

    d) Knowledge of a result may increase stress.

    'With this information, what is your view about having the antibody test?'

5. *The patient's greatest concern should be identified early on in the session, and be ranked alongside other concerns.* This helps to reduce anxiety to manageable proportions. The use of hypothetical, future-orientated questions helps to prepare the patient for the possibility of a positive test result (Bor & Miller 1988). No pre-test counselling is ever complete until this has been done, irrespective of the level of the patient's risk.

    'If you were HIV antibody positive, what might be your greatest concern?'
    'Of all your concerns about having the test, which is the greatest?'
    'What would help you most to make a decision about having the test?'

6. *Clarify with the patient how she normally copes* with uncertainty and problems. Identify who else there is to support her. Discuss past strategies for coping with difficult situations.

    'What has helped you make difficult decisions in the past?'
    'If your partner knew you were contemplating having the test, what might his views be? If his views differ from yours, how will you handle this?'
    'If you decide to have the test, who would you want to tell?'
    'If you were anti-HIV positive, who and what would help you most?'

7. Towards the end of the session an opportunity should be made for the *patient to ask questions.*

    'Are there any questions you would like to ask, or anything that you would like to say that you haven't had a chance to say during our talk?'

8. Before the patient leaves, a *decision* will have to be made about testing by the patient as well as the health care staff. For the latter, a decision is derived from an assessment of the risk, the patient's main concerns, her mental state and her level of social support. Staff may also ask themselves if the pre-test counselling was adequate, and whether a referral to an AIDS counsellor might be indicated. If staff consider that there is a risk for HIV, and the patient refuses to have the test, she should be considered positive for infection control purposes, and all attempts should be made to offer further counselling.

9. *A follow-up appointment* is always given. This provides a further opportunity to discuss concerns. The decision not to offer a further appointment should be reached by mutual agreement and the reasons documented in the medical notes.

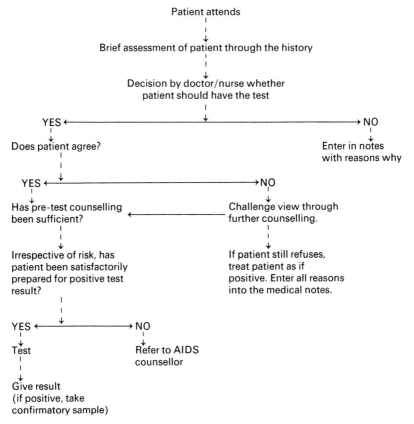

Fig. 2.1   Flow chart showing possible steps to be taken for pre-test HIV counselling and antibody testing in the antenatal clinic.

EXAMPLES OF DIFFICULT COUNSELLING SITUATIONS

(The cases described have been altered in order to preserve confidentiality.)

1. HIV screening a low risk woman

Description of the situation

Mrs J, aged 27, is 12 weeks pregnant and booking into the antenatal clinic for the first time. She was referred by her family doctor. She is accompanied by her mother, who waits outside during the interview.

Principal issues to be addressed
—   How to introduce the subject of HIV infection to a woman who appears to be at low risk.
—   Give the patient reasons for offering the HIV antibody test, and describe it.

— Assumptions should not be made about her risk or her knowledge about HIV.
— The opportunity can be used for checking knowledge and giving information.
— Insurance issues may be raised by the patient.
— Decisions have to be made about whether the test should be carried out.

An extract from an interview to illustrate how to address some of these issues

Doctor: Mrs J, as you might know, in this clinic we test all expectant mothers for HIV. What do you understand about why we might do this?
Mrs J: Not very much, as I am not at risk. My husband is my only partner. So it doesn't apply to me.
Doctor: You say that you don't understand much about the test. Can you tell me what you do understand?
Mrs J: Well, it's a test for AIDS.
Doctor: That is not quite correct. It is a test to see whether you have been infected by the virus, but it will not tell if you will develop AIDS. What do you know about how AIDS is transmitted?
Mrs J: Through sleeping with many people, and through blood and dirty needles.
Doctor: Yes, you are right, but it can also be passed from an infected mother to her child before birth, and that is why we offer the test to all expectant mothers. We also like to take the opportunity to see that people are well informed because some people fear that they can get AIDS in ways that do not present any risk, such as by sharing toilets. Others may not understand that their activities are risky, such as anal intercourse.
Mrs J: If I have the test, what about insurance problems?
Doctor: If the test is offered for routine screening for HIV and the result is negative, most insurance companies will now not load this against you. This is the same as for blood donors.
Mrs J: I suppose you might as well have the test, but I will worry until I get the result.
Doctor: Whilst you are waiting for the result and worrying, who might you talk to about it?
Mrs J: Well, not my mother. But maybe my husband, but he too will start wondering and worrying.
Doctor: Perhaps you would like to come with your husband to discuss this. If you have any questions or additional worries between now and next week when we have the result, you can contact us during office hours. Would you be able to discuss this with your family doctor?
Mrs J: He wouldn't think that I had any risk. I suppose I could talk to him.

Summary

The implications resulting from opening this type of discussion are far reaching and complex. The patient's views were challanged and she was helped to consider aspects that she had not previously considered. The opportunity was taken to check knowledge and give information. It was acknowledged that even for a patient with a low risk of infection, having the test and awaiting the result can be anxiety provoking.

2. An expectant mother at high risk who refuses to have the HIV antibody test

Description of the situation

Miss T, aged 23, is 12 weeks pregnant and has been referred to the clinic for antenatal care by her general practitioner. He reports that she has had a past history of injecting drugs. For the first time she has a steady boyfriend, the father of the child, and they intend to marry.

Principal issues to be addressed

— The importance of HIV screening for the present and future care of the mother, her infant and her sexual partner.
— The patient's knowledge should be checked and information given so that she can make informed decisions about testing, continuation of pregnancy and transmission of HIV to her sexual partner.
— Her main concerns should be identified early in the session so that the maximum time can be given to discussion about them.
— Decisions about infection control procedures should be raised if applicable in the setting. In some clinics, measures are taken for all patients, but in others there is more attention to detail when there is known to be an HIV risk.
— An assessment must be made of the patient's social and emotional situation because of past drug usage.

Extracts from an interview to illustrate how to address some of these issues

Doctor: How might you be infected with HIV?
Miss T: I used to mix with a crowd who injected drugs.
Doctor: What do you understand about the risk to your child if you were infected with HIV?
Miss T: I know there is some chance, but I will take that chance. I want this baby and I don't want that test.
Doctor: You say that you do not want the HIV antibody test. What do you fear most about having the test?
Miss T: That my boyfriend will find out about my past and that he will leave me.
Doctor: If you were positive, what difference might it make to your decision to continue with the pregnancy? What are your views about termination? Do you think that your boyfriend has had any risk for HIV?
Miss T: I hadn't thought about that.
Doctor: You say that you have finally found the right person, and you do not want the relationship to break up. What if you were positive and passed HIV on to him? If you are worried about a past risk, what can you do to now protect your boyfriend, if you indeed were infected?
Miss T: I would have to tell him if I suddenly asked him to use condoms.
Doctor: If your boyfriend did leave you, how might you cope?
Miss T: Maybe my family would be a help.
Doctor: What does your family know about you and drugs?

Miss T: I think I will have to risk talking to my boyfriend, but I still don't want to.
Doctor: These are difficult decisions. Should you have any further questions, or change your mind, who might you turn to? In any event, because of the discussion we've had, I would like to see you in a week, together with one of our counsellors.

Summary

There will be women who refuse to have the test because the risk to personal well-being and relationships is too great to contemplate. Contact should be maintained with them, particularly through their general practitioner who is in a position to monitor the health of the whole family. Occasionally a doctor may make a decision to inform a sexual partner if there is evidence that somebody has deliberately been put at risk for HIV. All attempts should be made to persuade the woman to do so herself before such action is taken.

3. Having children where one of the partners is anti-HIV positive

Description of the situation

Mr Adams, aged 35, has haemophilia and has known that he has been anti-HIV positive for 6 years. He has come with his wife, aged 34, to discuss their wish to have a child before it is too late for his wife. Mr Adams has a low T4 lymphocyte count, predictive of a poor prognosis.

Principal issues to be addressed

— The risk of HIV transmission to Mrs Adams
— The risk of HIV to the unborn child
— The effect on their relationships if:
    a) they have a child;
    b) the mother becomes infected, unwell or dies;
    c) the father becomes unwell or dies;
    d) the child is infected and becomes unwell and dies;
    e) they choose not to have children.
Other ways of having children should be discussed, such as artificial insemination by donor. If the couple are determined to have a child, advice should be given about reducing the risk of infection by confining penetration to the fertile period.

Some examples of questions that can be used to address the issues

'Which of the two of you most wants a child?'
'Are there any issues apart from HIV that might influence your decisions to have a child?'

'If you were unable to have a child because of AIDS or anything else, how do you see your relationship in the future?'
'If you decided to take the risk and have a child, and one or both of you became ill and even died, who would take care of the child?'

Summary

Despite all the risks involved, many couples still choose to have a child. It is important that they are adequately counselled, on an ongoing basis, about possible outcomes. Once pregnancy is embarked upon, there should be careful monitoring and follow-up of mother, child and father (Black & Levy 1988). Preparation for possible future major events, such as illness and death, is best achieved through hypothetical, future-orientated questions, i.e. 'What if . . .' questions.

CONCLUSION

The ripple effect of AIDS first had an impact on staff in sexually transmitted disease clinics and haemophilia centres (Miller et al 1989). With the recent evidence of the spread of HIV to the heterosexual population, antenatal and family planning clinics, and general practitioners' surgeries are important settings in which AIDS issues have to be addressed. Some staff in antenatal clinics may be reluctant to take on this counselling role.

It is important to recognize that staff in these clinics may have anxieties about exposure to HIV in their workplace. They must feel reassured about their safety before they are able to offer optimal care to their patients (Sherr 1987). A special feature is that many staff are themselves young and family-orientated and may identify with the women that they see. For this reason their outlook may differ from those of staff in sexually transmitted disease clinics and haemophilia care settings.

The first step is to identify the concerns, if any, of the staff. These may relate to safety in the workplace or inadequate skills in talking to patients about sensitive issues. If a range of professional staff in these clinics are able to share the counselling, this may reduce staff stress. Counselling that is done jointly, in other words with the doctor *and* counsellor, can increase the confidence and expertise of the antenatal clinic staff. Regular sessions for updating on knowledge about AIDS for staff should be provided.

There is a case for making available the skills and expertise of a trained AIDS counsellor. This could be on the basis of consultation-liaison, or of sessional work alongside the consultant and nurses during antenatal clinic sessions.

In conclusion, staff may find that they further facilitate and open up communication between themselves and their patients by discussing AIDS. Some women may be relieved to be able to talk about their fears and concerns in the context of the antenatal clinic rather than in other settings.

One effect of AIDS counselling for pregnant women should be to raise public awareness about AIDS and concomitantly reduce social stigma and the risks of transmission.

REFERENCES

Black P, Levy E 1988 HIV infection during pregnancy: psychosocial factors and medical legal implications—introductory remarks. In: Schinazi R, Nahmias A (eds) AIDS in children, adolescents and heterosexual adults. Elsevier: New York

Bor R, Miller R, Perry L 1988 Systemic counselling for patients with AIDS/HIV infections. Family Systems Medicine 6(1): 21–39

Bor R, Perry L, Miller R, Jackson J 1989 Strategies for counselling the 'Worried well' in relation to AIDS. Journal of the Royal Society of Medicine 82 (in press)

Bor R, Miller R 1988 Addressing 'dreaded issues': a description of a unique counselling intervention with patients with AIDS/HIV. Counselling Psychology Quarterly 1(4): 397–406

Bradbeer C 1989 Women and HIV. Editorial. British Medical Journal 298: 342–343

Hudson C N, Sharp F (eds) (1988) AIDS and obstetrics and gynaecology. Proceedings of the Nineteenth Study Group of the Royal College of Obstetricians and Gynaecologists, London

Johnson M A 1989 Human immunodeficiency virus infection in women. British Journal of Obstetrics and Gynaecology 96: 11–14

Marteau T M, Johnston M, Plenicdar M, Shaw R W, Slack J 1988 Development of a self-administered questionnaire to measure women's knowledge of prenatal screening and diagnostic tests. Journal of Psychometric Research 32: 403–408

Marteau T M, Johnston M, Shaw R W, Slack J 1989 Factors influencing the uptake of screening for Down's Syndrome. British Journal of Obstetrics and Gynaecology (in press)

Marteau T M, Kidd J, Cook R, Johnston M, Michie S, Shaw R W, Slack J 1988 Screening for Down's Syndrome. British Medical Journal 297: 1469

Miller R, Bor R 1988 AIDS: a guide to clinical counselling. Science Press, United Kingdom

Miller R, Goldman E, Bor R, Kernoff P 1989 Counselling children and adults about HIV: the ripple effect on haemophilia care settings. Counselling Psychology Quarterly 2: (1) 65–72

Mills A 1988 Human immunodeficiency virus antibody testing in pregnancy. Unpublished thesis submitted to the University of London in part fulfilment for requirements of MSc in Community Medicine

Novick B, Rubinstein A 1987 AIDS: the paediatric perspective. AIDS: 1: 3–7

Pinching A 1988 Prophylactic and maintenance therapy for opportunistic infections in AIDS. AIDS 2: 335–343

Sherr L 1987 The impact of AIDS in obstetrics and obstetric staff. Journal of Reproductive and Infant Psychology 5: 87–96

Tedder R 1988 HIV testing: problems and perceptions. British Medical Bulletin 44(1): 161–169

PART TWO

Obstetrics

3. The uteroplacental and fetoplacental circulations in clinical practice

Kevin P. Hanretty   Martin J. Whittle

The placenta provides respiratory, nutritional and excretory functions for the fetus and is anatomically defined by the eighth week of pregnancy. By term it is a substantial structure weighing, on average, 600 g, or just over a fifth of the fetal weight. The development of the placental circulation is complex, the mesoderm of primary villi giving rise to the ultimate placental vasculature which is appropriately rich and interconnected. The primitive fetoplacental circulation is formed about halfway through the second post-conceptional (PC) week and the fetal heart circulates blood from about the fourth (PC) week (Moore 1982). Placentation invokes a series of processes at the implantation site which have important implications for the maternal supply to the developing pregnancy. Invasion of the decidua by the syn-cytiotrophoblast is an early event which ensures a secure nutrient supply for the developing blastocyst (Pijnenborg et al 1983). This process continues until, early in the second trimester, cytotrophoblast invades the maternal spiral arteries. This invasion proceeds until about 24–26 weeks, by which time the normally tortuous and narrow resistance vessels have lost their muscularis layer. This results in the formation of flask-shaped low resistance vessels which provide a rich and unimpeded maternal blood supply to the bed of the growing placenta (Brosens et al 1977, Sheppard & Bonnar 1981, Moll et al 1975).

Even though fetal condition is absolutely dependent upon both the uteroplacental circulation and fetoplacental circulations, knowledge about their function and control remains limited. The interaction of these physically separate but contiguous circulations is undoubtedly complex (Fig. 3.1) and there is increasing evidence that changes in one circulation may modulate changes in the other. Certainly, the fetoplacental circulation should not be regarded as passive. The placental circulation will respond to a number of vasoactive substances such as 5-hydroxytryptamine and angiotensin II (AII), and vessel tone appears to be controlled by a number of systems, one of which is cyclo-oxygenase dependent. In addition, AII and atrial natriuretic peptide (ANP) and ANP receptors have been located, and appear to be active, in the placental vessel walls (Kingdom et al 1989).

33

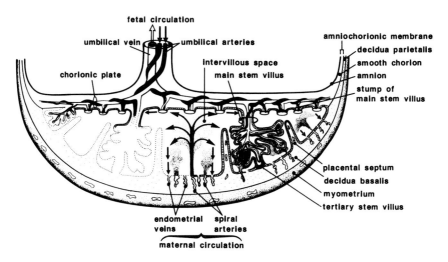

Fig. 3.1   The intimate relationship between the maternal uteroplacental and fetoplacental circulations. Exchange of nutrients and waste products relies on the adequate and complementary functions of both circulations.

The role of paracrine systems remains unclear, but endothelium-derived relaxing factor (EDRF) has been isolated from cord endothelium and an effector mechanism has been shown to be present. The role of these systems in maintaining the placental vessel tone remains speculative but it is conceivable that they regulate shunting of fetal blood within the placenta to optimize gas and nutrient transfer. Some evidence that events on the maternal side may influence the fetoplacental unit come from experiments using microsphere embolization of the uterine circulation in sheep, the fetal response to the resultant diminished maternal blood supply being a parallel reduction in umbilical flow (Clapp et al 1980).

This chapter discusses some determinants of uteroplacental and fetoplacental blood flow and some of the methods which have been used to gain a greater understanding of the vascular physiology and pathology of placentation.

METHODS OF ASSESSING UTEROPLACENTAL BLOOD FLOW

Although pathological disturbances in uterine blood flow have been implicated in some pregnancies complicated by essential hypertension, pregnancy-induced hypertension (PIH) and intrauterine growth retardation (IUGR), no direct data exist because of the difficulties in measurement. However, a number of strategies have been developed over the years, including clearance rates of endocrine and radio-isotope markers and, more recently, Doppler ultrasound velocimetry.

The findings of Browne & Veall (1953), which were later confirmed by Dixon et al (1963), did suggest that there was a reduction in uteroplacental perfusion in some complicated pregnancies. The methods used measured the rate at which radio-isotopes disappeared from the choriodecidual space, this change correlating with the extent of perfusion. The use of radio-isotopic methods of assessing placental perfusion in humans is no longer acceptable, not only because of concerns about radioactivity but also because of technical problems and physiological phenomena which tended to make results uninterpretable. For example, it has been shown in monkeys that the blood supply from the spiral arteries is patchy rather than uniform, which might invalidate some of the radio-isotope data. However, recently, Nylund et al (1983), using more sophisticated methods, have demonstrated the feasibility of studying normal and complicated pregnancies using very low radiation dosages although, because of the nature of these investigations, their methods have not found widespread acceptance.

Direct measurement of uterine blood flow has been performed using electromagnetic flow meters and has provided interesting physiological data. However, the studies were performed on pregnancies being terminated by hysterotomy (Assali et al 1960) and could not be used for routine investigation. Another invasive method, not yet applied to the pregnant uterus, is the use of thermistor techniques (Randall et al 1988, Hauksson et al 1988), but the possible role for such an approach remains unclear.

The introduction of Doppler methods to study the uterine circulation by Campbell et al, in 1983, offered the prospect of a non-invasive and repeatable method of studying ongoing pregnancies. Conceptually, Doppler only provides an indirect measure of flow, but it has been considered useful in assessing the uteroplacental circulation because of the relationship between vascular resistance and Doppler indices. Although this relationship in the uterine circulation has recently been questioned (Clewell et al 1988), Doppler methods do provide a qualitative technique for describing flow velocity waveforms which have been widely used to investigate uteroplacental perfusion.

The indices commonly used to describe Doppler flow velocity wave-forms, which were previously developed for use in study of peripheral vascular disease, are the resistance index, pulsatility index and systolic/diastolic ratio. All are highly correlated, reproducible and comparable, regardless of whether a continuous wave or pulsed Doppler system is used. High values for any of these indices reflect increased vascular resistance to flow. Numerous studies have shown the uteroplacental circulations to be characterized by low resistance waveforms in normal pregnancy, and high resistance patterns have been described in some complicated pregnancies. However, because of the non-uniform perfusion of the uteroplacental bed, the value of the Doppler technique in this circulation is doubtful. The use of Doppler colour flow mapping may be helpful since uteroplacental vessels can be more clearly identified, although this expensive method has still to be adequately evaluated.

METHODS OF ASSESSING FETOPLACENTAL BLOOD FLOW

The fetoplacental circulation is established early in gestation and, like the uteroplacental circulation, is characterized by low vascular resistance.

Invasive methods of measuring fetal blood flow using electromagnetic flow meters are of interest, and Assali et al (1960) demonstrated a flow rate of 110 ml/min in the umbilical artery in fetuses being terminated at hysterotomy, which is about 50% of the total cardiac output and highlights the dynamic nature of this circulation. Clearly these methods are not appropriate for the study of continuing pregnancies, and FitzGerald & Drumm (1977) and McCallum et al (1978), the pioneers of Doppler velocimetry in obstetrics, suggested that information obtained using Doppler would contribute to the understanding of complications such as PIH and IUGR. Doppler methods permit non-invasive methods of assessing fetoplacental perfusion but, as with the uteroplacental circulation, only qualitative measurements can be made.

PREGNANCY COMPLICATIONS AND THE MEASUREMENT OF UTEROPLACENTAL AND FETOPLACENTAL BLOOD FLOW

Assessment of uteroplacental and umbilical artery blood flow may provide important information concerning both the physiology and pathology of these circulations, and the availability of non-invasive techniques such as Doppler are potentially of enormous value. Other aspects to be discussed include the role of the evaluation of these circulations as a method of pregnancy assessment both as a screening tool and in the direct deter-mination of the fetal condition in defined disease states. In addition, these methods may provide an insight to the effect of maternal (and fetal) therapy.

UTEROPLACENTAL BLOOD FLOW IN HYPERTENSIVE PREGNANCIES

Brosens et al (1977) indicated that in pregnancies complicated by hyper-tension the physiological invasion of the spiral arteries was incomplete. This led to a failure to convert the maternal vasculature to a low resistance system with the implication that blood flow is thereby reduced and in-adequate to sustain a pregnancy (Gerretsen et al 1981).

The concept of placental ischaemia as a factor in the pathogenesis of pre-eclampsia had previously led Browne & Vealle (1953) to investigate the maternal blood flow using Na24 clearance rates. While the definitions of hypertension that they used would not be acceptable today, these workers showed that perfusion was reduced in some hypertensive pregnancies. They later confirmed their findings using larger numbers and also observed that the changes in blood flow were related to the degree of hypertension, being most marked in proteinuric pre-eclampsia. Using a different isotope, Xe133, Kaar et al (1980) confirmed that a reduction in intervillous blood flow occurred in pre-eclampsia, although there was a wide variation both in normal and complicated pregnancies.

Further support for reduced flow in hypertension comes from the study of clearance rates of C19 steroids, which have been shown to correlate with uterine blood flow (Edman et al 1981, Senner et al 1985). Gant et al (1971) showed a reduced metabolic clearance of dehydroisoandrosterone sulphate in pregnancies complicated by pre-eclampsia and also demonstrated that this reduction preceeded clinically detectable disease.

The possibility of identifying changes in perfusion in advance of clinical signs prompted Campbell et al (1986) to use Doppler studies of maternal arcuate arteries as a screening test for high risk pregnancy. This group had previously used Doppler to study uteroplacental flow velocity waveforms during the third trimester in a number of complicated pregnancies and had demonstrated patterns associated with high resistance vessels (Campbell et al 1983). Subsequently, in a study of 126 consecutive women attending their antenatal clinic at 16–18 weeks gestation, they showed a higher incidence of IUGR and PIH in women with abnormal, compared with normal, uteroplacental Doppler waveforms. The very high incidence of abnormal waveforms demonstrated in this series, and in a later study reported by Steel et al (1988), may be spurious and suggests that the normal ranges obtained initially were possibly inappropriate for the general population. Other workers, who have shown differences in uterine artery waveforms from either side of the uterus, have suggested that this may represent abnormal placentation which might be associated with hypertension (Schulman et al 1987, Kofinas et al 1988), although the basis for this hypothesis is unclear. Unfortunately most studies of Doppler uteroplacental waveforms in hypertensive pregnancies have studied mixed populations of patients receiving varieties of antihypertensive agents which themselves have unknown effects on Doppler indices. In a recent controlled study of untreated cases of PIH, the pulsatility index was no different from controls (Hanretty et al 1988). Although the method of obtaining the waveforms has been criticized (Pearce & McParland 1988), it was apparent that markedly different waveforms may be obtained from the uteroplacental vessels, a finding which probably relates to the focal nature of the placental pathology in PIH. Figure 3.2 shows two such waveforms, one highly abnormal and the other normal, obtained simultaneously in opposite channels, from the uteroplacental vessels. These waveforms, which were unequivocally uteroplacental in origin, were obtained from a patient with

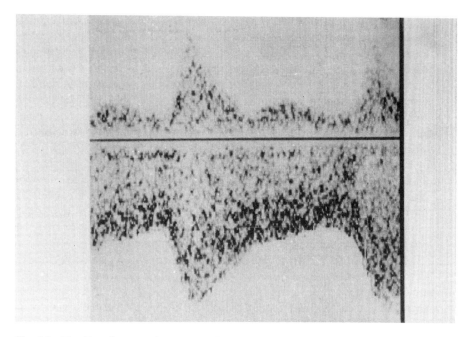

Fig. 3.2 Two Doppler uteroplacental waveforms are shown. These were obtained synchronously from arteries flowing in opposite directions within the uteroplacental circulation. The upper waveform represents a high resistance system whilst the lower pattern represents low resistance to flow. (Reproduced with permission of The Editor, The Lancet).

severe PIH. However, uniformly abnormal uteroplacental waveforms may be significant, and this was observed in one of the two perinatally related deaths in the series, suggesting that the vascular pathology was widespread and severe.

Doppler colour flow mapping of the uterine vasculature may provide useful information but is still to be fully evaluated. The clear identification of vessels and direction of flow afforded by this method is, however, promising.

In general, therefore, it does appear that, in hypertensive pregnancy, maternal perfusion of the placenta is reduced, as demonstrated by a number of different techniques. Doppler waveforms appear to be abnormal in some hypertensive pregnancies and may help to distinguish cases of essential hypertension from those with severe PIH, but the value of the technique both as a screening procedure and in the assessment of the clinically affected pregnancy is as yet unproven, and there seem to be major methodological problems which may limit the application of this technique.

Fetoplacental blood flow in hypertensive pregnancies

Almost all of the data concerning fetoplacental blood flow have been obtained from studies using Doppler velocimetry. However, a recent in vitro study has investigated umbilical flow to the placenta in a series of ten pregnancies complicated by hypertension (Abitbol et al 1987). Although only pregnancies at around term were included, suggesting that the disease was relatively mild, these workers showed reduced umbilical blood flow compared with uncomplicated pregnancies. Placental angiography was also performed and showed 'functional' normality in 79% of cotyledons from the control placentas compared with 51% in the study group. This highly significant difference also highlighted the focal nature of the pathology on the fetal side of the placenta.

Extensive in vivo studies have been performed using Doppler to obtain flow velocity waveforms in PIH. A number of groups have shown high resistance patterns and reduced diastolic flow velocities in some cases, but the definitions of PIH used and the inclusion criteria for study have not always been consistent.

Ducey et al (1987) classified the types of hypertension complicating pregnancy as chronic, PIH and pre-eclampsia and showed abnormal umbilical artery waveforms more commonly associated with the last diagnosis. However, Cameron et al (1988), in a prospective study of well-defined cases of pre-eclampsia, have shown normal Doppler indices in 70% of cases, with no clear correlation between Doppler indices and the absolute level of hypertension.

Nevertheless, clinical outcome appeared to correlate with the waveform as, in cases with an abnormal pattern, growth retardation, fetal distress and admission to the neonatal intensive care unit were commoner.

The mechanism whereby these abnormal waveforms occur is uncertain, although it presumably relates to increased downstream impedance within the placental vascular tree. This may be the result of obliteration of tertiary stem villus arterioles (Giles et al 1985), but whether this is the end result of prolonged vasoconstriction or intravascular coagulation is not clear. Other factors such as increased blood viscosity may also be important.

Nevertheless, repeated embolization of the fetoplacental circulation in the sheep fetus has been shown to produce Doppler waveforms similar to those seen in severely compromised hypertensive pregnancies (Trudinger et al 1987). The production of these waveforms was not associated with fetal compromise as evidenced by retarded growth, so it is possible that Doppler methods tell us more about the health of the placenta than fetal well-being directly.

Uteroplacental blood flow in IUGR

The study by Kaar (1980) already mentioned also included a group of babies whose birth weights were less than the tenth centile for gestational age and showed a reduction in perfusion in these cases. More recently, Nylund et al (1983), in a study of small-for-gestational age babies and matched controls, used intravenous indium[113] and demonstrated reduced scintillation counts over the placental site. A uterine blood flow index was derived and in the small-for-gestational age babies was less than half of the values obtained from controls. This difference remained significant when a group of pre-eclamptics, in which reduced flow might be attributable to the hypertension, were removed from the series. Six of 30 cases were complicated, unfortunately, by fetal abnormality, and although there was no difference in blood flow index between the normally formed and abnormal small-for-dates fetuses, it remains unclear what proportion of otherwise unexplained IUGR is associated with reduced uterine blood flow.

Although Doppler waveform indices in the uteroplacental circulation also appear to be abnormal in some cases of IUGR (McCowan et al 1988), the results are variable and the methodological criticisms mentioned in relation to hypertension make the observations of dubious significance in clinical practice. However, it would not be surprising if widespread pathology in the spiral arteries was associated with severe IUGR and waveform abnormalities.

Fetoplacental circulation in IUGR

Redistribution of blood flow within the fetal circulation is a likely feature of 'placental insufficiency', which may result in IUGR. Whether increased vascular resistance in the placenta is a cause or consequence of this re-distribution is not clear but, as with some cases of hypertension, abnormal Doppler waveforms have been described from the umbilical arteries of growth-retarded fetuses. Erskine & Ritchie (1985) demonstrated abnormal waveforms in a small series of severely growth retarded fetuses, and considerable interest was aroused in the potential use of Doppler to identify IUGR. Furthermore, from their work it seemed that Doppler might identify cases of genuine growth retardation with fetal compromise rather than fetuses which, although small-for-dates, show normal growth velocity and are well.

One problem in the evaluation of Doppler velocimetry in the identifi-cation of the small-for-dates fetus is the appropriateness of the end-point. Thus many studies are faulted by the use of birthweight charts not derived from the population under study. Not surprisingly the data from Doppler studies are conflicting: in 168 high risk cases Berkowitz et al (1988) demonstrated a sensitivity of 45% when using umbilical artery Doppler to identify fetuses weighing less than the tenth centile at birth. Mulders et al (1987), in a smaller series, obtained a corresponding figure of 53%. In contrast, Gaziano et al (1988) showed abnormal waveforms in 79% of such cases. It is possible that Doppler may be more useful in identifying the fetus which has failed to reach its growth potential but is not necessarily small-for-dates, and preliminary data from an ongoing study of umbilical artery

Doppler in an unselected population tend to confirm this (Hanretty et al 1989).

However, most studies strongly suggest that umbilical flow abnormalities detected by Doppler in the already small-for-dates fetus may identify those at increased risk for perinatal morbidity and mortality (Berkowitz et al 1988, Reuwer et al 1987).

Nevertheless, the clinical value of umbilical artery Doppler in screening for IUGR, though promising, has still to be evaluated in controlled trials.

Doppler assessment of umbilical artery blood flow and the identification of fetal well-being in high risk pregnancy

Doppler study of the umbilical circulation may play some role in monitoring the identified high risk pregnancy, including not only the familiar problems of hypertension and growth retardation, but also less common conditions such as rhesus disease (Rightmire et al 1986), lupus inhibitor (Trudinger et al 1988) and diabetes (Bracero et al 1986), and the categorization of pregnancies complicated by severe oligohydramnios and fetal abnormality may also be aided by Doppler evaluation of the umbilical artery (Hsieh et al, 1988).

There is a need for a method which identifies all pregnancies at risk in early pregnancy, and initially Doppler study of the umbilical artery appeared promising, although many of the previously reported studies are difficult to interpret as end-points used to define fetal compromise tend to be ill-defined and vary between studies. In spite of reservations about the use of Doppler velocimetry of the umbilical artery, it does seem that, in general, normal results are associated with a normal perinatal outcome. The situation is less clear when velocimetry indicates reduced, absent or reversed diastolic flow. Some reports suggest that the finding of absent or reversed velocity implies imminent fetal demise, indicating the need for immediate delivery (Woo et al 1987). Others, whilst agreeing that such abnormal waveform patterns do indeed signify fetal compromise, suggest that they indicate a need for intensive supervision, using established monitoring techniques, rather than urgent intervention, and have shown that the interval between the finding of abnormal waveforms and the necessity for delivery can vary from hours to weeks (Rochelson et al 1987, Johnstone et al 1988).

The use of Doppler study to evaluate high risk pregnancy has been studied in a controlled trial by Trudinger et al (1987). Three hundred pregnancies were studied, but the only difference in outcome parameters between the report and control groups related to a reduction in the numbers of caesarean sections performed during labour in the former. The conclusion was that decision-making had been improved by knowledge of the Doppler results, leading to a better selection of patients suitable for labour. However, this is not supported by the simultaneous observation of no difference in rates of induction of labour or elective caesarean section between groups.

It is likely that either larger studies with similar inclusion criteria or studies of higher risk pregnancies would be required to have sufficient power to demonstrate a difference in fetal and neonatal outcome attributable to the availability of Doppler results.

UTEROPLACENTAL AND FETOPLACENTAL BLOOD FLOW AND CLINICAL PHARMACOLOGY

Drugs and the uteroplacental circulation

Antihypertensives

The initial radio-isotope studies of the uteroplacental circulation by Dixon et al (1963) appeared to show a reduction in perfusion associated with the use of antihypertensives, and traditionally it has been a cause for concern among obstetricians that drug treatment might adversely affect the already compromised circulation in pregnancies complicated by hypertension. A number of studies have now been performed which suggest that this is not the case.

From the work of Lunell et al (1983) it seems that infused dihydralazine has no effect on uterine blood flow, determined using indium[113], despite a significant reduction in blood pressure. This finding was supported by Jouppila et al (1985), who reached the same conclusion using xenon[133].

The data regarding beta blockers are conflicting. Montan et al (1987) showed an increase in uteroplacental vascular resistance using Doppler in seven patients receiving atenolol. In a controlled study we have shown no difference in Doppler indices in patients established on atenolol for PIH (Hanretty et al 1988). The combined alpha-/beta-blocker, labetalol, appears to have no effect on uterine blood flow (Jouppila et al 1986), and a recent report on the calcium channel blocker, nifedipine, has also shown no effect despite significant reductions in blood pressure (Lindow et al 1988).

More speculative treatment have also been assessed. Jouppila et al (1985) showed no effect of the potent vasodilator, prostacyclin, on uteroplacental blood flow despite evidence of redistribution of maternal blood flow.

Beta mimetics

Jouppila et al (1985) studied the effect of ritodrine on uterine blood flow and showed no alteration of uterine haemodynamics during short-term treatment. In contrast, Brar et al (1988) have shown a significant reduction in Doppler indices of resistance. Whether this significantly increased volume blood flow to the uterus is not known, and the changes in Doppler waveform could be an effect of an increase in maternal heart rate, though a reduction in vascular resistance coupled with this might be expected to increase blood flow.

Epidural anaesthesia

The increasing use of conductive anaesthesia in labour has led to concern that the haemodynamic changes associated with its use might affect uterine blood flow. The results of Doppler studies have been conflicting: Giles et al (1987) found that epidural anaesthesia for elective caesarean section improved uteroplacental perfusion, although in a more recent report Long & Spencer (1988) found no change in uteroplacental perfusion in the absence of maternal hypotension.

It seems that the uteroplacental blood supply remains remarkably resistant to drug-induced changes and that locally active factors are responsible for this.

Table 3.1 Synopsis of uteroplacental and fetoplacental perfusion

	Uteroplacental	Fetoplacental
PIH		
In vitro	Not known	41% reduction in umbilical blood flow
Steroid clearance	Reduced metabolic clearance rates representing reduced perfusion precede clinical disease.	Not known
Radio-isotopes	Reduced blood flow of up to 60% demonstrated. No clear evidence that antihypertensives change perfusion.	Not known
Doppler: screening	Similar incidence of PIH in those with normal and abnormal uteroplacental waveforms when screened at 24 weeks.	Not known
Doppler: diagnosis	Waveforms representing high resistance to flow seen in some cases but methodological problems significant.	Abnormal umbilical artery Doppler waveforms appear to be a feature of fetal compromise rather than diagnostic of PIH.
IUGR		
Radio-isotopes	Uterine blood flow index 44% of normal in cases of IUGR.	Not known
Doppler: -screening	Four-fold increase in small-for-dates cases with abnormal waveform compared with normals at 24 weeks.	Sensitivity of 45% in detecting small-for-dates fetuses, but within this group Doppler does identify some cases at increased risk of morbidity and neonatal mortality.

Drugs and the fetoplacental circulation

Doppler remains the only method of assessing drug effects on the fetal circulation. The study by Montan et al showed no change in umbilical artery flow velocity waveforms following atenolol, and we have obtained similar results and also shown no change when nifedipine is the only therapy for PIH (Hanretty et al 1989). However, interpretation of results from investigating the umbilical artery only is fraught with difficulty. It seems unlikely that a drug that induces no change in the umbilical artery is having a significant effect elsewhere in the fetal circulation, but any apparent reduction in resistance to umbilical flow may reflect shunting from, for example, the cerebral circulation, and further investigation of drug effects on the fetus must be targeted at individual vessels.

Clearly, a greater understanding of drug effects on the fetal circulation itself is required before we accept that any treatment is having an adverse or beneficial effect as determined by Doppler.

Uteroplacental and fetoplacental circulations—the future

The ability to examine the uteroplacental and fetoplacental circulations with non-invasive techniques has increased our knowledge concerning their pathophysiology. However, local and systemic control mechanisms governing uteroplacental and umbilical blood flow remain largely un-explored in human pregnancy, and more information is required in these areas. Some of the available information concerning these circulations in disease has been discussed and is summarized in Table 3.1. Despite the enormous advances over the last 10 years, our knowledge is far from comprehensive and much remains to be done. The application of new ultrasound technology and more detailed investigation of blood flow regulation at the molecular level should open out new areas of investigation.

REFERENCES

Abitbol M M, LaGamma E F, Demeter E, Cipollina C M 1987 Umbilical flow in the normal and pre-eclamptic placenta. Acta Obstetricia et Gynecologica Scandinavica 66: 689–694

Assali N S, Rauramo L, Peltonen T 1960 Measurement of uterine blood flow and uterine metabolism. American Journal of Obstetrics and Gynecology 79: 86–98

Berkowitz G S, Chitkara U, Rosenberg J et al 1988 Sonographic estimation of fetal weight and Doppler analysis of umbilical artery velocimetry in the prediction of intrauterine growth retardation: a prospective study. American Journal of Obstetrics and Gynecology 158: 1149–1153

Berkowitz G, Mehalek K, Chitkara U, Rosenberg J, Cogswell C, Berkowitz R L 1988 Doppler umbilical velocimetry in the prediction of adverse outcome in pregnancies at risk for intrauterine growth retardation. Obstetrics and Gynecology 71: 742–746

Bracero L, Schulman H, Fleischer A, Farmakides G 1986 Umbilical artery velocity waveforms in diabetic pregnancy. Obstetrics and Gynecology 68: 654–658

Brar H S, Medearis A L, DeVore G R, Platt L D 1988 Maternal and fetal blood flow velocity waveforms in patients with preterm labor: effects of tocolytics. Obstetrics and Gynecology 72: 209–214

Brosens I, Dixon H G, Robertson W B 1977 Fetal growth retardation and the arteries of the placental bed. British Journal of Obstetrics and Gynaecology 84: 656–664

Browne J C M, Veall N 1953 The maternal placental blood flow in normotensive and hypertensive women. Journal of Obstetrics and Gynaecology of the British Empire 60: 141–147

Cameron A D, Nicholson S F, Nimrod C A, Harder J R, Davies D M 1988 Doppler waveforms in the fetal aorta and umbilical artery in patients with hypertension in pregnancy. American Journal of Obstetrics and Gynecology 158: 339–345

Campbell S, Diaz-Recasens J, Griffin D R et al 1983 New Doppler technique for assessing uteroplacental blood flow. Lancet i: 675–677

Campbell S, Pearce J M F, Hackett G, Cohen-Overbeek T, Hernandez C 1986 Qualitative assessment of uteroplacental blood flow: early screening test for high risk pregnancies. Obstetrics and Gynecology 68: 649–653

Clapp J F, Szeto H H, Larron R, Hewitt J, Munn L J 1981 Umbilical blood flow responses to embolisation of the uterine circulation. American Journal of Obstetrics and Gynecology 138: 60–67

Clewell W H, Hackett G, McCooke H B, Hanson M A, Campbell S 1988 Physiological interpretation of the Doppler waveform in the uterine artery of the sheep. In: C T Jones (ed) Fetal and neonatal development. Perinatology Press, New York

Dixon H G, Browne J C M, Davey D A 1963 Choriodecidual and myometrial blood flow. Lancet ii: 369–373

Ducey J, Schulman H, Farmakides G et al 1987 A classification of hypertension in pregnancy based on Doppler velocimetry. American Journal of Obstetrics and Gynecology 157: 680–685

Edman C D, Toofanian A, MacDonald P C, Gant N F 1981 Placental clearance rate of maternal plasma androstenedione through placental oestradiol formation: an indirect method of assessing uteroplacental blood flow. American Journal of Obstetrics and Gynecology 141: 1029–1036

Erskine R L A, Ritchie J W K 1985 Umbilical artery blood flow characteristics in normal and growth retarded fetuses. British Journal of Obstetrics and Gynaecology 92: 605–610

FitzGerald D E, Drumm J E 1977 Non invasive measurement of the human fetal circulation using ultrasound: a new method. British Medical Journal 2: 1450–1451

Gant N F, Hutchinson H T, Siiteri P K, MacDonald P C 1971 Study of the metabolic clearance of dehydroisoandrosterone sulfate in pregnancy. American Journal of Obstetrics and Gynecology 111: 555–561

Gaziano E, Knox E, Wager G P, Bendel R P, Boyce D J, Olson J 1988 The predictability of the small-for-gestational-age infant by real time ultrasound derived measurements combined with pulsed Doppler umbilical artery velocimetry. American Journal of Obstetrics and Gynecology 158: 1431–1439

Gerretsen G, Huisjes H J, Elema J D 1981 Morphological changes of the spiral arteries in the placental bed in relation to pre-eclampsia and fetal growth retardation. British Journal of Obstetrics and Gynaecology 88: 876–881

Giles W B, Trudinger B J, Baird P J 1985 Fetal umbilical artery flow velocity waveforms and placental resistance: pathological correlation. British Journal of Obstetrics and Gynaecology 92: 31–38

Giles W B, Lah F X, Trudinger B J 1987 The effect of epidural analgesia for caesarean section on maternal uterine and fetal umbilical artery flow velocity waveforms. British Journal of Obstetrics and Gynaecology 94: 55–59

Hanretty K P, Whittle M J, Rubin P C 1988 Doppler uteroplacental waveforms in pregnancy induced hypertension: a re-appraisal. Lancet i: 850–852

Hanretty K P, Whittle M J, Rubin P C 1988 Influence of atenolol on human umbilical and uteroplacental flow velocity waveforms. Clinical Science 74(suppl 18): 64

Hanretty K P, Primrose M H, Neilson J P, Whittle M J 1989 Pregnancy screening by Doppler uteroplacental and umbilical artery waveforms. British Journal of Obstetrics and Gynaecology (in press)

Hanretty K P, Whittle M J, Howie C A, Rubin P C 1989 The effect of nifedipine on Doppler flow velocity waveforms in severe pre-eclampsia. British Medical Journal (in press)

Hsieh F J, Chang F M, Ko T M, Chen H Y, Chen Y P 1988 Umbilical artery flow velocity waveforms in fetuses dying with congenital anomalies. British Journal of Obstetrics and Gynaecology 95: 478–482

Hauksson A, Akerlund M, Melin P 1988 Uterine blood flow and myometrial activity at menstruation and the action of vasopressin and a synthetic antagonist. British Journal of Obstetrics and Gynaecology 95: 898–904

Johnstone F D, Haddad N G, Hoskins P, McDicken W, Chambers S, Muir B 1988 Umbilical artery Doppler flow velocity waveform: the outcome of pregnancies with absent end diastolic flow. European Journal of Obstetrics Gynecology, and Reproductive Biology 28: 171–178

Jouppila P, Kirkinen P, Koivula A, Ylikorkala O 1985 Effects of dihydrallazine infusion on the fetoplacental blood flow and maternal prostanoids. Obstetrics and Gynecology 65: 115–118

Jouppila P, Kirkinen P, Koivula A, Ylikorkala O 1985 Failure of exogenous prostacyclin to change placental and fetal blood flow in pre-eclampsia. American Journal of Obstetrics and Gynecology 151: 661–665

Jouppila P, Kirkinen P, Koivula A, Ylikorkala O 1986 Labetolol does not alter the placental and fetal blood flow or maternal prostanids in pre-eclampsia. British Journal of Obstetrics and Gynaecology 93: 543–547

Jouppila P, Kirkinen P, Koivula A, Ylikorkala O 1985 Ritodrine infusion during late pregnancy: effects on fetal and placental blood flow, prostacyclin and thromboxane. American Journal of Obstetrics and Gynecology 151: 1028–1032

Kaar K, Jouppila P, Kuikka J, Luotola J, Toivanen J, Rekonen A 1980 Intervillous blood flow in normal and complicated late pregnancy measured by means of an intravenous Xe133 method. Acta Obstetricia et Gynecologica Scandinavica 59: 7–10

Kingdom J, Jardine A, Gilmore D H et al 1989 Atrial natriuretic peptide in the human fetus. British Medical Journal (in press)

Kofinas A D, Penry M, Greiss F C, Meis P J, Nelson L H 1988 The effect of placental location on uterine artery flow velocity waveforms. American Journal of Obstetrics and Gynecology 159: 1504–1508

Lindow S W, Davies N, Davey D A, Smith J A 1988 The effect of sublingual nifedipine on uteroplacental blood flow in hypertensive pregnancy. British Journal of Obstetrics and Gynaecology 95: 1276–1281

Long M G, Spencer J A D 1988 Uteroplacental perfusion after epidural analgesia in elective caesarean section. British Journal of Obstetrics and Gynaecology 95: 1081–1082

Lunell N O, Lewander R, Nylund L, Sarby B, Thornstrom S 1983 Acute effect of dihydrallazine on uteroplacental blood flow in hypertension during pregnancy. Gynecologic and Obstetric Investigation 16: 274–282

McCallum W D, Williams C S, Napel S, Daigle R E 1978 Fetal blood velocity waveforms. American Journal of Obstetrics and Gynecology 132: 425–429

McCowan L M, Titchie K, Mo L Y, Bascom P A, Sherret H 1988 Uterine artery flow velocity waveforms in normal and growth retarded pregnancies. American Journal of Obstetrics and Gynecology 158: 499–504

Moll W, Kunzel W, Herberger J 1975 Hemodynamic implications of hemochorial placentation. European Journal of Obstetrics, Gynecology, and Reproductive Biology 5: 67–74

Montan S, Liedholm H, Lingman G, Marsal K, Sjoberg N, Solum T 1987 Fetal and uteroplacental haemodynamics during short term atenolol treatment of hypertension in pregnancy. British Journal of Obstetrics and Gynaecology 94: 312–317

Moore K L 1982 The developing human, 3rd ed. W B Saunders, Philadelphia

Mulders L G M, Wijn P F F, Jongsma H W, Hein P R 1987 A comparative study of three indices of umbilical blood flow in relation to prediction of growth retardation. Journal of Perinatal Medicine 15: 3–12

Nylund L, Lunell N O, Lewander R, Sarby B 1983 Uteroplacental blood flow index in intrauterine growth retardation of fetal or maternal origin. British Journal of Obstetrics and Gynaecology 90: 16–20

Pearce J M, McParland P 1988 Lancet (letter) i: 1287

Pijnenborg R, Bland J M, Robertson W B, Brosens I 1983 Uteroplacental arterial changes related to interstitial trophoblast migration in early human pregnancy. Placenta 4: 397–414

Randall N J, Beard R W, Sutherland I A, Figueroa J P, Drost C J, Nathanielsz P W 1988 Validation of thermal techniques for measurement of pelvic organ flows in the non pregnant sheep: comparison with transit time ultrasonic and microsphere measurements of blood flow. American Journal of Obstetrics and Gynecology 158: 651–658

Reuwer P J H M, Sijmons E A, Rietman G W, Van Tiel M W M, Bruinse H W 1987
Intrauterine growth retardation: prediction of perinatal distress by Doppler ultrasound.
Lancet ii: 415–418

Rightmire D A, Nicolaides K H, Rodeck C H, Campbell S 1986 Fetal blood velocities in Rh
isoimmunisation: relationship to gestational age and to fetal hematocrit. Obstetrics and
Gynecology 68: 233–236

Rochelson B, Schulman H, Farmakides G et al 1987 The significance of absent end diastolic
velocity in umbilical artery waveforms. American Journal of Obstetrics and Gynecology
156: 1213–1218

Schulman H, Ducey J, Farmakides G et al 1987 Uterine artery Doppler velocimetry: the
significance of divergent systolic/diastolic ratios. American Journal of Obstetrics and
Gynecology 157: 1539–1542

Senner J W, Stanczyk F Z, Fritz M A, Novy M J 1985 Relationship of uteroplacental blood
flow to placental clearance of maternal plasma C19 steroids: evaluation of mathematical
models. American Journal of Obstetrics and Gynecology 153: 573–575

Sheppard B L, Bonnar J 1981 An ultrastructural study of uteroplacental spiral arteries in
hypertensive and normotensive pregnancy and fetal growth retardation. British Journal of
Obstetrics and Gynaecology 88: 695–705

Steel S A, Pearce J M, Chamberlain G V 1988 Doppler ultrasound of the uteroplacental
circulation as a screening test for severe pre-eclampsia with intra-uterine growth
retardation. European Journal of Obstetrics, Gynecology and Reproductive Biology 28:
279–287

Trudinger B J, Stevens D, Connelly A et al 1987 Umbilical artery flow velocity waveforms
and placental resistance: the effects of embolisation of the umbilical circulation. American
Journal of Obstetrics and Gynecology 157: 1443–1448

Trudinger B J, Cook C, Giles W B, Connelly A, Thompson R S. Umbilical artery flow
velocity waveforms in high risk pregnancy. Lancet i: 188–190

Trudinger B J, Stewart G J, Cook C, Connelly A, Exner T 1988 Monitoring lupus
anticoagulant positive pregnancies with umbilical artery flow velocity waveforms.
Obstetrics and Gynecology 72: 215–218

Woo J S K, Liang S T, Lo R L S 1987 Significance of an absent or reversed end diastolic flow
in Doppler umbilical artery waveforms. Journal of Ultrasound in Medicine and Biology 6:
291–297

4. Scleroderma and pregnancy

Carol M. Black   Salvatore Lupoli

INTRODUCTION

Scleroderma is a term which includes a heterogenous group of limited and systemic conditions causing hardening of the skin (Rodnan & Jablonska 1985). Systemic sclerosis (SSc) implies involvement of both skin and other sites, particularly certain internal organs.

Systemic sclerosis is an uncommon connective tissue disease, although the current estimates of 4.5–12 new cases/million population/year are probably low (Rodnan et al 1979). It is distributed both geographically and racially. The milder forms are often difficult to identify, and Raynaud's phenomenon, a frequent forerunner and common disorder in women, can be all too easily dismissed. It is a disease with a female preponderance—3F 1M—this figure rising to 8–10:1 in the reproductive years. Sex is the strongest genetic marker, but regrettably the role of the female hormones in scleroderma is unexplored and a much neglected research area. Scleroderma is a disease which can affect any age group, and is relatively less common during the early reproductive years. Thus the previous trend towards early third decade pregnancies has kept the incidence of pregnancy in scleroderma low. Now, with the recent trend in pregnancies later in life (Stein 1985), the co-occurrence may increase.

Because of the low incidence of SSc in association with pregnancy, individual clinicians or units are only likely to have experience of a very small number of cases, and, regrettably, published work on pregnancy and scleroderma is sparse. Most reports deal with only a single case, often reporting a complicated pregnancy, the successful ones rarely being described. There are a few larger series, and with rare exceptions the observations have been retrospective and uncontrolled.

This chapter will seek to summarize the disease and outline the changes which occur in the connective tissue. Such an outline is essential to an understanding of the disorder. The chapter will also review the literature—obstetric and otherwise—on scleroderma and pregnancy, suggest some guidelines for management and indicate the authors' own experience.

THE CONNECTIVE TISSUE

Systemic sclerosis is a disease in which uncontrolled and irreversible proliferation of what appears to be normal connective tissue occurs (Rodnan 1979, LeRoy 1982) along with striking vascular changes (Campbell & LeRoy 1975, Kahaleh et al 1979).

The connective tissue proteins known to be produced in excess are primarily collagen and, to a lesser extent, proteoglycans, fibronectin and laminin (LeRoy 1974, Bailey & Black 1988). The interrelationship between these extracellular matrix proteins in scleroderma is as yet unknown. It is currently believed that the excess collagen is the result of an overproduction of the protein by a certain subset of fibroblasts (Botstein et al 1982).

The earliest lesions in pre-sclerodermatous skin are vascular and inflammatory with collections of lymphocytes, monocytes and macrophages (Fleischmajer et al 1977a, b), and many of these cells are located in the perivascular region. The relationship between these inflammatory cells, their mediators and the subsequent fibrosis may be critical in the initial stages of scleroderma.

The initiating factors are unknown. One reasonable hypothesis derived from the results of numerous workers is that environmental agents such as chemicals (polyvinyl chloride, epoxy resins) (Black et al 1983, Yamakage et al 1980) and drugs (bleomycin, pentazocine) (Finch et al 1985) might cause or initiate defective immunoregulation with the development of autoantibodies and cellular autoimmunity (Postlethwaite et al 1984).

A subsequent widespread reaction of antigen-sensitive T cells with foreign or autoantigens would then lead to the release of mediators. These could facilitate the development of the fibrotic and vascular abnormalities of systemic sclerosis, as they do in chronic graft-versus-host disease. Chronic graft-versus-host disease is an important model for scleroderma: both humans and mice, after receiving a bone marrow transplant, may develop a scleroderma-like illness with Raynaud's, sclerosis and vascular lesions (Furst et al 1979, Deeg & Storb 1984, Janin-Mercier et al 1984). The concept of a foreign graft initiating disease will be discussed later in the chapter when the fetus (or graft) will be viewed as a possible initiator of the mother's (or host's) scleroderma.

CLINICAL FEATURES

The fibrous thickening affects the skin, muscles, joints, tendons, nerves and certain internal organs, especially the oesophagus, intestinal tract, lungs, heart and kidneys (Rodnan et al 1979).

The vascular changes are confined to the small blood vessels of many organs. These lesions are characterized by injury to the endothelium with subendothelial fibrin deposition, increased permeability, thickening of the basement membrane, myointimal cell proliferation, reduplication or fraying of the internal elastic lamina, and periadventitial fibrosis. In capillaries which have no myointimal cells, there is a reduction in their number and they undergo dilatation and telangiectatic change (LeRoy 1982).

The processes of fibrosis and vascular change considerably impair the normal physiological functions of many organs and can make the process of pregnancy difficult (see Table 4.1).

The spectrum of disease within the designation SSc is considerable, ranging from widespread involvement of the skin with diffuse visceral

Table 4.1   Clinical features of scleroderma and the additional problems of pregnancy

Organ	Disorder	Additional problems in pregnancy
Skin	Sclerosis of many areas	Microstomia: anaesthetic problem. Flexion contractures of arms: venous access. Tight abdominal wall: compression of abdominal viscera. Sclerosis of lower legs: painful limbs. Painful flexed hands: problems handling baby
Skeletal muscle	Wasting and weakness of both limb girdle and trunk muscle	Additional fatigue
Tendons	Contractures Friction rubs	Venous access; handling baby
Joints	Polyarthralgias Polyarthritis	Stiff painful joints
GI tract		
Oesophagus	Dysphagia Oesophageal stricture	Reflux oesophagitis and dysphagia worse
Small bowel	Diarrhoea Malabsorption Ileus	Possible malnutrition
Large bowel	Alternating diarrhoea and constipation Rarely: obstruction, perforation ulceration	Additional constipation
Heart	Arrhythmias Conduction defects Pericarditis Congestive cardiac failure Angina	Cardiac failure
Lungs	Dyspnoea Pulmonary fibrosis Pulmonary hypertension	Increasing dyspnoea Sudden pulmonary hypertension
Kidney	Proteinuria Hypertension Renal failure Microangiopathic haemolytic anaemia	Malignant hypertension and irreversible renal failure

Table 4.2 Classification of systemic sclerosis

Sub-group	Additional features
Diffuse cutaneous scleroderma Symmetrical rapidly progressing sclerosis It is advancement proximal to elbow which distinguishes it from the more limited variety Approx. 40%	Delayed or absent Raynaud's Joint and tendon involvement Early visceral involvement (within months to few years) (GI tract, lungs, heart, kidneys) Serum: anti Scl-70 antibodies
Limited cutaneous scleroderma Skin involvement limited to the distal extremities (fingers, e.g. sclerodactyly)— extending to dorsum of hand and face. Some only puffy fingers. Approx. 60%	Raynaud's Calcinosis Telangiectasias Very slow: often many years before visceral involvement, notably pulmonary hypertension and primary biliary cirrhosis Serum: anticentromere antibodies When sclerodactyly and Raynaud's phenomenon are associated with calcinosis, telangiectasia and oesophageal involvement, the acronym 'CREST' is used.

disease to the limited form. Classification is difficult but the most useful method to date is based on location, degree and extent of skin thickening, and a number of reliable clinical, laboratory and natural history associations with skin sclerosis have been made (Medsger 1985; see Table 4.2). The laboratory data include autoantibodies, and their detection in connective tissue diseases is not merely a theoretical exercise—it may help classification and prognosis (Tan et al 1980). In SSc, two antibodies are of importance: scleroderma 70 (Scl-70), which is associated with diffuse disease (Douvas et al 1979, Catoggio et al 1983), and anticentromere antibodies (ACA) (Tan et al 1980, Tuffannelli et al 1983) linked to the more limited form. Autoantibodies also have relevance in the management of pregnant patients with connective tissue diseases, particularly SLE (Scott & Taylor 1985). Following the association of Ro/SS-A antibodies with the neonatal lupus syndrome (Provost 1983, Scott et al 1983), and anticardiolipin antibodies with the increased thrombosis, abortions and intrauterine deaths especially found in SLE (Conley & Hartmann 1952, Carreras et al 1981, de Wolf et al 1982, Nilsson et al 1975), it was natural to study other connective tissue diseases. Scleroderma has no known associated neonatal syndrome, and several series (Seibold et al 1986, Rosenbaum et al 1988) have reported an absence of anticardiolipin antibodies in the disease, suggesting that the vascular damage is mediated via a different mechanism.

SCLERODERMA AND PREGNANCY

The co-occurrence of pregnancy and scleroderma is unusual. This is due to a combination of factors: scleroderma is an uncommon disease, it peaks in

Table 4.3 Summary of case reports of patients with co-existing scleroderma and pregnancy

Authors		Age of patients	Duration of disease (yrs)	No. of patients	Disease class.	No. of preg.	No. of abortions	Perinat. deaths	Toxaemia	Maternal deaths	Change of disease						
											S	R	P	DD	R/P	P/R	NR
Gunther	(1964)	21/22/24	4/5/7	1	dcSSc	3	–	–	–	–	–	2	1	–	–	–	–
Spellacy	(1964)	18/20	1/3	1	dcSSc	2	1	1	–	–	2	–	1	–	–	–	–
De Carle	(1964)	27/29/36	1/3/10	1	dcSSc	3	–	–	–	1	1	–	1	1	–	–	–
Fear	(1968)	26	6	1	dcSSc	1	–	1	1	1	–	–	1	–	–	–	–
Sood	(1970)	25	2	1	dcSSc	1	–	1	1	1	–	–	1	–	–	–	–
Znupp	(1971)	40	8	1	dcSSc	1	–	–	–	–	–	–	1	–	–	–	–
Karlen	(1974)	26	1	1	dcSSc	1	–	–	1	1	–	–	1	–	–	–	–
Woodhall	(1976)	24	1	1	dcSSc	1	–	–	–	1	–	–	1	–	–	–	–
Ehrenfeld	(1977)	20	1	1	lcSSc	1	–	–	1	1	–	–	1	–	–	–	–
Palma	(1981)	27	1	1	dcSSc	1	–	–	1	1	–	–	1	–	–	–	–
Sivanesaratnam	(1982)	31	2	1	dcSSc	1	–	–	1	–	–	–	–	–	–	1	–
Smith	(1982)	25	4	1	dcSSc	1	–	–	–	1	–	–	1	–	–	–	–
Thompson	(1983)	25	4	1	lcSSc	1	–	1	–	–	1	–	–	–	–	–	–
Goplerud	(1983)	NR	NR	1	lcSSc	1	–	–	–	–	–	–	–	–	–	–	1
Bellucci	(1984)	27	NR	1	dcSSc	1	–	–	–	–	1	–	–	–	–	–	–
Ballon	(1984)	24/26	5/7	1	dcSSc	2	–	–	1	–	2	–	–	–	–	–	–
Moore	(1985)	31	4	1	dcSSc	1	1*	–	–	–	–	–	–	–	1	–	–
Younker	(1985)	24	2	1	dcSSc	1	–	1	–	1	–	–	1	–	–	–	–
Scarpinato	(1985)	21	3	1	lcSSc	1	–	–	–	–	1	–	–	–	–	–	–
Luiz	(1986)	28	2	1	dcSSc	1	–	–	–	1	1**	–	–	–	–	–	–

*The abortion was therapeutic.

**The death was not related to scleroderma.

S – stable; R – regressed; P – progressed; DD – developed during pregnancy; R/P – regressed during and progressed after pregnancy; P/R – progressed during and regressed after pregnancy; NR – not recorded; dcSSc – diffuse cutaneous scleroderma; lcSSc – limited cutaneous scleroderma.

the third to fifth decade, and patients possibly exhibit a secondary infertility. There is unfortunately no reliable statistical information regarding the incidence or outcome for either the mother or the fetus. There have been numerous single case reports (see Table 4.3), three or four largely retrospective studies (Johnson et al 1964, Slate & Graham 1968, Weiner et al 1986, Black & Lupoli, unpublished) and recently three retrospective case-controlled reports (Giordano 1985, Silman & Black 1988, Steen et al 1988).

Over 100 cases can be found within the world literature, but some contain only minimal information. The first case was reported by Anselmino & Hoffmann in 1932. It is difficult to assess the effect of scleroderma on pregnancy and vice versa, because the natural history of the disease is variable, the cases reported do not represent the general scleroderma population and, as mentioned earlier, most of the series are retrospective. There appears to be general agreement that SSc can adversely affect both the fetus and the mother, but at the present time accurate prediction is impossible and prospective controlled data are sorely needed.

CASE REPORTS

These cases allow only individual observations and no epidemiological conclusions can be drawn. Bearing this in mind, in the 21 well-documented case reports outlined in Table 4.3, the age of the patients ranged from 18 to 40 years, although most were under 30. Their disease duration ranged from a few months to 10 years, although in most it was less than 5 years. Seventeen of the patients had the diffuse form of scleroderma and four, the limited cutaneous type. Eight out of nine deaths were in patients with the diffuse form and one death occurred in a patient who, at initial examination at the twentieth week of pregnancy, had disease limited to the hands. It was only in the last trimester that visceral complications occurred and the patient died of renal failure.

Effect of disease on pregnancy

There were 27 pregnancies in these 21 patients. No conclusions concerning fertility can be made as there was little available information. There were 2 abortions, 5 perinatal deaths (1 intrauterine death undelivered, 1 still-born, 3 early neonatal deaths). Of the three deaths in the early neonatal period, one was due to multiple congenital abnormalities (Thompson & Conklin 1983); the mother of this child had been taking chlorambucil until the tenth week of pregnancy. One was due to prematurity at 28 weeks (Spellacy 1964) and one other was due to multiple congenital abnormalities (Younker & Harrison 1985). Twenty out of 23 live-born infants survived. We have not reported on prematurity in these pregnancies because of the sporadic and insufficient information available.

Table 4.4 Summary of series of patients with co-existing scleroderma and pregnancy

Author	No. of patients	Disease classification	No. of pregnancies	Abortions	Perinatal deaths	Toxaemia	Maternal deaths	S	R	P	DD	NR
Johnson (1964)	NR	lcSSc	36	3	1	—	—	14	8	8	6	—
Slate (1968)	6	NR	17	13	2	—	1	—	—	—	—	17
Weiner (1986)	14	11 dcSSc	21	3	1	1	—	15	1	3	2	—
		3 lcSSc	9	1	—	—	—	—	—	9	—	—
Black	12	7 dcSSc	12	4	—	3	1	3	—	8	1	—
		5 lcSSc	6	—	1	2	—	2	2	2	—	—

S – stable; R – regressed; P – progressed; DD – developed during; NR – not reported; dcSSc – diffuse cutaneous scleroderma; lcSSc – limited cutaneous scleroderma.

Effect of pregnancy on the disease

The variable course of SSc with its exacerbations and remissions and the individual nature of the cases makes it difficult to assess accurately the effect of a superimposed pregnancy. In the 27 cases reported, the disease appeared unchanged in 9, regressed in 2, progressed in 12, developed during the pregnancy in 1, remitted during and progressed after the pregnancy in 1, progressed during and remitted after the pregnancy in 1, and was not recorded in 1. Nine patients developed toxaemia, and of these, 5 died of subsequent renal failure. There were nine maternal deaths in total: of the 5 who died of renal failure, all had biopsy findings compatible with renal scleroderma. One patient died of pulmonary hypertension, sepsis and gastrointestinal haemorrhage, two from viral pneumonia and one from an unknown cause, although the patient had established disease.

These single case histories present a depressing picture of both fetal and maternal wastage (see Table 4.3). However, as discussed later, this could be due to case selection.

SERIES REPORTS

Looking at the three reported series (two papers and one abstract) and our own experience, which is as yet unreported, there were 101 pregnancies

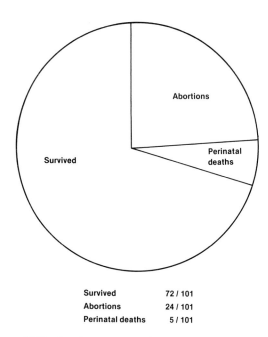

Survived	72 / 101
Abortions	24 / 101
Perinatal deaths	5 / 101

Fig. 4.1 Outcome of 101 scleroderma pregnancies.

(Table 4.4). The patients' ages ranged from 20 to 40 years. The length of disease was available in two series and ranged between 0 and 8 years (Johnson et al 1964) and 2 months to 8 years (Black & Lupoli, in preparation). Most of the patients had a limited form of scleroderma. There were 101 pregnancies but information on fertility is minimal. There were 24 spontaneous abortions, 5 perinatal deaths [3 still-born, 2 early neonatal deaths (Table 4.4; Fig. 4.1)], 6 cases of toxaemia and 2 maternal deaths.

Reviewing the 101 pregnancies, the disease was stable following 34 pregnancies, remitting in 11, progressive in 30, and developed during pregnancy in 9; for the remaining 17, the disease state is unknown (Table 4.4; Fig. 4.2). These figures would appear to compare favourably with the single case reports. Not surprisingly perhaps, the patients recorded in the larger series have less complicated pregnancies and a better prognosis than those reported in the single cases, presumably selected for their severity. However, this could be due to uncertainty about the number of unreported cases with normal outcome, lack of controlled data and selection of patients. Most of the patients in the single case reports had diffuse disease whereas the majority in the large series were limited.

CASE-CONTROLLED STUDIES

There are three recent case-controlled studies in the world literature.

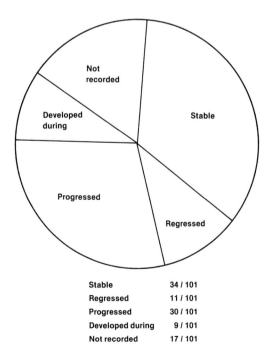

Stable	34 / 101
Regressed	11 / 101
Progressed	30 / 101
Developed during	9 / 101
Not recorded	17 / 101

Fig. 4.2   Disease states following pregnancy.

Italian study

A retrospective study by Giordano et al from Naples (1985) has produced some interesting information about the spontaneous abortion rate in scleroderma versus healthy controls. They analysed 86 married women with systemic sclerosis and 86 healthy normal controls. Only six of the 86 patients and four of the normal controls did not become pregnant.

The 80 SSc patients had a total of 299 pregnancies and 50 (28 women) of these were interrupted by spontaneous abortion. The 82 control women had 332 pregnancies, 32 (24 women) of which were interrupted by spontaneous abortion. The abortions were not therefore to be found in a few habitual aborters. The percentage of abortion in SSc patients was found to be significantly higher than that of controls ($x^2 = 6.36, P < 0.05$). The rate of abortions was not statistically different between the diffuse and limited forms of scleroderma. Unfortunately, accurate information was not available as to the exact time of onset of the scleroderma in relationship to the pregnancies. This study would also refute the suggestion by Ballou et al (1984) that pregnancy is uncommon in scleroderma: only 6 of their 86 patients did not get pregnant. There was, however, a lower total number of pregnancies ($n = 299$) in scleroderma as compared with controls ($n = 332$). These figures do not reach statistical significance.

The British study

A recent case-controlled study by Silman & Black (1988) used a postal questionnaire to obtain pregnancy and reproductive history in 155 cases of SSc and compared the results with that of 155 matched normal controls. The study showed that women destined to develop scleroderma have twice the rate of spontaneous abortion (relative risk 2:1) and three times the rate of fertility problems (relative risk 3:0—no successful pregnancy by the age of 35) of the control women. The SSc women were also more likely to have had recurrent abortions. The results of this study suggest for the first time that an adverse reproductive history may precede the clinical diagnosis of scleroderma, in some cases by many years.

These studies, together with the evidence from a recent large family study in scleroderma (Pereira et al 1987), where many women dated their symptoms to pregnancy, and also other features of the disorder including the similarities between it and graft-versus-host disease, suggest a hypothesis that transplacental transfer of cells between mother and fetus could lead to a state of 'micro-chimaerism' and that activation of such cells could lead to a syndrome similar to chronic graft-versus-host disease (Pereira, unpublished data).

The American study

A recent study by Dr Steen and colleagues (1988) was designed to determine the frequency of maternal morbidity, miscarriages, prematurity and fetal death by studying pregnancy outcome in a largely retrospective population using a case control design, the scleroderma patients being matched to neighbourhood controls and patients with chronic rheumatoid arthritis. There were 223 case-controlled pairs and their results showed an increased risk of prematurity and intrauterine growth retardation but no statistical increase in the rate of miscarriages, fetal death, maternal morbidity or mortality. Nor was any relationship found between pregnancy and disease onset. They noted that in those SSc pregnancies with adverse outcomes, births occurred a mean of 3.7 years (range 0.5–11.0 years) prior to disease expression. It may, however, not require an adverse outcome and it may take a longer time than was observed for this chronic disease to express itself; therefore this particular conclusion should be viewed with caution. In this study they did not address the problem of fertility.

The information available from single cases, larger series and case-controlled studies provides some interesting data but above all points to the need for careful long-term prospective studies on these patients and careful monitoring of all patients.

RENAL DISEASE AND SCLERODERMA

The data highlight the occurrence of renal involvement. Kidney disease and hypertension are not the only major cause of death in patients with SSc (Rodnan 1963, Cannon et al 1974, Medsger & Masi 1973) but are also the major cause of maternal death in the scleroderma pregnancies reviewed here.

Renal involvement is uncommon when scleroderma is first diagnosed. The average interval between diagnosis of scleroderma and the onset of renal disease is 3.2 years (Alfrey 1981). Renal involvement is thought to occur in up to 58% of patients with SSc (Cannon et al 1974, D'Angelo et al 1969). The presentation of renal involvement in scleroderma may take several forms. One group are those who, previously stable, present with the sudden onset of malignant hypertension, sometimes with microangiopathic haemolytic anaemia (Salyer et al 1973). Renal function deteriorates rapidly (Cannon et al 1974, Couser et al 1983), and prior to the introduction of captopril, minoxidil and enalapril therapy (Smith et al 1984, Thurm & Alexander 1984, Beckett et al 1985), most of these patients died within a 1–2 month period. A second group are normotensive or have well-controlled hypertension and present with rapidly progressive renal failure (Couser et al 1983). This group's prognosis is similar to the first. Thirdly, there is a group of patients in which renal involvement is manifest by proteinuria and/or azotaemia (Beigelman et al 1953, Heptinstall 1983). These patients appear to have prolonged survival times and follow a chronic course.

Histologically, the most prominent abnormalities are in the vessel walls. The interlobular arteries (150–500 μm in diameter) show intimal thickening as a result of deposition of mucinous or finely collagenous material, and concentric proliferation of intimal cells. These changes may resemble those seen in malignant hypertension, haemolytic-uraemic syndrome, idiopathic post-partum renal failure and acute tubular necrosis. It has been stressed that, in scleroderma, the alterations are not always associated with hypertension and are restricted to vessels 150–500 μm in diameter.

Hypertension, however, occurs in 30% of patients with scleroderma and in 7–10% is malignant. In hypertensive patients vascular changes are more pronounced and are often associated with fibrinoid necrosis, involving the arterioles together with thrombosis and infarction. When this occurs it becomes difficult to differentiate the lesions of scleroderma from those of other types of malignant hypertension. Glomerular changes are non-specific and mainly consist of slightly increased cellularity of the mesangium and localized irregular thickening of the basement membrane. Some of these changes may be related to the hypertension (Robbins et al 1984).

The renal disease of scleroderma that begins in pregnancy is a difficult, confused and challenging area. It can appear at any stage of the pregnancy and usually presents as hypertension. The differential diagnosis must include idiopathic hypertension, primary renal disease, renal scleroderma (perhaps hitherto not clinically apparent) or accelerated hypertension of the non-toxaemic variety appearing early in the post-partum period, and to the unaware physician this may masquerade as pre-eclamptic toxaemia. It is usually refractory to all kinds of therapy. In all but the most typical case of pre-eclampsia or eclampsia, especially a case not responding to conventional treatment, renal scleroderma should be given a prominent place in the differential diagnosis. This is important because the therapy and prognosis are different from those of pre-eclampsia. The post-partum period can be a particularly vulnerable one, something perhaps hitherto not fully recognized. It is also possible that the patient may have two of the above conditions, for example toxaemia and renal scleroderma.

In most reported cases there is no prior history of renal disease. This was so in the 21 cases reported in Table 4.3. None had hypertension at the onset of the pregnancy. Ten patients developed it during the pregnancy and one immediately afterwards. Nine of the patients had toxaemia and in seven patients there was biopsy-proven renal scleroderma. Five or possibly seven of the nine deaths in the series were due to renal disease.

From the evidence available to date, pregnancy in known renal scleroderma should be avoided. If a pregnancy is started, monitoring should be meticulous and a sustained fall in renal function should lead to consideration of therapeutic termination.

DRUG THERAPY IN SCLERODERMA

The treatment of scleroderma is difficult if not impossible. As there are no known satisfactory therapies for the disease, the use of drugs, particularly those which attempt to modify the disease, is naturally controversial. The drugs used in scleroderma fall into three main categories: those given for minor problems such as muscular and articular aches and pains and gastro-oesophageal reflux, those to improve the circulation, and those which attempt to modify the disease.

Non-steroidal anti-inflammatory drugs (NSAIDs)

The 'classical' NSAIDs, especially aspirin and indomethacin, have been used for decades in the treatment of connective tissue diseases without any teratogenicity being proven in man (Buckfield 1973, Turner & Collins 1975, Sloane et al 1976), and in low intermittent doses of less than 3 g daily they do not have any effect on the nursing infant. Amongst the newest NSAIDs (proprionic and acetic acid derivatives, fenemates and oxicams), naproxen, ketoprofen, ibuprofen and furbiprofen have been shown not to be teratogenic in man (Sloane et al 1976) and safe for breast-feeding mothers.

When NSAIDs are used to control musculo-skeletal problems during pregnancy, only drugs whose effects on pregnancy and the fetus are known to be innocuous should be prescribed. Intermittent dosage and the lowest possible dose should be used. Prostaglandin synthetase inhibitors may delay parturition and NSAIDs therefore should be avoided in late pregnancy. Well-motivated women with moderate symptoms may be managed with no therapy or simple analgesics, paracetamol being the drug of choice.

Corticosteroids

Corticosteroids are rarely indicated in the treatment of established scleroderma and should be avoided in pregnancy unless severe myositis is present or the patient develops the rampant oedematous inflammatory phase of the disorder. Their use in other connective tissue diseases has shown them to be free of teratogenicity in man (Hawkins 1983).

D-penicillamine

D-penicillamine is probably the most commonly used disease-modifying drug in SSc and its use in pregnancy is a controversial issue (Needs & Brooks 1985, Byron 1986). Its use in pregnancy has been associated with the development of a generalized connective tissue defect similar to the Ehlers–Danlos syndrome in three babies (Mjolnerod et al 1971, Solomon et al 1977, Linares et al 1979). Many normal children, however, have been born to mothers taking penicillamine for Wilson's disease (Scheinberg &

Sternlieb 1975, Walshe 1977) and it was proposed that in this disease the fetus was protected from the effect of penicillamine by the excessive maternal pool of copper. However, in another survey, one ventricular septal defect was the only abnormality reported in 27 pregnancies in patients with rheumatoid arthritis and cystinuria (Lyle 1978). Nevertheless, penicillamine should not be used during pregnancy and breast-feeding, and if the pregnancy occurs when the patient is receiving penicillamine, it should be slowly withdrawn (Lyle 1978).

Cytotoxic drugs

Antimetabolites and alkylating agents may be teratogenic and mutagenic, and even if used after the first trimester of pregnancy, the fetus is susceptible to infection, haemorrhage and bone marrow depression (Barber 1981). As they have no proven efficacy in scleroderma, they should not be used.

Raynaud's phenomenon often improves considerably during pregnancy due to the increased blood flow. Vasodilator therapy should be avoided and the patient educated in practical ways of keeping warm, for example thermal clothing, hand warmers and electrically heated gloves.

ANAESTHETIC PROBLEMS IN SCLERODERMA

The pregnant scleroderma patient is not only a potential anaesthetic problem but also a challenge because of her potential for precipitous cardiopulmonary and renal insufficiency. Some pathophysiological aspects of scleroderma pose problems for the anaesthetist, regardless of the type of anaesthetic and whether obstetric delivery is by the vaginal route or caesarean section (Younker & Harrison 1985, Thompson & Conklin 1983, Roelofsee & Shipton 1985).

The fibrosed skin, along with the vasoconstriction, frequently makes venous access difficult, and venous cut-down or central venous catheterization may be necessary. Flexion contractures combined with vasoconstriction may interfere with blood pressure monitoring by the usual methods, and pressures may need monitoring via arterial catheterization. Catheterization of the smaller peripheral arteries has been associated with spasm and subsequent necrosis; therefore these vessels should be avoided (Eisele 1981).

The anaesthetic risk to patients with SSc may be increased because of visceral involvement. Oesophageal involvement may produce an incompetent lower oesophageal sphincter, and cardiac, pulmonary and renal problems may be severe. Pulmonary hypertension is a known, albeit infrequent, finding in patients with the 'CREST' form of scleroderma (see Table 4.2), and pulmonary fibrosis (often sub-clinical) is common. Renal disease decreases renal perfusion and is accompanied by systemic hypertension, and cardiac function is compromised because of pericarditis conduction defects and heart failure.

The problems above are common to any patient with scleroderma. The type of anaesthetic and obstetric delivery will obviously be a very individual decision, but the pre-anaesthetic screen must be very comprehensive.

If regional anaesthesia is used for labour and delivery, smaller doses than usual of local anaesthetics are suggested because scleroderma patients may exhibit prolonged motor and sensory blockade afterwards (Eisele 1981). The regional anaesthesia, as well as giving pain relief, provides peripheral vasodilatation and increased skin perfusions in the lower limbs, which is helpful in relieving Raynaud's phenomenon. Other measures to prevent Raynaud's include warm delivery rooms, warm intravenous solutions and thermal socks. If a general anaesthetic is to be given, the patient's eyes should be protected as some patients suffer from kerato-conjunctivitis sicca and the cornea may be damaged. Microstomia can make intubation difficult if not impossible, nasal or oral telangiectasias may bleed if traumatized, and oesophageal dysmotility and sphincter incompetence can lead to aspiration. Finally, it may be desirable to insert a pulmonary artery catheter, especially if impaired renal function, pulmonary hypertension or cardiac problems are suspected. With invasive monitoring, the haemodynamic effect of both volume shifts and anaesthetic agents can be rapidly assessed and the efficacy of therapy determined.

ADVISING PATIENTS WITH SCLERODERMA

Review of an almost exclusively retrospective literature, where much of the information is inadequately documented, plus our own experience forms the basis for the current recommendations.

Will pregnancy be possible?

It is possible that the ability to get pregnant may be less in patients with scleroderma (Silman & Black 1988), and the abortion rate is also considered by some to be increased (Giordano et al 1985, Slate & Graham 1968, Silman & Black 1988). Other authors disagree with this (Johnson et al 1964, Steen et al 1988), showing no increase in spontaneous abortions. SSc women may also have recurrent abortions (Silman & Black 1988), although the American experience would disagree with this (Steen et al 1988).

Will pregnancy be complicated?

The prospective mothers must be counselled about the risks outlined earlier. There are no good prognosticators as yet. It would appear, looking at the available evidence (see Tables 4.3 and 4.4), that the extent of systemic involvement may be more important than the length of the disease, and that limited, mild disease carries a better prognosis.

The third trimester is a dangerous period with the risks of rapidly developing hypertension and renal failure and of interruption of the pregnancy, should one of the vital organs become compromised.

Patients should also be made aware of the effect the enlarging uterus can have on the abdominal skin and other viscera. Since the sclerosis usually spares the abdomen, this is rarely a problem, but there is one report (Moore et al 1985) of hydronephrosis presumed secondary to thickened skin and decreased abdominal wall compliance in a twin pregnancy complicated by polyhydramnios.

Reflux oesophagitis may increase but can usually be controlled with the appropriate dietary advice and antacids. Small bowel involvement and malabsorption potentially could present problems leading to malnutrition. The changes of pregnancy might also result in increased constipation in an already diseased large bowel.

Will the baby be healthy?

The answer is a qualified yes. Patients should be informed that the risks are certainly greater than in a normal pregnancy. The patient's fear concerning any hereditary tendency can be allayed. The recent genetic predisposition described by Welsh & Black (1988) shows a low relative risk. There are only three reports in the world literature of areas of sclerosis in the newborn (Anselmino et al 1932, Etterich & Mall 1955, Ohtaki et al 1986). Two of these cases were reports of sclerosis on the upper thighs and buttocks and were transient; they could of course have represented sclerema neonatorum (Winkelmann 1965). The third case was an infant boy born to a mother with systemic lupus erythematosus. This boy developed annular erythematosus lesions and multiple morphoea. The former were considered to be the lesions of neonatal lupus erythematosus and faded within 7 months. The latter progressed until the age of 6 months and was then stable until last observed at the age of 3 years.

Will the pregnancy adversely affect the underlying disease?

It may. Again the literature is conflicting. Tables 4.3 and 4.4 show that there is worsening of the disease in many patients. It would appear from our own experience that those with diffuse disease tend to fare worse. However, this is not always the case and those with limited disease may develop life-threatening involvement. Recent evidence from an American study gives a more hopeful picture and they found no significant deterioration in the disease after pregnancy.

MANAGEMENT OF PREGNANCY

A review of the literature provides no consensus of opinion. However, bearing in mind personal preference, the following are guidelines for management.

Pre-pregnancy advice

Ideally, the woman with scleroderma should have advice before embarking upon pregnancy. It should ideally represent a combined view of both a physician and an obstetrician who have special interest in, and experience of, the field.

Ante-natal care

1. A complete evaluation should be made as early in the pregnancy as possible.
2. If there is evidence of renal disease, pulmonary hypertension or myocardial fibrosis, a therapeutic abortion should be offered.

    In the absence of significant visceral involvement, the patient should be informed that there is always the possibility of the development of such complications, however mild the scleroderma, and that they cannot be predicted. With this information the patient may elect to terminate the pregnancy.
3. If the patient chooses to proceed with the pregnancy, ante-natal examinations should be fortnightly until the third trimester, and weekly thereafter.
4. Routine serial ante-natal observations should be supplemented by:
    (a) cardiopulmonary examination
    (b) monitoring of blood pressure for early detection of hypertension and assessment of its severity
    (c) careful assessment of renal function, urine examination and, if indicated, 24-hour clearance and creatinine
    (d) attention should be paid to weight, oesophageal and intestinal symptoms, and nutritional status
    (e) checks for oedema
5. Symptomatic treatment should be provided for musculo-skeletal problems and appropriate nutritional supplements should be provided for the patient.

Post-natal management

The post-natal period should be monitored carefully as acute hypertension with renal and cardiac failure may occur.

CONCLUSION

Experience with pregnancy in patients with systemic sclerosis is limited, confusing and controversial, thus making it difficult to give dogmatic advice to patients with this uncommon disease. However, there appears to be general agreement that:

1. Systemic sclerosis can adversely affect pregnancy, although the incidence of such interactions cannot be ascertained from the multiple anecdotal reports and uncontrolled series available for review.
2. Pregnancy may adversely affect the course of systemic sclerosis, renal disease being a particular high and lethal risk.

We conclude that information derived from the literature and our own experience suggests that there is a complex interaction between SSc and pregnancy and emphasizes the need to study and define this relationship.

REFERENCES

Alfrey C 1981 The renal response to vascular injury. In: Brenner B M, Rector F C Jr (eds) The kidney: W B Saunders, Philadelphia, pp 1680–1684

Anselmino K J, Hoffmann F 1932 Uber Sklerodermie und Schwangerschaft. Zeitschrift fur Geburtshilfe und Gynakologie 103: 60–66

Bailey A J, Black C M 1988 The role of the connective tissue in the pathogenesis of scleroderma. In: Black C M, Jayson M I V (eds) Systemic sclerosis: scleroderma. John Wiley, Chichester, pp 75–105

Ballou S P, Morley J J, Kushner I 1984 Pregnancy and systemic sclerosis. Arthritis and Rheumatism 27: 295–298

Barber H R K 1981 Foetal and neonatal effects of cytotoxic agents. Obstetrics and Gynecology 58 (suppl 5) 50: 41–47

Beckett V L, Donadio J V, Brennan Jr L A et al 1985 Use of captopril as early therapy for renal scleroderma: a prospective study. Mayo Clinic Proceedings 60: 763–771

Beigelman P M, Goldner F, Bayless J B 1953 Progressive systemic sclerosis (scleroderma). New England Journal of Medicine 249: 45–58

Bellucci M J, Coustan D R, Plotz R D 1984 Cervical scleroderma: a case of soft tissue dystocia. American Journal of Obstetrics and Gynecology 150: 891–892

Black C M, Welsh K I, Walker A E et al 1983 Genetic susceptibility to scleroderma-like syndrome induced by vinyl chloride. Lancet i: 53–55

Black C M, Lupoli S Paper 1989 In preparation

Botstein G R, Sherer G K, LeRoy E C 1982 Fibroblast selection in scleroderma. An alternative model of fibrosis. Arthritis and Rheumatism 25: 189–195

Buckfield P 1973 Major congenital faults in newborn infants: a pilot study in New Zealand. New Zealand Medical Journal 78: 195–204

Byron M J 1987 Prescribing in pregnancy. Treatment of rheumatic diseases. British Medical Journal 294: 236–238

Campbell P M, LeRoy R C 1975 Pathogenesis of systemic sclerosis: a vascular hypothesis. Seminars in Arthritis and Rheumatism 4: 351–368

Cannon P J, Hassar M, Case D B et al 1974 The relationship of hypertension and renal failure in scleroderma (progressive systemic sclerosis) to structural and functional abnormalities of the renal cortical circulation. Medicine 53: 1–46

Carreras L O, Defreyn G, Machin S J 1981 Arterial thrombosis, intrauterine death and 'lupus' coagulant. Detection of immunoglobulin interfering with prostacyclin formation. Lancet i: 244–246

Catoggio L J, Bernstein R M, Black C M et al 1983 Serologic markers in progressive systemic sclerosis. Arthritis and Rheumatism 23: 617–625

Conley C L, Hartmann R C 1952 A haemorrhagic disorder caused by circulating anticoagulant in patients with disseminated lupus erythematosus. Journal of Clinical Investigation 31: 621–622

Couser W G, Salant D J, Adler S et al 1983 Acute renal failure associated with renal vascular disease, vasculitis, glomerulonephritis and nephrotic syndrome. In: Brenner B M, Lazarus J M (eds) Acute renal failure. Saunders, Philadelphia, pp 343–344

D'Angelo W A, Fries J F, Masi A T et al 1969 Pathologic observations in systemic sclerosis (scleroderma). American Journal of Medicine 46: 428–440

DeCarle D W 1964 Pregnancy associated with scleroderma. Case report of a patient with three successful pregnancies. American Journal of Obstetrics and Gynecology 89: 356–361

Deeg H J, Storb R 1984 Graft-versus-host disease: pathophysiological and clinical aspects. Annual Review of Medicine 35: 11–24

de Wolf F, Carreras L O, Moerman P et al 1982 Decidual vasculopathy and extensive placental infarction in a patient with repeated thrombo-embolic accidents, recurrent foetal loss and a lupus coagulant. American Journal of Obstetrics and Gynecology 142: 829–834

Douvas A S, Achten M, Tan E M 1979 Identification of a nuclear protein (Scl-70) as a unique target of human antinuclear antibodies in scleroderma. Journal of Biochemistry 254: 10514–10522

Eisele J H 1981 Connective tissue diseases. In: Katz J, Benumof J, Kadis L (eds) Anesthesia and uncommon diseases. Saunders, Philadelphia, pp 518–521

Ehrenfeld M, Licht A, Stessman J, Yanko L, Rosenmann E 1977 Post-partum renal failure due to progressive systemic sclerosis treated with chronic hemodialysis. Nephron 18: 175–181

Etterich M, Mall M 1955 Sklerodermie and Schwangerschaft. Gynecologia 139: 236–239

Fear R E 1968 Eclampsia superimposed on renal scleroderma: a rare cause of maternal and fetal mortality. Obstetrics and Gynecology 31: 69–74

Finch W R, Buckingham R B, Rodnan G P et al 1985 Scleroderma induced by bleomycin. In: Black C M, Myers A R (eds) Systemic sclerosis (scleroderma). Gower, New York, pp 114–121

Fleischmajer R, Perlish J S, Reeves I R T 1977a Cellular infiltrates in scleroderma skin. Arthritis and Rheumatism 20: 975–984

Fleischmajer R, Perlish J S, West W P 1977b Ultrastructure of cutaneous cellular infiltrates in scleroderma. Archives of Dermatology 113: 1661–1666

Furst D E, Clements P J, Graze P, Gale R, Roberts N 1979 A syndrome resembling progressive systemic sclerosis after bone marrow transplantation: a model for scleroderma? Arthritis and Rheumatism 22: 904–910

Giordano M, Valentini G, Lupoli S et al 1985 Pregnancy and systemic sclerosis. Arthritis and Rheumatism (letter) 28: 237–238

Goplerud C P 1983 Scleroderma. Clinical Obstetrics and Gynecology 26: 587–591

Gunter R E, Harer B W 1964 Systemic sclerosis in pregnancy—report of a case. Obstetrics and Gynecology 24: 98–100

Hawkins D F 1983 Drug treatment of medical disorders in pregnancy. In: Hawkins D F (ed) Drugs and pregnancy. Churchill Livingstone, Edinburgh, pp 76–92

Heptinstall R H 1983 Pathology of the kidney, (3rd edn). Little Brown, Boston, pp 938–953

Janin-Mercier A, Devergie A, Van Cawemberge D et al 1984 Immunohistologic and ultrastructural study of the sclerotic skin in chronic graft-versus-host disease in man. American Journal of Pathology 115: 296–306

Johnson T R, Banner E A, Winkelmann R K 1964 Scleroderma and pregnancy. Obstetrics and Gynecology 23: 467–469

Kahaleh M B, Sherer G K, LeRoy E C 1979 Endothelial cell injury in scleroderma. Journal of Experimental Medicine 149: 1326–1335

Karlen J R, Cook W A 1974 Renal scleroderma and pregnancy. Obstetrics and Gynecology 44: 349–354

Knupp M Z, O'Leary J A 1971 Pregnancy and scleroderma. Systemic sclerosis. Journal of the Florida Medical Association 58: 28–30

LeRoy E C 1974 Increased collagen synthesis by scleroderma skin fibroblasts in vitro: a possible defect in the regulation or activation of the scleroderma fibroblast. Journal of Clinical Investigation 54: 880–889

LeRoy E C 1982 Pathogenesis of scleroderma (systemic sclerosis). Journal of Investigative Dermatology 79 (suppl): 87–89

Linares A, Zarranz J J, Rodriguez-Alarcon J, Diaz-Perez J L 1979 Reversible cutis laxa due to maternal D-penicillamine treatment (letter). Lancet ii: 43

Luiz D A, Moodley J, Naicker S N, Pudifin D 1986 Pregnancy in scleroderma. A case report. South African Journal of Medicine 69: 642–643

Lyle W H 1978 Penicillamine in pregnancy. Lancet i: 606–607

Medsger T A Jr, Masi A T 1973 Survival with scleroderma II. A life table analysis of clinical and demographic factors in 358 male US veteran patients. Journal of Chronic Diseases 26: 647–660

Medsger T A Jr 1985 Comment on scleroderma criteria cooperative study. In: Black C M, Myers A R (eds) Current topics in rheumatology—systemic sclerosis (scleroderma). Gower, New York, pp 16–17

Mjolnerod O K, Dommerud S A, Rasmussen K et al 1971 Congenital connective tissue defect probably due to D-penicillamine treatment in pregnancy. Lancet i: 673–675

Moore M, Saffran J E, Baraf H S et al 1985 Systemic sclerosis and pregnancy complicated by obstructive uropathy. American Journal of Obstetrics and Gynecology 153: 893–894

Needs C J, Brooks P M 1985 Anti-rheumatic medication in pregnancy. British Journal of Rheumatology 24: 282–290

Nilsson I M, Astedt B, Hedner U et al 1975 Intrauterine death and circulating anticoagulant ('anti-thromboplastin'). Acta Medica Scandinavica 197: 153–159

Ohtaki N, Miyamoto C, Orita M et al 1986 Concurrent multiple morphoea and neonatal lupus erythematosus in an infant boy born to a mother with SLE. British Journal of Dermatology 115: 85–90

Palma A, Sanchez-Palencia A, Armas J R et al 1981 Progressive systemic sclerosis and nephrotic syndrome. An unusual association resulting in postpartum acute renal failure. Archives of Internal Medicine 141: 520–521

Pereira R S, Black C M, Welsh K I et al 1987 Autoantibodies and immunogenetics in 30 patients with systemic sclerosis and their families. Journal of Rheumatology 14: 760–765

Postlethwaite A E, Stuart J M, Kang A H 1984 The cell-mediated immune system in progressive systemic sclerosis: an overview. In: Black C M, Myers A (eds) Proceedings of the second conference on systemic sclerosis. Gower, New York, pp 319–325

Provost T T 1983 Commentary neonatal lupus erythematosus. Archives of Dermatology 119: 619–622

Robbins S L, Cotran R S, Kumar V 1984 Diseases of immunity. In: Pathologic basis of disease. Saunders, Philadelphia, pp 158–213

Rodnan G P 1963 The natural history of progressive systemic sclerosis (diffuse scleroderma). Bulletin on the Rheumatic Diseases 13: 301–304

Rodnan G P, Jablonska S, Medsger T A Jr 1979 Classification and nomenclature of progressive systemic sclerosis (scleroderma). Clinics in the Rheumatic Diseases 5: 5–13

Rodnan G P, Jablonska S 1985 Classification of systemic and localized scleroderma. In: Black C M, Myers A R (eds) Current topics in rheumatology: systemic sclerosis (scleroderma). Gower, New York, pp 3–6

Roelofse J A, Shipton E A 1985 Anaesthesia in connective tissue disorders. South African Medical Journal 67: 336–339

Rosenbaum J, Pottinger B E, Woo P et al 1988 Measurement and characterisation of circulating anti-endothelial cell IgG in connective tissue diseases. Clinical and Experimental Immunology 72: 450–456

Salyer W R, Salyer D C, Heptinstall R M 1973 Scleroderma and microangiopathic hemolytic anemia. Annals of Internal Medicine 73: 895–897

Scarpinato L, Mackenzie A H 1985 Pregnancy and progressive systemic sclerosis. Case report and review of the literature. Cleveland Clinical Quarterly 52: 207–211

Scheinberg I H, Sternlieb I 1975 Pregnancy in penicillamine-treated patients with Wilson's disease. New England Journal of Medicine 293: 1300–1301

Scott J S, Maddison P J, Taylor P V et al 1983 Connective tissue disease antibodies to ribonucleoprotein and congenital heart block. New England Journal of Medicine 309: 209–212

Scott J S, Taylor P V 1985 Pregnancy and the connective tissue diseases. Seminars in Dermatology 4: 127–135

Seibold J R, Knight P J, Peter J B 1986 Anticardiolipin antibodies in systemic sclerosis (letter). Arthritis and Rheumatism 29: 1052–1053

Silman A, Black C M 1988 Increased incidence of spontaneous abortion and infertility in women with scleroderma before disease onset: a controlled study. Annals of the Rheumatic Diseases 47: 441–444

Sivanesaratnam V, Chong H L 1982 Scleroderma and pregnancy. Australian and New Zealand Journal of Obstetrics and Gynaecology 22: 123–124

Slate W G, Graham A B 1968 Scleroderma and pregnancy. American Journal of Obstetrics and Gynecology 101: 335–341

Sloane D, Heinonen O, Kaufman D W, Shapiro S 1976 Aspirin and congenital malformations. Lancet i: 1373–1375

Smith C A, Pinals R S 1982 Progressive systemic sclerosis and postpartum renal failure complicated by peripheral gangrene. Journal of Rheumatology 9: 455–458

Smith C D, Smith R D, Korn J H 1984 Hypertensive crisis in systemic sclerosis: treatment with the new oral angiotensin converting enzyme inhibitor MK 421 (enalapril in captopril-intolerant patients. Arthritis and Rheumatism 27: 826–828

Solomon L, Abrams G, Dinner M, Berman L 1977 Neonatal abnormalities associated with D-penicillamine treatment during pregnancy. New England Journal of Medicine 296: 54–55

Sood S V, Kohler H G 1970 Maternal death from systemic sclerosis (report of a case of renal scleroderma masquerading as pre-eclamptic toxaemia). Journal of Obstetrics and Gynaecology of the British Commonwealth 77: 1109–1112

Spellacy W N 1964 Scleroderma and pregnancy — report of a case. Obstetrics and Gynecology 23: 297–300

Steen V D, Conte C, Day N et al 1988 Pregnancy in systemic sclerosis (in press)

Stein Z A 1985 A woman's age child-bearing and child-rearing. American Journal of Epidemiology 121: 327–342

Tan E M, Rodnan G P, Garcia I et al 1980 Diversity of antinuclear antibodies in progressive systemic sclerosis. Arthritis and Rheumatism 23: 617–625

Thompson J, Conklin K A 1983 Anesthetic management of a pregnant patient with scleroderma. Anesthesiology 59: 69–71

Thurm R H, Alexander J C 1984 Captopril in the treatment of scleroderma renal crisis. Archives of Internal Medicine 144: 733–735

Tuffannelli D L, McKeon F, Kleinsmith A M et al 1983 Anticentromere and anti-centriole antibodies in the scleroderma spectrum. Archives of Dermatology 119: 560–565

Turner G, Collins E 1975 Fetal effects of regular salicylate ingestion in pregnancy. Lancet ii: 338–340

Walshe J M 1977 Brief observations on the management of Wilson's disease. Proceedings of the Royal Society of Medicine 70 (suppl 3): 1–3

Weiner R S, Brinkmann C R, Paulus H E 1986 Scleroderma, CREST syndrome and pregnancy. Arthritis and Rheumatism 29(4): S51

Welsh K I, Black C M 1988 Environmental and genetic factors in scleroderma. In: Black C M, Jayson M I V (eds) Systemic sclerosis: scleroderma. John Wiley, Chichester, pp 33–47

Winkelmann R D 1965 Scleroderma and pregnancy. Clinical Obstetrics and Gynecology 8: 280–285

Woodhall P B, McCoy R C, Gunnells J C et al 1976 Apparent recurrence of progressive systemic sclerosis in a renal allograft. Journal of the American Medical Association 236: 1032–1034

Yamakage A, Ishikawa M, Saito Y et al 1980 Occupational scleroderma-like disorders occurring in men engaged in the polymerization of epoxy resins. Dermatologica 161: 33–44

Younker D, Harrison B 1985 Scleroderma and pregnancy. Anaesthetic consideration. British Journal of Anaesthetics 57: 1136–1139

5. Calcium channel blockers in pregnancy

Mark Brincat   Peter McParland

INTRODUCTION

Since the introduction of calcium-channel blockers to clinical practice in the early seventies (Fleckenstein 1971), there has been an escalation in the number of potential clinical applications. Calcium channel blockers now have an established role in the treatment of non-gravid hypertension, angina and supraventricular tachycardia. There is also evidence that these agents may be useful in a diverse range of disorders such as Raynaud's phenomenon, migraine, hypertrophic cardiomyopathy, oesophageal spasm, cyclosporin A nephrotoxity, reducing neurological deficit after subarachnoid haemorrhage, and reducing cell death due to calcium overload after cardiac arrest (Feely et al 1988).

Transmembrane calcium flux plays a crucial role in many important physiological functions, and it is not surprising that calcium channel blockers have widespread clinical use. The wide variety of effects are thought to be mediated by reducing the influx of calcium into cells, thus reducing smooth muscle contractility and causing arteriolar vasodilatation. Although these agents were termed 'calcium antagonists', they do not directly antagonize the effects of calcium. Rather, they inhibit the entry of calcium into cells or its mobilization from intracellular stores and, as such, have been termed 'calcium channel blockers'. The ability of these agents to regulate smooth muscle activity suggests that they could be useful in pregnancy, in the treatment of preterm labour and pregnancy-induced hypertension.

PHYSIOLOGY OF MUSCLE CONTRACTION

Calcium ions are essential for the contraction of both skeletal and smooth muscle. The latter is activated by nerves of the autonomic nervous system or by hormones. The events leading to muscle contraction are regulated within a very narrow range of intracellular calcium ion concentration, with very small fluctuations in intracellular calcium ion concentration sharply affecting smooth muscle tone. Thus, in resting muscle the intracellular calcium concentration is maintained below 10^{-7} M. An increase in

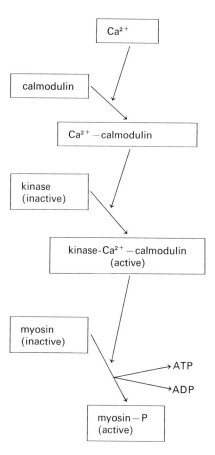

Fig. 5.1   The cascade of reactions by which the contraction of smooth muscle is activated in the presence of Ca^{2+}.

threshold concentration to 10^{-6} M is required to initiate contraction (Hartshorne & Mrwa 1981). This calcium can be derived from several sources—the extracellular medium, the cell membrane, the sarcoplasmic reticulum and possibly the mitochondria. Smooth muscle contractions are initiated by electrical activity with depolarization leading to a change in voltage across the cell membrane, causing calcium channels to open, permitting extracellular calcium to enter, and resulting in a cascade of reactions (Fig. 5.1). It is generally assumed that this inflow occurs through two different channels in the cell membrane—the potential sensitive channel and the receptor-operated channel. The potential sensitive channel allows the passage of calcium ions when the electric potential across the cell membrane is reduced to a certain level by an action potential. The receptor-operated channel is controlled by drugs acting via membrane receptors. This type of activation, corresponding to pharmaco-mechanical coupling, enables effects on mechanical activity without associated electrical activity.

In order to reach the concentrations needed for contractile activation, calcium may also be released from intracellular stores such as the sarcoplasmic reticulum and mitochondria (Carsten 1979, Bolton 1979). The signal from the action potential is transferred to the sarcoplasmic reticulum, which is an intracellular sheath of anastomosing flattened vesicles derived from the endoplasmic reticulum. The sarcoplasmic reticulum then releases large amounts of calcium ions into the cytoplasm. These calcium ions bind to calmodulin, a small protein. Calmodulins binding to calcium ions can be compared to haemoglobin binding to oxygen, with each additional calcium ion increasing the affinity of the molecule for the next calcium ion. Three or four binding sites must be occupied before calmodulin activates the target protein myosin—a light chain kinase (Leimback & Varner 1985). Activation of the myosin kinase results in phosphorylation of the light chain of myosin, allowing it to interact with actin and leading to 'cross bridging' and muscle contraction. During relaxation, myosin and actin filaments are sliding freely past each other. The final regulator of activity of these contractile proteins appears to be the concentration of cytoplasmic-free calcium concentration.

MODE OF ACTION

Calcium channel blockers are characterized by their ability to inhibit calcium influx through potential sensitive channels and possibly also through receptor-operated channels. By blocking the movement of calcium into vascular smooth muscle cells, angina is relieved by coronary artery dilatation, and hypertension is relieved by reduction in arteriolar resistance. The effect of inhibiting contraction in non-vascular smooth muscle may therefore be of benefit in asthma and oesophageal and bladder motility disorders, as well as in dysmenorrhoea and premature labour.

INHIBITION OF UTERINE ACTIVITY

Premature delivery is undoubtedly the single most important cause of perinatal mortality and morbidity (Rush et al 1976), and although successful tocolysis is not the complete solution, an improvement in morbidity and mortality would be expected with effective suppression of uterine contractions. A wide variety of drugs have been used in attempts to suppress uterine contractility. Figure 5.2 demonstrates the site of action of some of these drugs. Although various claims have been made about the efficacy of these agents, the recent Royal College of Obstetricians and Gynaecologists' report on preterm labour concluded that 'the current available evidence does not demonstrate an effect of beta mimetic tocolysis on perinatal mortality or morbidity and this can certainly be broadened to other tocolytic agents for which there is even less information available'

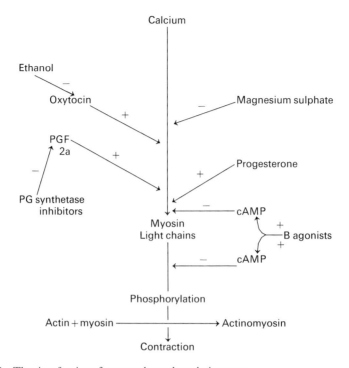

Fig. 5.2   The site of action of commonly used tocolytic agents.

(Calder & Patel 1985). This underlines the need for a more effective drug which theoretically calcium channel blockers could provide. However, as Hendricks et al (1961) have pointed out, it may be naive to expect to arrest a process which has presumably evolved over weeks, months or even years of programming once it has become fully developed. Nevertheless, initial reports on the benefit of calcium channel blockers have been encouraging.

Animal studies

The efficacy of calcium channel blockers as tocolytic agents in various animals has been reported, and the data are summarized in Table 5.1. Csapo et al (1982) demonstrated that nicardipine arrested and prolonged labour in a dose-dependent manner when given during spontaneous labour and during experimentally induced preterm labour in rats. Nicardipine also demonstrated a potent tocolytic effect when administered to pregnant rabbits in premature labour induced by prostaglandin F_2 (Lirette et al 1985). Nifedipine has also been shown to have a significant tocolytic effect in animals (Roebuck et al 1985, Golichowski et al 1985).

Although all studies demonstrate a tocolytic effect, some report haemodynamic effects with a significant increase in maternal and fetal heart

Table 5.1 Summary of published data on the use of calcium channel blockers as tocolytic agents in pregnant animals

Author	Drug	Animal	No.	Type of uterine activity	Tocolytic effect
Csapo et al (1982)	Nicardipine	Rats	22	Postpartum spontaneous uterine activity	Delayed onset of spontaneous uterine activity
			7	Induced pre-term labour	Delayed delivery
			20	Spontaneous labour	Labour arrested
Roebuck et al (1985)	Nifedipine	Sheep	15	Oxytocin-induced contractions	Arrested uterine activity
Lirette et al (1985)	Nicardipine	Rabbits	20	Prostaglandin-induced premature activity	Potent tocolytic effect
Golichowski et al (1985)	Nifedipine	Ewes	10	Dexamethasone-induced labour Postpartum uterine activity	Inhibited advanced labour
Lirette et al (1987)	Nicardipine	Rabbits	9	Prostaglandin-induced term labour	Effective tocolysis
Ducsay et al (1987)	Nicardipine	Rhesus monkeys	4	Spontaneous uterine contractions	Effective decrease in strength and frequency of contraction
Holbrook et al (1988)	Diltiazem	Rabbits	7	Oxytocin-induced term contractions	Effective tocolysis

rate and possibly a reduction in uteroplacental blood flow (Lirette et al 1987)—see under 'Adverse effects' (p. 81–82).

Human studies

In vitro studies have been performed on human myometrial strips obtained from women undergoing hysterectomy because of menorrhagia, and from pregnant women undergoing caesarean section because of cephalo-pelvic disproportion (Forman et al 1979). These strips were mounted in organ baths filled with Krebs' solution at body temperature, and the effects of various calcium antagonists on spontaneous uterine contractility as well as contractions induced by various different agents were investigated. In preparations from non-pregnant patients, nifedipine inhibited spontaneous contractility in a dose-dependent manner (Forman et al 1979). Nifedipine was also able to suppress contractions induced by vasopressin and potassium depolarization (Forman et al 1979).

In the pregnant strips of myometrium, nifedipine inhibited spontaneous contractility and oxytocin-induced contractions (Forman et al 1979). These results have been confirmed (Maigaard et al 1985) and similar studies performed with nicardipine (Maigaard et al 1983) and nitrendipine (Maigaard et al 1986) with similar conclusions. These results support the view that calcium influx through potential sensitive channels is a necessary step in activation of spontaneous contractions in human myometrium.

Both nicardipine and nifedipine were more potent in relaxing potassium-induced contractions in myometrial tissue in vitro from term-pregnant than from non-pregnant women (Forman et al 1979, Maigaard et al 1983). This may reflect pregnancy-induced differences in sensitivity to calcium entry blockade.

The effects of nifedipine on uterine motility in pregnancy have been evaluated in patients undergoing late therapeutic abortion and also in the early postpartum period where the characteristics of the uterus are closely related to the intrapartum situation. Contractile activity induced by prostaglandin F_2 in second trimester pregnancy can be inhibited by nifedipine (Andersson et al 1979). Moreover, spontaneous contractions, and contractions produced by oxytocin, prostaglandin F_2 and ergometrine in the postpartum uterus, were reduced or abolished by oral administration of 20–30 mg nifedipine (Forman et al 1982a, b). These results suggest that unwanted spontaneous and drug-induced uterine activity may be treated by this drug. Nicardipine may prove an even more effective alternative as this drug was more potent than nifedipine in reducing potassium-induced contractions in preparations from term-pregnant myometrium (Maigaard 1983).

Several clinical studies on calcium channel blockers in preterm labour have been published. Nifedipine was administered to ten patients with preterm labour, who did not respond to bed rest. In all subjects, successful delay in delivery was achieved (Ulmsten et al 1980). A further study by the same group, again using nidefipine, in 28 patients achieved an average delay of 12 days from the commencement of treatment, with 80% of deliveries being delayed for more than 3 days, during which time corticosteroids could be given to accelerate fetal lung maturation (Ulmsten 1984).

In the only controlled study nifedipine was compared with ritodrine and a control group who received no treatment. Nifedipine (20 mg 8 hourly) was significantly more effective than ritodrine or with holding treatment and was free of serious side-effects (Read & Wellby 1986). Both ritodrine and nifedipine caused a similar significant rise in the fetal heart rate but only ritodrine caused a significant rise in maternal heart rate. Whilst these studies are encouraging, caution must be exercised in the interpretation of these results, mainly due to the small numbers involved. However, they do justify further trials, preferably on a coordinated multicentre basis.

Although this chapter is primarily concerned with the use of calcium channel blockers in pregnancy, it is of interest that these agents may have a beneficial effect in the treatment of dysmenorrhoea. Contractile activity of the human uterus varies during the menstrual cycle and is most pronounced with the onset of menstruation (Akerlund 1979). In primary dysmenorrhoea, uterine ischaemia and pain is a suggested consequence of the hypertonic menstrual uterine contractions (Ylikorkala & Dawood 1978). As a result, attempts at treatment have focused on methods of inducing myometrial relaxation. When tested on day 1–3 of the menstrual cycle in healthy volunteers, nifedipine (20–30 mg) reduced or virtually abolished uterine contractile activity when this was recorded with micro-transducers to measure intrauterine pressure (Ulmsten et al 1978). The same group has assessed the effects of nifedipine in women with pronounced dysmenorrhoeic pain and myometrial hypertonic contractile activity (Andersson & Ulmsten 1978). Oral nifedipine (20–30 mg) induced marked inhibition or disappearance of the uterine contractions with simultaneous pain relief.

The clinical effectiveness of nifedipine in dysmenorrhoea has been tested in two further series (Sandahl et al 1979, Mondero 1983). Many patients had almost immediate pain relief, possibly as a result of sublingual absorption. Although hormonal contraceptives and prostaglandin-synthetase inhibitors should remain the treatment of choice for dysmenorrhoea, calcium channel blockers merit further evaluation.

CALCIUM CHANNEL BLOCKERS AND HYPERTENSION IN PREGNANCY

Theoretical basis

The efficacy of nifedipine in the treatment of non-gravid hypertension by lowering peripheral resistance both acutely (Kuwajima et al 1978) and in the long term (Guazzi et al 1980) has been proven. One advantage of calcium channel blockers in the treatment of hypertension is that the fall in blood pressure is related to the degree of hypertension. Using the same dose of nifedipine, patients with mild hypertension have smaller drops in blood pressure than those with severe hypertension, with all patients tending towards a common mean.

Nifedipine has a rapid onset of action when taken orally and this property would be advantageous in simplifying the management of hypertension in pregnancy. Similar results have been described for verapamil (Leary et al 1979, Midtbok et al 1980).

Pre-eclampsia is characterized by vascular hyper-responsiveness and generalized vasospasm. In normal pregnancy the pressor response to angiotensin II (AII) infusion is significantly reduced when compared with non-pregnant controls (Chesley et al 1965). This relative refractoriness to AII is absent in patients with pre-eclampsia, in whom there is a sensitivity to AII similar to non-pregnant patients. Indeed this knowledge has been used to predict the later development of pre-eclampsia (Gant et al 1973, Oney & Kaulhausen 1982). Vascular insensitivity to AII can be restored in pre-eclamptic women by administration of theophylline (Everett et al 1978). This effect is thought possibly to be the result of theophylline-induced inhibition of phosphodiesterase, which causes an increase in intra-cellular cyclic AMP and subsequent decreased levels of free intracellular calcium ions. Studies in pregnant sheep have shown that nitrendipine reduces the sensitivity to various humoral agents inducing angiotension II (Lawrence & Broughton-Pipkin 1987a).

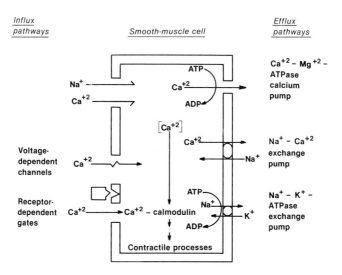

Fig. 5.3 There are three important influx pathways for calcium ions and two major efflux pathways for them.

Calcium channel blockers have been shown to be potent vasodilators of the coronary arteries (Stone et al 1970) as well as of other arterial systems. The effect of calcium channel blockers on arterial vasculature from various locations suggests that these agents may be effective in preventing generalized vasospasm of pre-eclampsia.

It is also possible that calcium channel blockers may have a role in the prevention of eclampsia. The precise mechanism by which eclamptic convulsions occur remains uncertain but may result as a direct result of cerebral vasospasm. Calcium channel blockers have vasodilatory effects on the cerebral vessels and have been shown to relieve cerebral vascular vasospasm (Edvinsson et al 1979). Pre-eclampsia is also characterized by inadequate trophoblastic invasion, rendering the spiral arteries musculo-elastic vessels subject to various vasoactive agents resulting in reduced uteroplacental perfusion. In vitro studies have demonstrated that calcium channel blockers cause vasodilatation in human pregnant uterine vessels as well as in fetal placental vessels (Maigaard et al 1984, 1986). Thus it may be anticipated that calcium channel blockers will at least maintain and possibly increase uteroplacental perfusion.

In pre-eclampsia, platelets are more likely to aggregate and release potent vasoactive substances such as thromboxane. Lawrence & Broughton-Pipkin (1987b) have demonstrated in women about to undergo elective termination of pregnancy that nitrendipine inhibited platelet aggregation, experimentally induced by sodium arachidonate. They suggested that this effect may be of some therapeutic relevance in pre-eclampsia.

In summary, calcium channel blockers possess properties that would suggest at least a theoretical benefit in the management of pre-eclampsia, in that they should relieve generalized vasospasm and thus control hypertension. They may also prevent platelet activation and aggregation and improve uteroplacental perfusion.

Clinical studies

All studies, both in pregnant animals and humans, have demonstrated that calcium channel blockers are effective antihypertensive agents both in the acute and chronic situation.

Ulmsten (1984) studied the effect of nifedipine in 28 patients in preterm labour, of whom eight patients had hypertension. Patients were treated with a loading dose of 30 mg orally followed by 20 mg 8-hourly. Blood pressure fell considerably in all eight patients within 2 hours of commencing therapy, and these patients remained normotensive until delivery.

Walters & Redman (1984) reported on the effect of nifedipine administered as first-time therapy to 21 women with acute episodes of severe hypertension during pregnancy or in the puerperium. A rapid and significant fall in blood pressure by an average of 26/20 mmHg was seen 20 minutes after oral ingestion of either 5 or 10 mg. Walker et al (1987) showed that a single dose of nicardipine (10 mg) was not successful in reducing diastolic blood pressures of 100 mmHg, but a higher dose of 20 mg achieved a fall of at least 10 mmHg (diastolic) within an hour and remained at this level for approximately 2 hours. Similar results were obtained by Allen et al (1987). They reported the acute effects of a single dose (20 mg) of nitrendipine in ten women with pregnancy-induced hypertension between 32 and 42 weeks gestation. A significant reduction in mean blood pressure to normal levels was achieved within 1 hour and maintained for 4 hours. After this time, blood pressure slowly increased to pretreatment levels. In a controlled study comparing a sublingual dose of nifedipine (5 mg) with placebo in the treatment of pregnancy-induced hypertension, there was a significant reduction in blood pressure in the active group when compared with placebo (Lindow et al 1988).

Other studies have assessed the use of calcium channel blockers as second-line therapy in pre-eclampsia. Constantine et al (1987) studied slow release nifedipine (40–120 mg/day) in 23 pregnant women with severe hypertension when atenolol or methyldopa had failed to reduce maternal blood pressure to 140/90 mmHg. The addition of nifedipine achieved control of blood pressure in 20 of the 23 women. Similar results in other uncontrolled studies have also been reported in a total of 24 patients (Rubin et al 1984, Dultizky et al 1987, Greer et al 1987).

A wide range of acute and chronic antihypertensive drugs are currently used in pregnancy (methyldopa, labetolol, atenolol, pindolol, metoprolol, hydralazine, diazoxide and sodium nitroprusside). The choice of a particular drug often seems to follow a local or personal preference rather than clear objective evidence that one drug is superior to another. Before another group of antihypertensive drugs are introduced, controlled studies are necessary. These studies should include investigation of haemo-dynamics as well as metabolic changes in both mother and fetus. Pharmacokinetic data should be a natural part of these studies which should be performed as joint projects in very well defined populations under controlled conditions. Finally, comparative studies with current drugs, in addition to assessing short- and long-term safety, should be performed before routine use of calcium channel blockers. The initial efficacy studies on calcium channel blockers in hypertension of pregnancy are promising and certainly justify further investigation.

CALCIUM CHANNEL BLOCKERS AND FETAL TACHYCARDIAS

The ability of calcium channel blockers, namely verapamil, to slow conduction and increase the refractory period in the atrioventricular node has been used in the treatment of some fetal tachycardias, mainly as second-line therapy.

The incidence of fetal tachycardias has been estimated at approximately 0.4–0.6% of all pregnancies (Southall et al 1980). Fetal tachycardia may be due to sinus tachycardia, atrial flutter or fibrillation or supraventricular tachycardia. The most frequent tachyarrhythmia is paroxysmal supraventricular tachycardia characterized by heart rates frequently exceeding 200 beats per minute. Persisting fetal supraventricular tachycardia can lead to high output cardiac failure in up to 70% of cases. Diagnosis is made by two-dimensional real-time M-mode recording of atrial and ventricular activity. The decision to institute antenatal treatment of supraventricular arrhythmia depends on the nature and seriousness of associated cardiac effects, the presence or absence of an abnormal karyotype, the gestational age and the presence of congestive heart failure or fetal hydrops.

Digoxin is generally considered the drug of choice in the treatment of fetal tachyarrhythmias; however, in refractory cases other drugs, including propranolol, procainamide, amiodarone, verapamil (Wladimiroff & Stewart 1985) and flecanide (Wren & Hunter 1988), have been reported to normalize fetal heart rate. Only limited experience in fetal tachyarrhythmia exists with the use of verapamil. Verapamil's main effect is to slow conduction and increase the refractory period in the atrioventricular node. It also decreases the rate of discharge in the sino-atrial node. Successful conversion of supraventricular tachycardia and atrial flutter has been obtained using a combination of digoxin and verapamil (Wolff et al 1980, Kleinman et al 1985, Maxwell et al 1988).

There is no clear consensus as to which drug should be used as second-line treatment. However, recent reports of cardiovascular collapse, when verapamil was given to five neonates (Kirk et al 1987), suggests that its administration should be under very careful supervision.

ADVERSE EFFECTS

Maternal side-effects

The major side-effects with calcium channel blockers are associated with excessive vasodilatation, a negative inotropic effect, depression of the sinus nodal rate, and A-V nodal conduction disturbances.

Excessive vasodilatation results in peripheral oedema, dizziness, transient headaches, hypotension, facial flushing, nausea, vomiting and sedation. These side-effects, which occur in 20% of patients, are usually benign and often abate with time or with adjustment of the dose.

Calcium channel blockers should not be used in patients with sick sinus syndrome, second- or third-degree atrioventricular block, severe bradycardia or heart failure.

Because of the muscle relaxant properties of calcium channel blockers, problems with delayed parturition, prolonged labour and an increase in postpartum haemorrhage might be anticipated. To date, no such effects have been observed.

Fetal side-effects

Although limited information on the use of calcium channel blockers in pregnancy is available to date, there have been no reports of major adverse fetal effects. However, animal data suggest that calcium channel blockers may decrease uterine blood flow—the opposite to what might be expected (Lirette et al 1985, Ducsay et al 1985, Harake et al 1987). The latter two studies showed a reduction in fetal oxygenation and pH with no alteration in maternal arterial pH or blood gases. Harake et al (1987) suggested that these changes were secondary to a fall in uterine blood flow. Uteroplacental peripheral resistance assessed by Doppler ultrasound appeared to increase, suggesting reduced uteroplacental blood flow in response to intravenous infusion of nicardipine in ten patients with pre-eclampsia (McParland et al 1988); however, sublingual nifedipine had no effect on uteroplacental blood flow when measured by a radio-isotope technique (Lindow et al 1988). The fall in uteroplacental blood flow seen in some of these studies may be caused by a regional uterine vasoconstriction and/or by a massive peripheral vasodilatation and diversion of blood to other regions. There is ample evidence that several vascular beds are affected by calcium channel blockers, including the pulmonary, coronary, hepatic, renal, cerebral, mesenteric and dermal beds (Braunwald 1982). Thus it is possible that such widespread vasodilatation diverts blood flow from the pregnant uterus to other organs. It is possible that the reduction in uteroplacental blood flow in some of these studies is short lived, reflexly mediated and not sustained during chronic therapy. Further studies are required to establish the effect of calcium channel blockers on uteroplacental blood flow and to determine whether these changes interfere with fetal well-being or the ability to tolerate stress.

SUMMARY

The calcium channel blockers, by virtue of their inhibition of trans-membrane calcium flux, have clinically important effects on the contractile process of cardiac and vascular smooth muscle. They already have an established role in the medical therapy of non-gravid hypertension and angina. At least 20 new calcium channel blockers are under development. Some of these may have more selective effects on certain regional vasculature.

There is sufficient evidence available that calcium channel blockers may be of use in premature labour and hypertensive disorders of pregnancy. However, before their introduction to routine clinical practice, further studies are required to clearly determine their short- and long-term safety. The pharmacokinetics and haemodynamic and metabolic changes with various calcium channel blockers need to be established. Until such time, calcium channel blockers should be used only as second-line therapy, under careful supervision, when traditional therapy has failed.

REFERENCES

Allen J, Maigaard S, Forman A et al 1987 Acute effects of nitrendipine in pregnancy-induced hypertension. British Journal of Obstetrics and Gynaecology 94: 222–226

Andersson K E, Ulmsten U 1978 Effects of nifedipine on myometrial activity and lower abdominal pain in women with primary dysmenorrhoea. British Journal of Obstetrics and Gynaecology 85: 142–148

Andersson K E, Ingemarsson I, Ulmsten U, Wingerup L 1979 Inhibition of prostaglandin-induced uterine activity by nifedipine. British Journal of Obstetrics and Gynaecology 86: 175–179

Akerlund M 1979 Pathophysiology of dysmenorrhoea. Acta Obstetricia et Gynecologica Scandinavica 87(suppl): 27–32

Antman E, Muller J, Goldberg S et al 1980 Nifedipine for coronary artery spasm. New England Journal of Medicine 302: 1269–1273

Bolton T B 1979 Mechanisms of action on transmitters and other substances on smooth muscle. Physiology Review 59: 606–718

Braunwald E 1982 Mechanism of action of calcium channel blocking agents. New England Journal of Medicine 307: 1618–1627

Calder A A, Patel N B 1985 Are betamimetics worthwhile in preterm labour? In: Beard R W, Sharp F (eds) 13th Study Group of the Royal College of Obstetricians and Gynaecologists, pp 209–218

Carsten M E 1979 Calcium accumulation by human uterine microsomal preparations: effects of progesterone and oxytocin. American Journal of Obstetrics and Gynecology 133: 598–601

Chesley L C, Talledo E, Bohler C S, Zuspan F P 1965 Vascular reactivity to angiotension II and norepinephrine in pregnant and non-pregnant women. American Journal of Obstetrics and Gynecology 91: 837–842

Constantine G, Beevers D G, Reynolds A L, Luesley D M 1987 Nifedipine as a second line antihypertensive drug in pregnancy. British Journal of Obstetrics and Gynaecology 94: 1136–1142

Csapo A I, Puri C P, Tarro S, Henzl M R 1982 Deactivation of the uterus during normal and premature labor by the calcium antagonist nicardipine. American Journal of Obstetrics and Gynecology 142: 483–491

Ducsay C A, Thompson J S, Wu A T, Novy M J 1987 Effects of calcium entry blocker (nicardipine) tocolysis in rhesus macaques: fetal plasma concentrations and cardiorespiratory changes. American Journal of Obstetrics and Gynecology 157: 1482–1486

Dulitzky M, Posenthal T, Barkai G, Mani A, Rabau E, Mastuach S 1987 Nifedipine in the treatment of hypertension in pregnancy and puerperium. Clinical and Experimental Hypertension B6: 235

Edvinsson L, Brandt L, Andersson K E, Bergtsson B 1979 Effect of a calcium antagonist on experimental constriction of human brain vessels. Surgical Neurology 11: 327–330

Everett R B, Worley R J, MacDonald P C, Gant N F 1978 Oral administration of theophylline to modify pressor responsiveness to angiotensin II in women with pregnancy induced hypertension. American Journal of Obstetrics and Gynecology 132: 359–362

Feely J, Pringle T, MacLean D 1988 Thrombolytic treatment and new calcium antagonists. British Medical Journal 296: 705–708

Fleckenstein A, Grun G, Tritthart H, Byon K 1971 Uterus-relaxation durch hochaktive Ca^{++}-antagonistische Hemmstoffe der elektro-mekanische Kopplung mit Isoptin (Vera-pamil, Iproveratril), Substanz D-600 und Segontin (Prenylamin). Klinische Wochenschrift 49: 32–41

Forman A, Anderson K E, Persson C G A, Ulmsten U 1979 Relaxant effects of nifedipine on isolated human myometrium. Acta Pharmacologica et Toxicologica 45: 81–86

Forman A, Anderson K E, Ulmsten U 1981 Inhibition of myometrial activity by calcium antagonists. Seminars in Perinatology 5: 288–294

Forman A, Gandrup P, Anderson K E, Ulmsten U 1982a Effects of nifedipine on spontaneous and methylergometrine-induced activity post partum. American Journal of Obstetrics and Gynecology 144: 442–448

Forman A, Gandrup P, Andersson K E, Ulmsten U 1982b Effects of nifedipine on oxytocin-

and prostaglandin F_2-induced activity postpartum uterus. American Journal of Obstetrics and Gynecology 144: 665–670

Gant N F, Daley G L, Chand S, Whalley P J, McDonald P C 1973 A study of angiotension II pressor response throughout primigravid pregnancy. Journal of Clinical Investigation 52: 2682–2689

Golichowski A M, Hathaway D R, Fineberg N, Peleg D 1985 Tocolytic and hemodynamic effects of nifedipine in the ewe. American Journal of Obstetrics and Gynecology 151: 1134–1140

Greer I A, Walker J J, Bjornsson S, Calder A A 1987 Second line therapy with nifedipine in severe pregnancy induced hypertension. Clinical and Experimental Hypertension B6: 78

Guazzi M D, Fiorentini C, Olivari M T, Bartolli A, Necchi G, Polese A 1980 Short and long term efficacy of a calcium antagonistic agent (nifedipine) combined with methyldopa in the treatment of severe hypertension. Circulation 61: 913–919

Harake B, Gilbert R D, Ashwal S, Power G G 1987 Nifedipine: effects on fetal and maternal hemodynamics in pregnant sheep. American Journal of Obstetrics and Gynecology 157: 1003–1008

Hartshorne D J, Mrwa U 1981 Regulation of smooth muscle actomyosin. Blood Vessels 19: 1–18

Hendricks C H, Cibils L A, Pose S T, Eskes T K 1961 The pharmacologic control of excessive uterine activity with isoxsuprine. American Journal of Obstetrics and Gynecology 82: 1064

Holbrook R H, Gibson R N, Voss E M 1988 Tocolytic and cardiovascular effects of the calcium antagonist diltiazem in the near-term pregnant rabbit. American Journal of Obstetrics and Gynecology 159: 591–595

Kirk C R, Gibbs J L, Thomas R, Radley-Smith R, Qureshi S A 1987 Cardiovascular collapse after verapamil in supraventricular tachycardia. Archives of Disease in Childhood 62: 1265–1266

Kleinman C S, Copel J A, Weinstein E M, Santulli T V, Hobbins J C 1985 In utero diagnosis and treatment of fetal supraventricular tachycardia. Seminars in Perinatology 9: 113–129

Kuwajima I, Ueda K, Kamata C et al 1978 A study on the effects of nifedipine in hypertensive crises and severe hypertension. Japanese Heart Journal 19: 455–467

Lawrence M R, Broughton-Pipkin F 1987a Effects of nitrendipine on cardiovascular parameters in conscious pregnant sheep. Clinical and Experimental Hypertension B6: 77

Lawrence M R, Broughton-Pipkin F 1987b Some observations on the effects of a calcium channel blocker, nitrendipine, in early human pregnancy. British Journal of Clinical Pharmacology 23: 683–692

Leary W P, Asmal A C 1979 Treatment of hypertension with verapamil. Current Therapeutics 25: 747–752

Leimbach W N, Varner M W 1985 Calcium's role in hypertension. In: Chamberlain G (ed) Contemporary Obstetrics and Gynaecology, Butterworths, London pp 184–202

Lindow S W, Davies N, Davey D A, Smith J A 1988 The effect of sublingual nifedipine on uteroplacental blood flow in hypertensive pregnancy. British Journal of Obstetrics and Gynaecology 95: 1276–1281

Lirette M, Holbrook R H, Katz M 1985 Effect of nicardipine HCL on prematurely induced uterine activity in the pregnant rabbit. Obstetrics and Gynecology 65: 31–36

Lirette M, Holbrook R H, Katz M 1987 Cardiovascular and uterine blood flow changes during nicardipine HCL tocolysis in the rabbit. Obstetrics and Gynecology 69: 79–82

McParland P, Steel S A, Pearce J M F 1988 The effect of a calcium channel blocker (nicardipine) on uteroplacental blood flow. Submitted to British Journal of Obstetrics and Gynaecology

Maigaard S, Forman A, Andersson K E, Ulmsten U 1983 Comparison of the effects of nicardipine and nifedipine on isolated human myometrium. Gynecologic and Obstetric Investigation 16: 354–366

Maigaard S, Forman A, Andersson K E 1984 Effects of nifedipine on human placental arteries. Gynecologic and Obstetric Investigation 18: 217–224

Maigaard S, Forman A, Andersson K E 1985a Differences in contractile activation between human non-pregnant myometrium and intramyometrial arteries. Acta Physiologica Scandinavica 124: 371–379

Maigaard S, Forman A, Andersson K E 1985b Different responses to prostaglandin F_2 and E_2 in human non-pregnant extra- and intramyone trial arteries. Prostaglandins 30: 599–607

Maigaard S, Forman A, Andersson K E 1986 Differential effects of angiotensin, vasopressin and oxytocin on various smooth muscle tissues within the human uteroplacental unit. Acta Physiologica Scandinavica 128: 23–31

Maigaard S, Forman A, Andersson K E 1986 Inhibiting effects of nitrendipine on myometrial and vascular smooth muscle in human pregnant uterus and placenta. Acta Pharmacologica et Toxicologica 59: 1–10

Maxwell D J, Crawford D C, Curry P V M, Tynan M J, Allan L D 1988 Obstetric importance, diagnosis, and management of fetal tachycardias. British Medical Journal 297: 107–110

Midtbok K, Hals O 1980 Verapamil in the treatment of hypertension. Current Therapeutics 27: 830–838

Mondero N A 1983 Nifedipine in the treatment of dysmenorrhea. Journal of the American Osteopathology Association 82: 704–708

Murphy M B, Scriven A J, Dollery C T 1983 Role of nifedipine in the treatment of hypertension. British Medical Journal 287: 257–259

Norris M C, Rose J C, Dewan D M 1986 Nifedipine or verapamil counteracts hypertension in gravid ewes. Anesthesiology 65: 254–258

Olivari M T, Bartorelli C, Polese A, Florentine C, Moruzzi P, Guazzi M D 1979 Treatment of hypertension with nifedipine, a calcium antagonist agent. Circulation 59: 1056–1062

Oney T, Kaulhausen H 1982 The value of the angiotensin sensitivity test in the early diagnosis of hypertensive disorders in pregnancy. American Journal of Obstetrics and Gynecology 142: 17–20

Read M D, Wellby D E 1986 The use of a calcium antagonist (nifedipine) to suppress preterm labour. British Journal of Obstetrics and Gynaecology 93: 933–937

Roebuck M M, Castle B M, Vojcek L, Weingold A, Dawes G S, Turnbull A C 1985 The effect of nifedipine administration on the fetus and the myometrium of pregnant sheep during oxytocin induced contractions. In: Jones C T, Nathanielsz P W. The Physiological Development of the Fetus and Newborn. Academic Press, London, 499–503

Rubin P C, McCabe R, Low R A 1984 Calcium channel blockade with nifedipine combined with atenolol in the management of severe pre-eclampsia. Clinical and Experimental Hypertension B3: 379

Rush R W, Karse M J, Howat P, Baum J D, Anderson A B, Turnbull A C 1976 Contribution of preterm delivery to perinatal mortality. British Medical Journal 2: 965

Sandahl B, Ulmsten U, Andersson K E 1979 Trial of the calcium antagonist nifedipine in the treatment of primary dysmenorrhoea. Archives of Gynecology 227: 147–151

Southall D P, Richard J, Hardwick R A et al 1980 Prospective study of fetal heartrate and rhythm patterns. Archives of Disease in Children 55: 506

Stone P H, Antman E M, Muller J E, Braunwald E 1980 Calcium channel blocking agents in the treatment of cardiovascular disorders. Part III. Haemodynamic effects and clinical applications. Annals of Internal Medicine 93: 886–904

Ulmsten U, Andersson K E, Forman A 1978 Relaxing effects of nifedipine on the non pregnant human uterus in vitro and in vivo. Obstetrics and Gynecology 52: 436–441

Ulmsten U 1984 Treatment of normotensive and hypertensive patients with preterm labor using oral nifedipine, a calcium antagonist. Archives of Gynecology 236: 69–72

Ulmsten U, Andersson K E, Wingerup L 1980 Treatment of premature labour with the calcium antagonist nifedipine. Archives of Gynecology 229: 1–5

Van Neuten J M, Vanhoutte P M 1981 Calcium entry blockers and vascular smooth muscle heterogenity. Federation Proceedings 40: 2862–2865

Veille J C, Bissonnette J M, Hohimer A R 1986 The effect of a calcium channel blocker (nifedipine) on uterine blood flow in the pregnant goat. American Journal of Obstetrics and Gynecology 154: 1160–1163

Walker J J, Bjornsson S, Greer I A, Cheyne H, McEwan H 1987 The use of a new calcium channel blocker, nicardipine, in the treatment of acute hypertension in pregnancy. Clinical and Experimental Hypertension B6: 76

Walters B N J, Redman C W 1984 Treatment of severe pregnancy-associated hypertension with the calcium antagonist nifedipine. British Journal of Obstetrics and Gynaecology 91: 330–336

Wladimiroff J W, Stewart P A 1985 Treatment of fetal cardiac arrhythmias. British Journal of Hospital Medicine 34: 134–140

Wolff F, Breuker K M, Schlensker K M, Bolte A 1980 Prenatal diagnosis and therapy of fetal heart rate anomalies; with a contribution on the placental transfer of verapamil. Journal of Perinatal Medicine 8: 203

Wren C, Hunter S 1988 Maternal administration of flecanide to terminate and suppress fetal tachycardia. British Medical Journal 296: 249

Ylikorkala O, Dawood M Y 1978 New concepts in dysmenorrhoea. American Journal of Obstetrics and Gynecology 130: 833–847

6. Posture in labour

Peter Stewart

INTRODUCTION

George Englemann, Professor of Obstetrics in the Missouri Medical School, published a treatise in 1883 on his observations of 'Labour among primitive peoples'. In it he stated that 'the care with which the parturient women of uncivilized people avoid the dorsal decubitus position is sufficient evidence that it is most undesirable for ordinary cases of confinement'. More recently, other obstetricians and midwives (Howard 1959, Newton & Newton 1960, McKay 1984) have suggested potential benefits from the so-called 'physiological positions', including a reduction in the duration of labour and a reduction in the need for episiotomies and forceps deliveries, together with an improvement in the condition of the neonate. Yet the majority of women in the western world labour and deliver their baby in the semi-recumbent position in a hospital bed. There is little doubt that this arrangement is the convention that most women expect. It also makes it easier for the midwife and doctor to monitor both fetus and mother, and since safety has a priority in obstetrics, it will require more than anecdotal observation to dramatically change current practice. Scientific evidence is required to show that alternative positions increase the efficiency of parturition, are not detrimental to the outcome of mother or baby, and are preferred by women in labour. The evidence to support claims for alternative positions, therefore, needs careful evaluation.

THEORETICAL CONSIDERATIONS

Uterine activity

The pioneer work of the effect of posture on uterine activity in labour was performed by Caldero-Barcia et al (1960). These workers used intrauterine pressure measurements in the first stage of labour and the patient acted as her own control. This showed that there was an increase in the frequency but a decrease in the intensity of uterine contractions in the supine position when compared with the lateral recumbent position. This resulted in an overall reduction in uterine activity, as measured by Montevideo units, when the patients were supine. As a result of this work, labouring patients are now always nursed in the lateral position or 'propped' dorsal position when in bed. Unfortunately, subsequent studies have often failed to take note of this original work and compared the supine position with other postures. Mendez-Bauer et al (1975), using similar techniques, demonstrated that the standing position produced more effective uterine activity than when the patient was supine. More recent work from the same group (Roberts et al 1983) has, however, demonstrated that the sitting position produced less effective uterine activity than both the lateral recumbent position and the standing position. They conclude that a simple change of position may be as effective as any one position itself in promoting efficient uterine activity as long as the supine position is avoided. The only study to consider the effect of posture on uterine activity in the second stage of labour used external tocography to measure contractions, thus rendering any information of the intensity of contractions invalid (Liu 1974).

Effect of Gravity

It is possible that in a more upright position gravity may aid the expulsion of the fetus and hence reduce the duration of the second stage. Mengert & Murphy (1933), carrying out measurements with a balloon placed in the vagina of non-pregnant women, suggested that the pressure in the vagina produced by voluntary muscular effort was increased by 20% when sitting or squatting as compared with the lateral recumbent position. Mendez-Bauer et al (1976) have suggested that in pregnancy this effect of gravity may be as much as 30 mmHg. We have carried out some studies to measure the pressure between the fetal head and the lower segment of the uterus in early labour. A catheter tip pressure transducer was inserted through the uterine cervix and positioned extra-amniotically 4 cm from the internal os. A baseline recumbent pressure was then recorded by taking the mean pressures obtained in the right and left lateral and supine positions. The patients were than asked to stand or sit. In the majority of patients there was a significant increase in pressure on adopting the more upright position (Fig. 6.1). These results do therefore support the idea that gravity may aid the descent of the presenting part in labour, but not to such an extent as suggested by Mendez-Bauer and his associates.

Pelvic moulding

It is reasonable to assume that the second stage would be reduced in duration if a specific position significantly increased the pelvic dimensions, thus decreasing the mechanical resistance to delivery. With the use of X-rays, Heyman & Lundqvist (1932) and Brooke et al (1934) studied patients throughout pregnancy and delivery. They concluded that separation of the pelvic joints occurred in early pregnancy and that there was no further increase during labour. Young (1940) investigated the

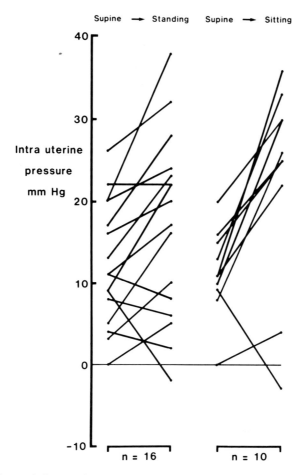

Fig. 6.1 Changes in intrauterine pressure between fetal head and cervix with varying posture—see text for experimental details (Stewart, unpublished data).

Walcher, or hanging leg position, which was reintroduced by its protagonist as a method of increasing the pelvic inlet. He failed to demonstrate any increase in pelvic dimensions. More recently, Russell (1969) did show that the squatting position produced a mean increase in the bispinous diameter of 7.6 mm when compared with the supine position, and a total increase of the pelvic outlet of 28%. Few patients, however, deliver in the true supine position and the hyperflexion and abduction of the hips which is responsible for producing this change in pelvic dimensions in the squatting position can readily be achieved in the propped dorsal position: the woman pulls her thighs onto her abdomen and the midwife pushes on her patient's feet to aid abduction—a practice adopted by many experienced midwives to aid a slightly more difficult delivery.

Soft tissue resistance

McKay (1984) has suggested that the squatting position for delivery provides more evenly distributed pressure on the vaginal opening and therefore reduces the need for episiotomies. Bankfield (1965) has, however, claimed that squatting or the thigh-on-abdomen position, both of which exhibit a similar anatomical relationship between lumbar spine, pelvis and thigh, may increase the possibility of perineal damage. She claims that as the skin and fascia overlying the perineal body are attached to the flexion creases of the thighs, then the hyperflexion of the hips will result in these tissues becoming excessively taut, thus narrowing the introitus and predisposing to perineal lacerations.

CLINICAL OBSERVATIONS

Clinical studies of the effect of posture on labour have tended to concentrate either on the first or second stage of labour independently. Those related to the first stage have compared ambulation with the recumbent position and those related to the second stage have compared delivery in a birth chair with the more conventional dorsal position.

First stage of labour

Duration of the first stage

Randomized trials of patients in the first stage of labour have produced varying results. The main outcomes studied have been the duration of the first stage and the need for analgesia. They can be roughly divided into those which demonstrated a benefit from ambulation (Mitre 1974, Diaz et al 1978, Flynn et al 1978) and those which did not (Chan 1963, McManus & Calder 1978, Williams et al 1980). It is not possible, however, to compare directly the various trials because of the different methodologies. What can perhaps be concluded is that there is unlikely to be a significant benefit from patients adopting one particular posture. This may well reflect the theoretical findings of Roberts et al (1983) which showed that efficiency of uterine activity was more related to changes in posture than any one specific position.

It is an inherent problem with randomized studies that inevitably patients will be entered into a trial group which would not have been their choice. This could perhaps influence the progress of their labour. It is of interest that in the study by Williams et al (1980), 87% of those patients allocated to be ambulant asked to return to bed when in active labour. Patients' choice may well be an important factor in determining the outcome of labour in these circumstances.

Patients' preference

In an observational study of 80 consecutive patients with uncomplicated labour, Carlsen et al (1986) showed that patients, given freedom of choice, tended to change position frequently in early labour, but then resorted to one position at the end of the first stage and the second stage. They also found that most patients adopted the more conventional positions of recumbency towards the end of labour. Stewart & Calder (1984) carried out a study to ascertain whether or not patients' choice had an effect on the outcome of labour. They found that many women, including those at high risk, preferred not to be confined to bed in the early stages. Analysis of their data on the basis of 'intention to treat', i.e. the original choice made by the patient, showed that those patients who were ambulant for only part of their labour did less well than those patients who opted for full ambulation or were in bed throughout labour. They concluded that although there was an association between prolonged periods of ambulation and favourable outcome in labour, it was not possible to ascribe a causal relationship. It may well have been that inherently easy labours allowed ambulation rather than ambulation producing easy labours.

Fetal monitoring

Several studies have established the effectiveness of fetal monitoring using radiotelemetry (Kelly et al 1980). There seems little reason to suggest that the need for continuous monitoring should prevent a patient with a high risk pregnancy from being ambulant.

Second stage of labour

Duration of the second stage

Some recent reports have enthusiastically endorsed the sitting position as beneficial in the second stage (Romney 1985, Kesby 1982, Haukland 1981). They were, however, uncontrolled studies. A randomized study by Stewart

Table 6.1 Details of second stage of labour in a randomized study comparing delivery in a birth chair with delivery in the conventional wedged dorsal position (from Stewart et al, unpublished data)

	Chair ($n = 125$)	Bed ($n = 125$)	Chair ($n = 125$)	Bed ($n = 125$)
Mean duration of second stage (min) ($\pm$ SD)	86 ($\pm$67)	80 ($\pm$55)	20 ($\pm$30)	22 ($\pm$21)
Mean duration of active pushing (min) ($\pm$ SD)	44 ($\pm$26)	50 ($\pm$25)	15 ($\pm$14)	19 ($\pm$15)

et al (1983) of 189 patients gave a suggestion that there may be a slight reduction in the duration of the second stage among patients using a birth chair for delivery. That initial study was expanded to include 500 patients, but no significant differences were demonstrable either in the overall duration of the observed second stage or the duration of active pushing (Table 6.1). Turner et al (1986), in another large randomized study, failed to demonstrate any reduction in the duration of the second stage. Hemminki et al (1986) reported a study of 175 women. They did not attempt to assess the durations of the first and second stages separately but found that the use of a birth chair actually increased the overall mean length of labour (9.9 vs 8.0 hours). However, if adjustments are made for other variables in the study groups, this difference, although persisting, becomes statistically insignificant.

It would appear therefore that, although there may be theoretical considerations which should suggest that a more upright position should reduce the duration of the second stage of labour, this is not borne out in clinical practice.

Mode of delivery

If the sitting or squatting position increases dimensions of the bony pelvis, it would be reasonable to assume that the use of a birth chair would result in a reduced incidence of instrumental delivery. Hemminki et al (1986) were unable to show any difference in the rate of forceps deliveries between their study and control groups. In our study of 500 women at Glasgow Royal Maternity Hospital, there was, however, an apparent difference in forceps delivery rate among primigravidae. This reached statistical significance when primigravidae with epidurals alone were considered (Table 6.2). The principle indication for the use of forceps was delay in the second stage, including the need for rotational forceps, and it is possible that a more upright position encourages rotation of the fetal head when the efficiency of

Table 6.2 Mode of delivery in primigravidae with epidural analgesia in a randomized study comparing delivery in a birth chair with delivery in the conventional wedged dorsal position (from Stewart et al, unpublished data)

	Chair ($n = 68$)	Bed ($n = 70$)
Spontaneous vaginal delivery	45	34
Forceps delivery	20	35
Caesarean section	3	1

$\chi^2 = 7.32; P < 0.05.$

the normal rotational mechanism of the pelvic floor musculature is decreased by the use of regional analgesia.

Hemminki et al (1986) unfortunately make no mention of the type of analgesia used in their study. Turner et al (1986), however, were unable to demonstrate any difference despite having an epidural rate of 26% in their series, so the effect of posture on the outcome of labour in patients with epidural analgesia remains uncertain. Without epidural analgesia there is certainly no evidence that a birth chair delivery reduces the need for operative intervention.

Perineal trauma

Our initial study suggested that the incidence of significant perineal trauma (episiotomies and second degree tears) was reduced by the use of a birth chair (Table 6.3). Turner et al (1986), however, came to the opposite conclusion, finding an increase in perineal trauma in their patients delivering in a birth chair. In a recent study using a new birth chair specifically designed to support the perineum during delivery, Stewart & Spiby (1989) failed to show any difference between groups delivering in a bed or the chair. Charles White an eighteenth century English obstetrician, stated that delivery in the upright position was potentially hazardous, frequently occasioning laceration of the perineum and sphincter ani (Atwood 1976). There seems little information from recent work to conclusively support or refute this historical viewpoint. It may well be that this aspect of midwifery is more dependent on individual patients and midwives than the actual position of delivery.

Fetal outcome

All studies carried out to date have failed to show any beneficial or deleterious effects on the fetus of delivering in an upright position. There is

Table 6.3 Perineal trauma in a randomized study comparing delivery in a birth chair with delivery in the conventional wedge dorsal position (from Stewart et al, unpublished data)

	Primigravidae		Multigravidae	
	Chair ($n = 125$)	Bed ($n = 125$)	Chair ($n = 125$)	Bed ($n = 125$)
None	24	11	39	33
1° Tear	24	4	48	37
2° Tear	16	12	20	17
Episiotomy	61	98	18	38

$\star \chi^2 = 28.3; P < 0.01$ $\star\star \chi^2 = 9.3; P < 0.05.$

no doubt, however, that the dorsal recumbent position should be avoided. Humphrey et al (1974) demonstrated a decrease in fetal pH during the second stage of labour when the mother lay in the dorsal position. A semi-recumbent or 'propped' position is now accepted labour ward practice. A small study by Aarnoudse et al (1984), using a continuous Po_2 electrode, failed to demonstrate any improved oxygenation of the fetus during the second stage of labour if the mother adopted an upright position.

Blood loss at delivery

John Burton (1710–1771), an English obstetrician, was cautious about delivery in the sitting position and stated that: '. . . if the patient be disposed to flood, this posture will increase it' (Atwood 1976). Recent studies tend to confirm that view. In a non-randomized study, Shannahan & Cottrell (1985) assessed blood loss at delivery by measuring haemoglobin and haematocrit levels before and after delivery. They concluded that delivery in a birth chair resulted in greater blood loss. Turner et al (1986) and Stewart et al (1983) found a greater rate of post-partum haemorrhage and greater blood loss respectively. The results of the former study could perhaps be explained by the increased rate of perineal lacerations they noted, as this is known to increase blood loss by up to 50% (Wallace 1967). This, however, was not the case in the latter study. All three groups of workers used a commercial birth chair for their studies. The chair gives no support to the perineum, thus increasing tissue congestion and prolapse (Goodlin & Frederick 1983). It is possible that minor trauma of the excessively congested perineum was responsible for the increased blood loss that was noted. The design of the birth chair used in the study by Stewart & Spiby (1989) was such as to provide good support to the perineum so as to overcome this problem. No difference was noted in the degree of perineal trauma, but delivery in the chair again resulted in significantly increased mean blood loss and incidence of post-partum haemorrhage. It has been suggested that blood loss at delivery is often underestimated. The potential hazard of delivery in a birth chair may therefore be greater than these results suggest.

Psychological effects

The reports of uncontrolled studies (Hawkland 1981, McKay 1984) suggest that mothers have a more positive approach to the use of alternative delivery positions than to conventional management. As these are self-selecting groups, this is to be expected. It would be extremely difficult to obtain a truly objective assessment of maternal preferences regarding their position for delivery. It may well be, however, that the mother's subjective opinions rather than experimental fact will determine the future interest in alternative positions for birth.

CONCLUSION

In the past, much dogma has been used by obstetricians and midwives to emphasize their own prejudices on this subject. Opinions have often been based on theoretical considerations rather than controlled clinical observations. More recently, many lay people and childbirth educators have been equally vociferous in expounding their views, particularly that ambulation in labour and alternative positions for delivery are beneficial. There appears, however, to be little good evidence at present to suggest that the posture a pregnant woman adopts for either the first stage of her labour or delivery has a major effect on the outcome for mother or baby. There are two exceptions. Firstly, there is the well-documented detrimental effect of the supine position which reduces uterine activity and produces fetal hypoxia via maternal hypotension. Secondly, the woman adopting the sitting position for delivery appears to have an increased tendency to excessive blood loss. This latter finding has been consistently noted in several studies. The exact reason for it remains to be elucidated but it would be prudent to warn women who wish to adopt this position for delivery that this potential hazard has been identified.

The experimental data, otherwise, have often been contradictory, and although many of the studies have flawed methodology it is unlikely that any other significant effects have been overlooked. The advice of the midwife or obstetrician to a pregnant woman in labour should perhaps be that she should adopt the position which she feels is most appropriate for her, assuming it does not prejudice the safety of herself or her baby.

REFERENCES

Aarnoudse J G, Romney M L, Gordon H 1984 Does the fetal oxygen supply improve in the birthing chair? Journal of Obstetrics and Gynaecology 4: 141–142
Atwood R J 1976 Parturitional posture and related birth behaviour. Acta Obstetrica et Gynecologica Scandinavica 57: 5–25
Blankfield A 1965 The optimum position for childbirth. Medical Journal of Australia 2: 666–668
Brooke R, Roberts R E, Bristow W R 1934 Discussion on the physiology and pathology of pelvic joints in relation to child bearing. Proceedings of the Royal Society of Medicine 27: 1211–1230
Caldeyro-Barcia R, Noriega-Guera L, Cibils L A et al 1960 Effect of position changes on the intensity and frequency of uterine contractions during labor. American Journal of Obstetrics and Gynecology 80: 284–290
Carlson J M, Diehl J, Sachtleben-Murray M, McRae M, Fenwick L, Freidman E 1986 Maternal position during parturition in normal labour. Obstetrics and Gynecology 68: 443–447
Chan D 1963 Positions in labour. British Medical Journal 1: 100–102
Diaz A G, Schwartz R, Fescina R, Caldeyro-Barcia R 1978 Position materna y trabajo del parto. Sepereata Prevista. Clinica e Investigacion en Ginecologia y Obstetrica 5: 101–109
Engleman G J 1882 Labour among primitive people. AMS Press, New York, 1935
Flynn A M, Kelly J, Hollins G, Lynch P F 1978 Ambulation in labour. British Medical Journal 2: 591–593
Goodlin R C, Frederick I B 1983 Postpartum vulval oedema associated with the birthing chair. American Journal of Obstetrics and Gynecology 143: 334

Haukeland I 1981 An alternative delivery position: new delivery chair developed and tested at Kongsberg Hospital. American Journal of Obstetrics and Gynecology 141: 115–117

Hemminki E, Virkkuen A, Makela A et al 1986 A trial of delivery in a birth chair. Journal of Obstetrics and Gynaecology 6: 162–165

Heyman J, Lundqvist A 1932 Symphysis pubis in pregnancy and parturition. Acta Obstetrica et Gynecologica Scandinavica 12: 191–226

Howard F H 1959 The physiological position for delivery. American Journal of Obstetrics and Gynecology 78: 1141–1143

Humphrey M D, Chang A, Wood E C, Morgan S, Hounslow D 1974 A decrease in fetal pH during the second stage of labour when conducted in the dorsal position. Journal of Obstetrics and Gynaecology of the British Commonwealth 80: 600–602

Kesby J 1982 A case for the birthing chair. Nursing Mirror 150: 37–38

Kelly J, Flynn A M, Hollins C 1980 Ambulant fetal monitoring. British Journal of Hospital Medicine 22: 449–451

Liu Y C 1974 Effects of an upright position during labour. American Journal of Nursing 74: 2202–2205

McKay S 1984 Squatting: an alternate position for the second stage of labour. American Journal of Maternal and Child Nursing 9: 181–183

McManus T J, Calder A A 1978 Upright posture and efficiency of labour. Lancet i: 72–74

Mendez-Bauer C, Arroyo J, Garcia Ramos C et al 1975 Effects of standing position on spontaneous uterine contractility and other aspects of labor. Journal of Perinatal Medicine 3: 89–100

Mendez-Bauer C, Arroyo J, Menendez A 1976 Effects of maternal positions during labour. In: Alqvist, Wiksell (eds) 5th European Congress of Perinatal Medicine, Uppsala, Stockholm, Sweden

Mengert W F, Murphy D P 1933 Intra-abdominal pressures created by voluntary muscular effort, II. Relation to posture in labour. Surgery, Gynecology and Obstetrics 57: 745–751

Mitre N 1974 The influence of maternal position on duration of the active phase of labour. International Journal of Gynaecology and Obstetrics 12: 181–183

Newton M, Newton N 1960 The propped position for the second stage of labour. Obstetrics and Gynecology 15: 28–34

Roberts J E, Mendez-Bauer C, Wodell D A 1983 The effects of maternal position on uterine contractility and efficiency. Birth 10: 243–249

Roberts J E, Mendez-Bauer C, Blackwell J, Carpenter M, Marchese T 1984 Effects of lateral recumbency and sitting in the first stage of labor. Journal of Reproductive Medicine 29: 477–482

Romney M L 1985 Chair versus bed. Nursing Mirror 160: 35–36

Russell J G B 1969 Moulding of the pelvic outlet. Journal of Obstetrics and Gynaecology of the British Commonwealth 76: 817–820

Shannahan M D, Cottrell B H 1985 Effect of the birth chair on the duration of the second stage of labour, fetal outcome and maternal blood loss. Nursing Research 34: 89–92

Stewart P, Hillen E, Calder A A 1983 A randomised trial to evaluate the use of a birth chair for delivery. Lancet i: 1296–1298

Stewart P, Calder A A 1984 Posture in labour: patients' choice and its effect on performance. British Journal of Obstetrics and Gynaecology 91: 1091–1095

Stewart P, Spiby H 1989 A randomised study of the sitting position for delivery using a newly designed obstetric chair. British Journal of Obstetrics and Gynaecology 96: 327–333

Turner M J, Romney M L, Webb J B, Gordon H 1986 The birthing chair: an obstetric hazard? Journal of Obstetrics and Gynaecology 6: 232–235

Wallace G 1867 Blood loss in obstetrics using a haemoglobin dilution technique. Journal of Obstetrics and Gynaecology of the British Commonwealth 74: 64–67

Williams R M, Thom M H, Studd J W 1980 A study of the benefits and acceptability of ambulation in spontaneous labour. British Journal of Obstetrics and Gynaecology 87: 122–126

Young J 1940 Relaxation of pelvic joints in pregnancy: pelvic arthropathy of pregnancy. Journal of Obstetrics and Gynaecology of the British Commonwealth 47: 493–524

7. The management of twin pregnancy

Judith B. Weaver

INTRODUCTION

Twin pregnancies resulting from spontaneous conception account for 1:80 births. Where ovulation has been induced or conception manipulated, however, multiple pregnancy is much more common. The perinatal mortality rate associated with twin pregnancy is four times that with singleton pregnancy and is related to the higher incidences of preterm delivery, fetal growth retardation, antepartum haemorrhage, maternal pre-eclampsia and fetal anomaly. In addition to the major complications of pregnancy, the mother is more likely to suffer from the so-called minor disorders of pregnancy (dyspepsia, varicose veins and dependent oedema).

ANTENATAL MANAGEMENT

Planned antenatal care commences with the definite diagnosis of a twin pregnancy.

Diagnosis

The clinical diagnosis of a twin pregnancy cannot be made by abdominal palpation until at least 24 weeks gestation, though it may be suspected earlier if the uterus is larger than the period of amenorrhoea or if the mother presents with severe hyperemesis. Relying on clinical diagnosis and clinical suspicion to identify mothers with a twin pregnancy is, however, fraught with error. In one series (Pridmore 1985) no twins were present in 50 mothers in whom a multiple pregnancy was suspected, and 22 sets of twins were delivered where there was no antenatal suspicion.

The routine use of ultrasound has been shown to not only increase the detection rate of twins but also to decrease the gestational age at which diagnosis can be made (Grennert et al 1978), with an associated improvement of perinatal outcome (Pridmore 1985, Hughey & Olive 1985).

The advent of first trimester ultrasound scanning has shown that twin gestations are at least twice the number of resultant twin births (Varma 1979). The 'vanishing' sac may be associated with no maternal

97

symptomatology, but in 25% the mother will have first trimester bleeding (Landy et al 1986, Gindoff et al 1986). When this early loss occurs, the outcome for the surviving fetus does not appear to be adversely affected. When the diagnosis of a twin pregnancy is made by ultrasound scan early in gestation, it is important that the mother is appraised of the possibility of the loss of one conceptus. This will enable her to accept a change in her pregnancy expectations, should this occur, more readily. It should also discourage her from too wide a degree of publication of the findings until the outcome is more predictable.

Ultrasound in the diagnosis of zygosity

The perinatal mortality rate in monozygous twins is higher than that associated with dizygous twins due to an increase in fetal anomaly and polyhydramnios. Determination of zygosity where possible may therefore influence pregnancy management.

Dizygous twins are four times more common than monozygous twins and can be identified in early pregnancy when the sacs are widely separate (Barss et al 1985). Later in pregnancy, sex differences may be apparent or two separate placentae may be identified.

The increase in monozygous twin perinatal mortality is associated with monochorionic twins where, in at least 85%, there is a vascular connection within the placentae. This may lead to discordant growth or twin-to-twin transfusion. Where possible it is therefore useful to try to identify this subgroup of twins.

When embryonic division occurs within 4 days of fertilization, dichorionic diamniotic twins will result. This occurs in about 25% of monozygotic twins.

If embryonic division occurs at the blastocyst stage later in the first week, the twins are monochorionic and diamniotic. Should division not occur until the blastocyst has implanted and the amnion has differentiated, the developing twins will be monochorionic and monoamniotic. Though this group only accounts for 3% of all twin pregnancies, they carry a high perinatal mortality rate from loss due to cord entanglement or conjoining.

Where the placentae abut, it is therefore helpful to try to identify the amnionicity and chorionicity of the pregnancy by looking for a membrane between the two fetuses. The membrane may be difficult to visualize such that a definite diagnosis of monoamniotic twins cannot be made unless cord entanglement is seen (Mahoney et al 1985). Conjoining may be evident if major structural connections are present but should be suspected if the fetal attitudes one to the other remain consistent.

Where the membrane is adequately identified, its thickness should be examined to either identify two or four layers (D'Alton & Dudley 1986) or to judge it as paper thin (monochorionic) or equivalent to one wall of the umbilical cord (dichorionic) (Barss et al 1985).

Antenatal advice

Following the diagnosis of a twin pregnancy it is important to explain the need for increased antenatal supervision. This allows the mother to make appropriate changes to her lifestyle such as increased rest and earlier cessation of employment. Adequate dietary advice should be given. Though it has been customary to ensure that a mother has haematinic supplements, including folic acid, the requirement for this has not been proven.

Detection of fetal abnormality

One of the commonest reasons for the finding of a raised serum alpha fetoprotein is a multiple pregnancy. This test therefore cannot be offered as a neural tube screening test. In singleton pregnancies an additional association with a raised serum alpha fetoprotein is the identification of mothers with structurally normal fetuses who have a poorer perinatal outcome. With twin pregnancies the perinatal outcome in association with a raised serum alpha fetoprotein is similar to those with a normal serum alpha fetoprotein (Patel et al 1985).

Structural fetal abnormalities may be identified by offering detailed mid-trimester scanning, or later in pregnancy, when further detailed ultrasound investigation has been prompted by the detection of polyhydramnios. When this is persistent with twins it has been shown that there is a 50% incidence of malformation in one of the twins (Hashimato et al 1986). It is, however, extremely uncommon for both twins to be affected by a structural abnormality (unless conjoined).

When a structural abnormality is detected, the management is usually directed to ensure that the well-being of the normal fetus is not compromised, this being particularly relevant at the time of parturition.

Selective feticide may be considered if it is the mother's wish. Before this is undertaken, however, it is important to identify the chorionicity of the pregnancy and hence the likelihood of placental vascular connections.

If vascular connections exist, intravascular emboli given to the abnormal twin to try to achieve fetal death could cross to the normal fetus and result in its death also. An alternative method of selective feticide is pericardial or pleural infusions to cause death by cardiac tamponade. Following death, however, there is the possibility of thromboembolic phenomena passing from the dead fetus to the living, resulting in a wide spectrum of defects (Hoyme et al 1981) including central nervous system defects and gut atresias. There are, however, reports of selective feticide being performed in association with twin-to-twin transfusions where the remaining twin has not been apparently compromised (Wittmann et al 1986). They do not, however, give any long-term follow-up to assess neurological development.

Maternal age is the commonest reason for either professionals offering or mothers requesting genetic screening of a pregnancy. When it is a twin pregnancy it is important to stress that it is highly unlikely that both fetuses would have a chromosomal anomaly, even if monozygotic. The mother would then have to consider what she would do if one twin were abnormal. Would she find the bringing up of a mongol child so abhorrent that she would consider the associated abortion of the normal fetus?

The other problem that is important to stress is that it is not always possible to test both fetuses, and hence the mother may not have the full information on which to base her decision (Elias et al 1980, Tabsh et al 1985). With this information the majority of mothers will opt not to have genetic screening unless they are at high risk by being themselves translocation carriers.

When the mother does opt for genetic screening, amniocentesis is still the procedure of choice. If the intra-amniotic membrane is easy to visualize and is in the midline, it is possible to aspirate fluid from each sac without the introduction of any confirmatory dye. Some authors have recommended the introduction of indigo carmine dye into the first sac to confirm that tapping of the same sac has not been carried out twice. Though no side-effects have been reported with indigo carmine, methylene blue should not be used (Cowett et al 1976).

Reduction of premature delivery

For many years compulsory hospitalization from 30 to 34 weeks gestation was advised to reduce the risk of premature delivery. It has been shown that for bed rest to have any effect at all it must be commenced before 25 weeks gestation (Hawrylyshyn et al 1982). Most obstetricians would now only advise hospitalization for selected mothers with pregnancy complications or excessive uterine irritability. Perhaps of more importance is the initial advice given regarding increased rest at home and earlier cessation of employment.

Cervical cerclage as a prophylactic measure is not effective in reducing preterm delivery (Weekes et al 1977). The use of prophylactic oral ritodrine has similarly not been found to affect outcome (O'Connor et al 1979).

Assessment of fetal growth

The birth weight of term twins is approximately 10% less than its singleton counterpart. Discordancy is said to exist if the difference between their weights exceeds 25% (Grumbach et al 1986), though others would say a difference of 250 g. This may relate to implantation site differences or twin-to-twin transfusion.

Clinical assessment of fetal growth in a twin pregnancy has even poorer correlation with fetal size than in a singleton. It is also impossible to detect discordant fetal growth. An overall clinical assessment should, however, include maternal weight gain, symphysis fundal height and maternal girth.

Having established the correct gestational age of a twin pregnancy by first- and second-trimester ultrasound measurements, it is helpful to commence serial ultrasound measurements from 25 weeks gestation. This is particularly important if the pregnancy is known to be monochorionic or the chorionicity has not been determined. The biparietal diameter alone is a poor predictor of fetal growth and of discordancy. This is related to both head sparing when looking for asymmetrical growth and dolichocephaly due to uterine compressions (Crane et al 1980, Redford 1984). Head circumference is a better measure of identifying discordancy. Abdominal circumference should be measured to identify asymmetrical growth retardation.

When discordant growth has been identified, umbilical artery waveforms using Doppler ultrasound have been used to differentiate between idiopathic growth retardation and twin-to-twin transfusion. In the latter the waveforms are identical, whereas if one twin is normal and the second twin growth retarded, the waveforms of only the smaller twin are abnormal (Giles et al 1985).

The identification of polyhydramnios with the larger twin and oligo-hydramnios with the smaller twin is also indicative of twin-to-twin transfusion (Chescheir & Seeds 1988).

Antepartum assessment of fetal well-being

Maternal assessment of fetal activity is a poor indicator of fetal well-being as one would be asking the mother to differentiate the activity of each fetus. Where ultrasound evidence of either discordant growth or concordant asymmetrical growth retardation has been found, antenatal cardiotoco-graphy should be employed, the frequency depending upon the growth characteristics, but usually three times per week. It may be helpful to identify the position of the fetal hearts by ultrasound prior to placing the transducer (Devoe 1985). The resultant cardiotocograph tracings should be compared to identify dissimilarity to be certain that both fetuses have been monitored.

When one twin is judged to be fit and one twin has suboptimal cardiotocograph tracings, the management decision is difficult and will depend upon gestational age and fetal size. In order to rescue the compromised fetus, is one doing a disservice to the well fetus such that it is likely to suffer from severe hyaline membrane disease? In this instance it may be helpful to perform an amniocentesis, taking fluid from the sac of the well fetus and assessing lung maturity (Hays & Smeltzer 1986).

Maternal assessment

In addition to close supervision of the fetuses it is necessary to supervise the mother because of her increased risk of pre-eclampsia. Placental position should be identified by ultrasound in view of the increased risk of placenta praevia. At each visit questioning should be directed to gain information regarding uterine irritability.

INTRAPARTUM MANAGEMENT

Elective caesarean section

Elective caesarean section may be employed for a variety of reasons but is most commonly associated with maternal pre-eclampsia and mal-presentation of the first twin (Crawford 1987). It is also recommended for the delivery of monoamniotic twins (Rodis et al 1987).

When delivery is performed under epidural analgesia, both twins are likely to be clinically similar at birth, whereas under general anaesthesia the twin in the best clinical condition is variable. With regard to biochemical aspects, twin one has less metabolic acidosis than twin two, irrespective of the anaesthesia employed (Crawford 1987).

Term labour

When both twins are presenting by the head and are appropriately grown, there is agreement that vaginal delivery is appropriate. Where the second twin is either transverse or in a breech position it has been suggested that caesarean section should be employed. A randomized trial of caesarean section compared with vaginal delivery (Rabinovici et al 1987) has shown no difference in outcome for the second twin even though breech extraction with or without internal podalic version was employed in a substantial number of cases. Malpresentation of the second twin should not be the reason for elective caesarean section.

Labour may occur spontaneously or may be induced. A commonly accepted indication for induction of labour is 40 weeks gestation, as past these dates for a twin pregnancy post maturity is considered to be present. Other indications for induction around term included growth retardation in either both or one of the twins.

Continuous electronic monitoring of both fetuses should be employed. This is particularly important if the twins are considered to be monozygous as twin-to-twin transfusion may become manifest during labour. Ideally a cardiotocograph machine, which allows two fetal heart rates to be simul-taneously recorded on a single paper print-out, should be employed. The first twin's heart rate is recorded from a fetal scalp electrode and the second twin by means of ultrasound. On a single tracing it is easier to be certain that both fetuses are being monitored.

Abnormalities in the fetal heart rate trace of twin one can, if of doubtful significance, be investigated in the usual way by employing fetal blood sampling. This cannot, however, be employed in twin two and in this circumstance the heart rate trace has to be interpreted in isolation. Where there is a suggestion of fetal compromise in either twin, caesarean section is employed.

Failure to progress in labour in association with poor uterine contractility is an indication for Syntocinon augmentation as is employed in a singleton pregnancy. Pre-existing polyhydramnios is a common finding in this situation.

The analgesia of choice for labour is epidural block (Crawford 1978, Jarvis & Whitfield 1981). Epidural block allows manipulative deliveries of twin two to be performed without the need for general anaesthesia.

During the early 1980s there has been an increase in the incidence of caesarean section being employed for delivery of the second twin (Constantine & Redman 1987, Patel et al 1985). This change has led to the view that not only should an anaesthetist be present during a twin delivery, but that the delivery should be conducted in either an operating theatre (Crawford 1987) or at least in a well-equipped operative delivery room with appropriate anaesthetic monitoring equipment.

Following the delivery of the first twin, the placental end of the cord should be left clamped as a precaution against placental anastomoses. If the second twin is lying longitudinally, the membranes should be kept intact until the presenting part is well within the pelvis. Too early rupture of the membranes of the second twin, leading to cord prolapse or impacted shoulder, is a common cause of requiring caesarean section. If uterine contractility is poor it may be aided with Syntocinon. The second twin should then be delivered appropriately.

Should the second twin be either oblique or transverse, two different options are available. External cephalic version may be employed or internal podalic version performed with intact membranes (Rabinovici et al 1988). The 'rediscovery' of internal podalic version may help in reducing the incidence of caesarean section for the second twin. Though with experience it is possible to identify a foot with certainty through intact membranes, the less experienced operator may feel happier employing ultrasound as an adjuvant to the procedure. Where version is employed it is important to perform this during the uterine quiescence that follows the delivery of twin one. In this circumstance accidental membrane rupture is less likely to occur.

An active policy of third stage management should be employed, as over-distention of the uterus leads to an increased risk of postpartum haemorrhage.

Preterm labour

Spontaneous preterm labour occurs in 30% of twin pregnancies and is associated with zygosity, being most common in association with mono-chorionic twins (Hall 1985). Once labour is established, it will proceed. The use of tocolytic agents such as beta mimetics in this situation do have the benefit of achieving short-term delay in delivery (King et al 1985). The major benefit is to allow transfer of the mother to a unit with adequate paediatric support services should this prove necessary. In a unit with a regional neonatal intensive care unit, of mothers whose only indication for transfer was threatened preterm delivery, 30% of the mothers transferred had a multiple pregnancy (Weaver 1988).

Some obstetricians believe that all twins of less than 36 weeks gestation should be delivered by caesarean section (Olofsson & Rydhstrom 1985). The more usual practice is to manage the labour in a similar way to that employed for mature twins but with a lower threshold for operative intervention. Even if the gestational age is such that caesarean section would not be considered (less than 26 weeks), it would still be appropriate to give the usual care and have a paediatric presence at the delivery.

PUERPERIUM

When both twins are born alive and survive, the mother requires the additional support necessary to allow her to gain experience in caring for two children.

Twin pregnancy has an increased risk of perinatal loss associated with prematurity and lethal congenital abnormality. This may result in the mother being left with only one surviving child. When this occurs it is important to encourage an appropriate grieving response even though she has to care for the survivor. A failure to grieve may result in long-term problems for the mother and may also have repercussions within the family unit (Lewis 1983).

REFERENCES

Barss V A, Benacerraf B R, Frigoletto F D 1985 Ultrasonographic determination of chorion type in twin gestation. Obstetrics and Gynecology 66: 79
Chescheir N C, Seeds J W 1988 Polyhydramnios and oligohydramnios in twin gestations. Obstetrics and Gynecology 71: 882
Constantine G, Redman C W 1987 Caesarean delivery of the second twin. Lancet 8533: 618
Cowett R, Hakanson D, Kocon R 1976 Untoward neonatal effect of intra-amniotic administration of methylene blue. Obstetrics and Gynecology (suppl) 48: 745
Crane J P, Tomich P G, Kopta M 1980 Ultrasonic growth patterns in normal and discordant twins. Obstetrics and Gynecology 55: 678
Crawford J S 1978 Principles and practice of obstetric anaesthesia, 4th edn. Oxford, Blackwell, p 218
Crawford J S 1987 A prospective study of 200 consecutive twin deliveries. Anaesthesia 42: 33
D'Alton M E, Dudley D K L 1986 Ultrasound in the antenatal management of twin gestation. Seminars in Perinatology 10: 30
Devoe L D 1985 Simultaneous antepartum testing of twin fetal heart rates. Southern Medical Journal 78: 380
Elias S, Gervie A, Simpson J L 1980 Genetic amniocentesis in twin gestations. American Journal of Obstetrics and Gynecology 50: 68
Giles W B, Trudinger B J, Cook C M 1985 Fetal umbilical artery flow velocity waveforms in twin pregnancies. British Journal of Obstetrics and Gynaecology 92: 490
Gindoff P R, Yeh M-N, Jewelewicz R 1986 The vanishing sac syndrome: ultrasound

evidence of pregnancy failure in multiple gestations, induced and spontaneous. Journal of Reproductive Medicine 31: 322

Grennert L, Persson P H, Gennser G 1978 Benefits of ultrasonic screening of a pregnant population. Acta Obstetricia et Gynecologica Scandinavica 8(suppl): 5

Grumbach K, Coleman B G, Arger P H, Mintz M L, Gabbe S G, Mennuti M T 1986 Twin and singleton growth patterns compared using ultrasound. Radiology 158: 237

Hall M H 1985 Preterm labour and its consequences. Proceedings of the thirteenth study group of the Royal College of Obstetricians and Gynaecologists, p 11

Hashimoto B, Callen P W, Filly R A, Laros R K 1986 Ultrasound evaluation of polyhydramnios and twin pregnancy. American Journal of Obstetrics and Gynecology 154: 1069

Hawrylyshyn P A, Barkin M, Berstein A 1982 Twin pregnancies: a continuing perinatal challenge. Obstetrics and Gynecology 59: 463

Hays P M, Smeltzer J S 1986 Multiple gestation. Clinics in Obstetrics and Gynaecology 29: 264

Hoyme H D, Higginbottom M C, Jones K L 1981 Vascular etiology of disruptive structural defects in monozygotic twins. Pediatrics 67: 288

Hughey M J, Olive D L 1985 Routine ultrasound scanning for the detection and management of twin pregnancies. Journal of Reproductive Medicine 30: 427

Jarvis G T, Whitfield M F 1981 Epidural analgesia and the delivery of twins. Journal of Obstetrics and Gynecology 2: 90

King J F, Keirse M J N C, Grant A, Chalmers I 1985 Preterm labour and its consequences. Proceedings of the thirteenth study group of the Royal College of Obstetricians and Gynaecologists, p 206

Landy H J, Weiner S, Corson S L, Batzer F R, Bolognese R J 1986 The 'vanishing twin': ultrasonographic assessment of fetal disappearance in the first trimester. American Journal of Obstetrics and Gynecology 755: 14

Lewis E 1983 Advances in Perinatal Medicine 3: 232

Mahoney B S, Filly R A, Callen P W 1985 Amnionicity and chorionicity in twin pregnancies: prediction using ultrasound. Radiology 155: 205

O'Connor M C, Murphy H, Dalrymple I J 1979 Double blind trial of ritodrine and placebo in twin pregnancy. British Journal of Obstetrics and Gynaecology 86: 706

Olofsson P, Rydhstrom H 1985 Management in the second stage of labour in term twin delivery. Acta Geneticae Medicae et Gemellologiae 34: 213

Patel N, Barrie W, Campbell D et al 1985 Scottish twin study 1983, preliminary report. Distributed by the Departments of Child Health and Obstetrics, University of Glasgow

Pridmore B R 1985 The role of ultrasound in the management of twin pregnancies. Australasian Radiology 29: 154

Rabinovici J, Barkai G, Reichman B, Serr D M, Mashiack S 1987 Randomised management of the second non vertex twin: vaginal delivery or Caesarean section. American Journal of Obstetrics and Gynecology 156: 52

Rabinovici J, Barkai G, Reichman B, Serr D M, Mashiack S 1988 Internal podalic version with unruptured membranes for the second twin in transverse lie. Obstetrics and Gynecology 71: 428

Redford D H A 1984 Early abnormal fetal growth—an ominous ultrasonic sign in twin pregnancy. Proceedings of the International Workshop on Twin Pregnancies. Malmo Sweden (abstract) 79

Rodis J F, Vintzileos A M, Cambell W A, Decton J L, Fumia F, Nochimsw D J 1987 Antenatal diagnosis and management of monoamniotic twins 157: 1255

Tabsh K M A, Crandall B, Lebherz T B, Howard J 1985 Genetic amniocentesis in twin pregnancy. Obstetrics and Gynecology 65: 843

Varma T R 1979 Ultrasound evidence of early pregnancy failure in patients with multiple conceptions. British Journal of Obstetrics and Gynaecology 86: 290

Weaver J B 1988 Birmingham Maternity Hospital Perinatal Report, p 25

Weekes A R L, Menzies D N, De Boer C H 1977 The relative efficacy of bed rest, cervical suture and no treatment in the management of twin pregnancy. British Journal of Obstetrics and Gynaecology 84: 161

Wittman B K, Farquharson D F, Thomas W D S, Baldwin J V, Wadsworth L D 1986 The role of feticide in the management of severe twin transfusion syndrome. American Journal of Obstetrics and Gynecology 155: 1023

8. The vacuum extractor

Jonathan Carter

INTRODUCTION

The vacuum extractor has gained wide popularity in the United Kingdom and Europe, but has not done so in the United States and Australia. The reason may rest with the obstetrician's greater familiarity with forceps.

The vacuum extractor has advantages over forceps for certain types of delivery, and if we refuse to employ it or at least evaluate it, we may do ourselves and our patients a disservice.

The advantages of the vacuum extractor include its ease of application, its encouragement of 'autorotation' of the malpositioned fetal head, and its safety for both mother and fetus. The maternal complications resulting from the use of the vacuum extractor are limited to vaginal and cervical tears usually caused by accidental inclusion of these tissues into the cup. They are preventable if appropriate attention is paid to application techniques.

The most obvious fetal injury is the formation of the chignon, the oedematous artificial caput formed beneath the vacuum cup. Abrasions and lacerations of the fetal scalp are also encountered after use with the vacuum extractor, but are usually minor and self limiting.

Cephalhaematomas are also more common after use of the vacuum extractor, but apart from causing neonatal jaundice are rarely of clinical significance.

The long-term outcome of infants delivered by vacuum extractor has been studied, and these infants have normal neurological development.

HISTORY

The first report of the use of a vacuum device as a traction instrument to assist delivery was by James Yonge in 1705. He had made an unsuccessful attempt to extract the fetus of a 30-year old primipara 'by a Cupping-Glass fixt to the scalp with an Air-Pump' (Sjostedt 1967).

The first instrument to be developed and made practicable and useful was presented by James Young Simpson (1849) in Edinburgh. Simpson's first cup was fitted with a piston, and consisted of a trumpet-shaped concave disc, covered with leather at its broader end. Simpson modified this design in 1855, his new device consisting of a slender brass syringe worked by a piston with a cup attached to its lower extremity. According to Simpson, a tractor like this was safer than forceps, because the instrument lay completely below the fetal head unlike forceps which took up a certain amount of space between the head and the birth canal—a feature leading to greater maternal trauma.

Modifications have continued on these instruments. Stillman (1875) made a more flexible cup attached to an air pump equipped with a set of cervical dilators. McCahey (1880) constructed various forms of tractors, some with a ball valve, some with an aircock, to which a rubber tube 3 or 4 feet long was attached. An air pump was connected to the other end of the tube so that the nurse could produce the desired vacuum.

Kuntzsch (1912) designed a cup made of metal and rubber which could be inserted into the vagina without using analgesia. The Gladish (1933) suction cup was a hollow elliptical cup made of flexible material. It had a detachable handle, which was hollow to allow the passage of air. Cornu (1934) modified the Gladish cup, altering its shape to that of a cone, and formed it into a single apparatus with the pump attached.

Over the next two decades a number of clinicians altered the design of the suction cup. Torpin's (1938) cup had a flexible rubber concave hemisphere designed to fit the fetal vertex closely. On the concave surface were rubber projections, the purpose of which was to keep the fetal scalp from blocking the opening that led to the vacuum pump.

Couzigou's (1947) instrument 'La Ventouse Eutocique' was operated with tapes attached to the cup. A vacuum was produced by an air–water electric pump. It incorporated for the first time a manometer to measure pressure. There was also a bottle between the cup and the pump, in a similar fashion to the Malmstrom design about 16 years later.

Korber, in 1950, devised a cup whereby the edges were fixed on a semi-solid disc and a hollow handle connected the cup concavity to an electrical air pump. A net inside the cup was inserted to improve safety by reducing caput formation.

Malmstrom of Gothenburg, Sweden, presented his vacuum extractor (the VE/53) to a meeting of the local medical society in 1953. He later modified this device, the VE/56 having a different height, diameter and hemispherical walls. Because of seal problems the cup edge had a smaller radius. Like the VE/53, the new model VE/56 had a traction chain passing through a rubber suction tube, and terminated in a metal handle. Malmstrom (1967) further developed his suction device (VE/67) so that the suction outlet was depressed in the cup, making the cup shallower and its introduction into the vagina easier.

Paul et al (1973) developed a novel plastic instrument, while in 1973 Kobayashi introduced a pliable silastic vacuum extractor which offered the potential advantage of less scalp trauma (Maryniak 1984, Pelosi 1984).

The most recent instrument designed by O'Neil has a traction chain linked to a ring on the cup. This allows the direction of traction to be changed during the procedure without loss of effective traction (O'Neil 1981).

INDICATIONS FOR USE OF THE VACUUM EXTRACTOR

Since the first descriptions of the vacuum extractor by Yonge & Simpson, the indications for its use have varied. The vacuum extractor was originally introduced as an alternative to forceps delivery at a time when high extractions were common. Such deliveries produced unacceptably high fetal and maternal morbidity and mortality. Simpson thought that the tractor would prove as useful when the head was at the brim as when it was at the outlet. He claimed it could enable the obstetrician 'to add a few pounds to every pain' and in this way make completion of delivery safer and faster in cases that would otherwise have progressed slowly.

James, who was a student of Simpson, reported in 1849 that a suction instrument could be used in uterine inertia or disproportion to deliver the high head to a low position in the pelvis where it might be within reach of forceps. Kuntzsch (1912) reported the use of this cup in breech presentations as well as cephalic presentations.

It was not until 1938 that the indications and conditions for the use of this instrument became the same as that for forceps, when Torpin reported a series of 600 vacuum deliveries without evidence of fetal brain haemorrhage or injury.

The indications for the use of the vacuum extractor are (i) fetal, (ii) maternal or (iii) obstetric reasons (Table 8.1).

Fetal indications

A number of authors have reported using the vacuum extractor for fetal

Table 8.1   Indications for use of the vacuum extractor

Fetal indications
Fetal distress in second stage
Prolapsed cord/fetal distress after 7 cm of cervical dilatation

Maternal indications
Maternal physical distress
To avoid maternal effort, e.g. in patients with hypertension, cardiac disease, respiratory
    disease, etc.

Obstetric indications
Problems with second twin (delay, fetal distress, prolapsed cord, etc.)
Borderline cephalopelvic disproportion (trial of VE)
Delay in second stage/prolonged labour
'Elective delivery'
Malrotations or attitudes of deflexion

---

distress. Roszkowski et al (1963) reported 521 deliveries by vacuum extraction, of which 40.6% were done for evidence of fetal distress. Their overall perinatal mortality for vacuum extraction deliveries was 1.34% as compared with 2.14% overall perinatal mortality. The perinatal mortality for infants delivered by vacuum extraction because of signs of fetal distress was 1.4%.

Similarly Ngan et al (1986) recently reviewed 1664 babies delivered by the vacuum extractor; fetal distress was suspected in 36.2% of patients who had meconium-stained liquor, abnormal fetal heart rate tracings or abnormal fetal blood pH. Their perinatal mortality rate of 0.6/1000 total births was low and similar to findings in other studies (Brat 1965, Nyirjesy 1963).

Surprisingly, Chamberlain (1980), in a review article, claims: 'the indications for vacuum extraction are found mostly in the first stage of labour. If fetal distress occurs after 7 cm of cervical dilatation in a multiparous patient, applying and using a vacuum extractor to dilate the cervix would be much quicker than a caesarean section'.

Altaras et al (1974) have reported the use of the vacuum extractor in the delivery of 30 infants with prolapsed cord in cases where the cervix was greater than 6 cm dilated. Their overall perinatal mortality was 10.0% as compared with a 10.7% perinatal mortality rate for infants with prolapsed cord delivered by caesarean section. Over 50% of the infants were delivered within 5 minutes of the diagnosis of prolapsed cord. The general perinatal mortality for prolapsed cord is 12% if delivered by caesarean section and 22.5% if delivered by forceps (Altaras et al 1974).

Operative vaginal delivery is more often performed for fetal distress in the second stage of labour. Many would argue against the use of the vacuum extractor, claiming it is much swifter to apply forceps under local anaesthesia than using a vacuum extractor. Certainly the modification of the vacuum extraction method introduced by Evelbauer & Beyer (1961) using an electric pump achieves a rapid, high and constant vacuum which enables rapid deliveries with the vacuum extractor.

Maternal indications

The maternal indications are often prophylactic. Instrumental intervention aims at accelerating the delivery. In the study by Ngan et al (1986) of 1526 deliveries completed by the vacuum extractor, maternal indications such as hypertension, previous lower segment uterine scar or maternal distress accounted for 11.1% of patients.

Likewise, Matheson et al (1968), in a review of 168 deliveries completed by the vacuum extractor, found maternal indications for decreasing the duration of the second stage in 12%. Seventeen patients had severe pre-eclampsia; and bleeding secondary to abruptio placenta occurred in two patients. The remaining patient had a previous caesarean section with subsequent vaginal deliveries.

Maternal distress is much harder to define than fetal distress but usually it means maternal exhaustion after a long or painful first stage. The patient is often frightened and has not had proper analgesia. Operative delivery with a vacuum extractor in this situation is very useful.

Obstetric indications

The vacuum extractor was introduced to overcome uterine inertia in combination with cervical dystocia. There is now considerable disagreement as to the place of the vacuum extractor for intervention during first stage.

The most common indication for use of the vacuum extractor had been that of prolonged labour (Sjostedt 1967, Ott 1975, Ngan 1986, Malmstrom 1965). The causation could be either inertia, malpresentation or malposition, contraction of the pelvis, an abnormally big baby or delayed dilatation of the cervix. Malmstrom stated that in over 50% of his patients, the indication for vacuum extraction was prolonged labour (Malmstrom 1965). He claimed that mild traction on the head, pressing it against the cervix, stimulated an increase in uterine contractions, thus facilitating delivery. Ngan et al (1986) agree. In their analysis of 1526 vacuum extraction deliveries, prolonged second stage or poor maternal effort was the indication for vacuum extraction delivery in 52.8% of patients.

In a comparative study of delivery by vacuum extractor and forceps, Schenker found 140 (46.6%) of cases delivered by the vacuum extractor. Intervention was decided upon because of lack of progress in labour either from secondary uterine inertia or maternal exhaustion.

However, in Wider's (1967) study of a series of 201 vacuum extraction deliveries, the instrument was used in the majority of cases (64%) for 'elective' delivery, whereas uterine inertia accounted for only 13% of the vacuum deliveries.

Malpresentation is a contraindication for delivery by vacuum extraction, although two of its most ardent supporters have documented delivery of a fetus with brow presentation (Chalmers 1960, Lillie 1960). Vacuum extraction of cases of breech presentation with delay in the second stage of labour has also been reported by authors (Chalmers 1960, Lillie 1960). I believe the use of the vacuum extractor in situations such as these will only occasionally be successful, and may increase the risk to both mother and fetus. In these circumstances the procedure should be discouraged.

Malrotations or attitudes of deflexion present the greatest difficulty in effecting successful delivery for the vacuum extractor. Initial results of the early 1960s were disappointing. Hammerstein & Gromotke (1962) in their series failed to deliver 50% of cases by vacuum extractor. Brey et al (1962) pointed out that in cases of deflexion and occipito-posterior position, it is much more difficult to expediate the delivery than in cases of vertex and occipito-anterior positions.

Bourne & Williams (1962) claimed that, in cases where the occiput is lateral or oblique, a good occipital application of the extractor cup will frequently lead to increased flexion which will be followed by spontaneous forward rotation of the occiput. Lancet (1963) claimed that the descent of the head following traction was accompanied by rotation, and that in most cases spontaneous rotation occurs by traction alone. Chalmers et al (1960) indicated that rotation of the occiput arrested in the posterior or transverse position could in most instances be more easily and more physiologically effected with the vacuum extractor than either manually or with forceps. Evelbauer, as early as 1956, had created the term of 'autorotation' for this occurrence.

Poor cup design hampered early attempts to deliver malpositions of the fetal head by the vacuum extractor. Further development and refinement of these cups has increased the success with these types of delivery. The O'Neil obstetric cup with its modified traction apparatus has dramatically improved the usefulness of this instrument for malpositions (O'Neil 1981).

CONTRAINDICATIONS FOR USE OF THE VACUUM EXTRACTOR

Any operative procedure, including vacuum extraction, is contraindicated when safety and success cannot be guaranteed. Another mode of delivery should then be sought. Over the years, with changing obstetric indications and improvement of general anaesthesia and safety of caesarean sections, the contraindications for vacuum extraction delivery have increased (Table 8.2).

There is no doubt that absolute cephalopelvic disproportion is a contra-indication to vaginal delivery by vacuum extraction. Another is an un-corrected face presentation since, according to Chalmers, 'apart from the risk of trauma to the eyes, the irregular bony contours of the face make it impossible to achieve a suitable vacuum' (Chalmers 1960).

In brow presentation the fetal head is extended, presenting the large mentovertical diameter and leading to absolute cephalopelvic disproportion. Many authors agree that the vacuum extractor is then

Table 8.2 Contraindications for use of the vacuum extractor

Malpresentations (face, brow, breech, transverse or oblique lie)
More than borderline cephalopelvic disproportion (trial of VE)
Cervix insufficiently dilated to permit application of a 50 mm cup to a single fetus or a first twin, or a 40 mm cup to a second twin
Uncooperative patient
Suspected fetal coagulopathy

contraindicated (Sjostedt 1967, Ngan 1986, Brat 1965). Surprisingly, a few of its most ardent supporters do not feel that brow presentation is a contraindication to the use of the vacuum extractor (Chalmers 1960, Bergman 1961, Chalmers 1969), as proper application of the cup may still produce a more flexed attitude.

The vacuum extractor was introduced initially to effect deliveries in high positions where forceps were considered dangerous to mother and fetus. Much is also written of its use in extracting infants though an incompletely dilated cervix. Malmstrom, in 1967, wrote: 'high station of the fetal head and a "bad cervix"—incompletely dilated or unmatured—must be considered as a contraindication. The time for "Trial of VE" is over'.

First-stage applications demand superior obstetric judgement as to the indication, pelvic architecture and fetal position and should be reserved for extreme situations, such as abruptio placentae, cardiac patients in failure, or tamponade in bleeding marginal placenta praevia. Per Lange (1964) reports a 20% perinatal mortality rate associated with deliveries where the instrument was applied when the cervix was 7 cm dilated or less and a 16% perinatal mortality rate when the station is 0 or above.

Some authors particularly mention that they never use the vacuum extractor in breech presentation (Bourne 1962, Bird 1982, Earn 1967). A number of investigators, though, have used the suction cup in breech presentation, fixing it to the anterior fetal buttock (Chalmers 1960, Evelbauer 1963) for increased traction. My views are similar to those of Chalmers (1969) who, after 2 years of using the vacuum extractor for breech presentations, ceased to do so and reverted to caesarean section. In my view the use of the vacuum extractor in this instance is no different to that of breech extraction, a procedure declining in routine breech deliveries.

Roseman (1969) and others have reported a higher perinatal mortality and morbidity when the vacuum extractor was used in premature deliveries (compared with forceps or spontaneous deliveries). Among 60 extractions of premature infants, all infants had scalp lesions, most had Apgar scores below 5, and relatively severe jaundice occurred in 15%. The perinatal mortality was 5% compared with matched term controls whose perinatal mortality was 3.3%. Sjostedt (1967) has reviewed the literature on the use of the vacuum extractor in premature infants and states that its use in premature infants is probably contraindicated. Surprisingly, Chalmers states that he has had excellent success with its use in these conditions (Chalmers 1969).

Fetal scalp blood sampling is a procedure increasing in popularity and demand for intrapartum diagnosis of fetal acidosis. Roberts & Stone (1978) described a case of acute fetal blood loss (45 ml) from a scalp puncture site during subsequent application of the vacuum extractor, a previously un-reported complication. For similar reasons to that in the case of Roberts & Stone, a fetus at risk of thrombocytopenia secondary to maternal ITP, or any inherited coagulation defect, should not be delivered by the vacuum extractor, even when vaginal delivery has been planned.

MECHANICS OF THE VACUUM EXTRACTOR

The vacuum cup affixes to the smooth fetal head, allowing traction to be applied. The suction raises an edged dome of the soft tissues of the scalp and the pull is on the overhang of this edge. One of the major advantages of the vacuum extractor is that when traction force is too great, the cup dislodges. This in-built safety factor avoids intracranial damage to the fetus.

Correct application of the cup to the occiput is necessary to enable flexion and synclitism to occur after the traction force has been applied. Rydberg (1954) has shown that the fetal head is completely flexed when its longest diameter—the mentovertical diameter—points in the direction of descent, and that this diameter ends posteriorly on the sagittal suture, 3 cm in front of the posterior fontanelle in the average case. It follows then that the cup is ideally positioned when its centre is over the posterior end of the mento-vertical diameter, or in practical terms, when it covers the posterior fontanelle with the sagittal suture pointing to the centre of the cup. The distance in centimetres between the anterior edge of the cup and the posterior angle of the bregma is termed the 'application distance' (AD). A paramedian application of the cup will determine if the extraction attitude will by synclitic or asynclitic.

Factors that effect proper application of the cup may have an effect on the success of the delivery. The position of the cup depends on the experience and dexterity of the operator, the level, attitude and position of the head when the cup is applied, and most importantly, the manoeuvrability of the cup.

The manoeuvrability of the cup depends on the depth and diameter of the cup and the position and pliability of the suction tube. By moving the suction tubing from its central position to an eccentric position, the 'anterior' and 'posterior' cups were developed.

Traction and compressive forces

The amount of traction force which the cup will accept before it comes off the scalp depends mainly on the shape, diameter and depth of the cup, the level of negative pressure in the cup and the direction of the applied force. Saling & Hartung (1978), using an electronic measuring device, observed that a 60 mm Malmstrom cup was pulled off the scalp in 10 out of the 22 deliveries when the traction force was 20 kg or more, and that detachment did not occur if the force was less than 20 kg. Moolgaoker et al (1979), also using electronic measuring equipment, found that a 50 mm Malmstrom cup with a negative pressure of 0.8 kg/cm^2 accepted pulls of up to 48 pounds

(21.8 kg), and in one patient the cup did not come off until a pull of 51 pounds (23.1 kg) had been applied.

All users of the vacuum extractor know that an oblique pull is more likely to dislodge the cup than a perpendicular one, and that this is often disadvantageous. Ability to withstand obliquely applied traction has been increased by fixing the traction chain to a deep depression in the base of the cup (Halkin), to the base of the cup as in the 'anterior' and 'posterior' models, or by special traction devices as in the O'Neil cup (O'Neil 1981). O'Neil claims his cup is safe and easy to use with single-handed control over a 70° range without any loss of effective traction.

For the vacuum extractor to be accepted as a method of operative delivery, proof of its safety for the baby is imperative. In an evaluation of fetal safety, one important aspect involves the amount of cerebral compression exerted by the instruments used for delivery, be they obstetric forceps or vacuum extractor. Holland's classic work has demonstrated the mechanism by which increasing cerebral compression induces rises in intracranial pressure which may result in cerebral haemorrhage and brain damage (Holland 1922). Theoretical estimations of the compressive force of obstetric forceps and the vacuum extractor have been determined mathematically by Mishell (1962) (Table 8.3).

It will be noted that when a pull of 22 pounds is exerted, the calculated compressive force is 20 times greater with forceps than with the vacuum extractor. Mishell & Kelly (1962) attempted to measure the amount of traction required to achieve vaginal delivery in 50 women by obstetric forceps and by vacuum extractor. The amount of pull was determined by a spring gauge attached to the handle of the forceps and the handle of the vacuum extractor. They found that the average single pull with Simpson forceps was 27.2 pounds, which was greater than on the vacuum extractor, being 17.0 pounds. This resulted in a total traction force for delivery by forceps of 67.5 pounds (approximately 40% greater than the 38.8 pounds by the vacuum extractor). Two possible explanations exist as to why less traction is required with the vacuum extractor. (i) The vacuum extractor does not affect the diameter of the presenting vertex, whereas with forceps the thickness of the blades increases the transverse diameter by 8%. More pull is thus required to overcome the resultant additional resistance. (ii) By virtue of its scalp traction, the vacuum extractor may be mechanically more efficient than the obstetric forceps and its malar eminence traction.

Table 8.3 Theoretical compressive forces in vacuum extraction and forceps delivery

Instrument	Theoretical compressive force (g/cm²)
Simpson forceps	1500
Vacuum extractor	75

Technique for use

Patient positioning depends on operator preference and expected degree of difficulty of delivery. Either the dorsal, lateral or lithotomy positions may be used. Where at least modest traction is expected, then lithotomy position is favoured. The patient is prepared and draped as for a standard vaginal delivery. Prior to the application of the vacuum cup, the cervix should be fully dilated and the position and station of the presenting part is determined. The bladder should be empty, and the head well engaged in the presence of good uterine contractions and without evidence of cephalopelvic disproportion.

Analgesia and anaesthesia are determined by patient needs and the obstetrician's requirements. No anaesthesia, local infiltration or regional anaesthetic blockage is preferred, while conduction and general anaesthesia is discouraged as it abolishes the sensation to 'bear down', necessary in vacuum extraction deliveries.

A 50 mm cup is suitable for most deliveries. After testing the equipment for leaks, the cup is placed in the vagina. Rarely, an episiotomy may be needed. The cup is placed as close as possible to the posterior fontanelle in the midline. If this is not possible then an application distance (AD) of at least 3.0 cm is needed to achieve a deflexing attitude. The AD is the distance from the posterior bregma to the leading edge of the cup.

A negative pressure of $-0.2\,kg/cm^2$ is applied, and the cup is rechecked for position and possible entrapment of maternal tissue. When satisfied, a vacuum of no greater than $-0.8\,kg/cm^2$ is produced either in increments or rapidly.

Traction in the direction of the birth canal is made with uterine contractions and as close to perpendicular to the cup as possible. Counter traction with the thumb of the non-pulling hand against the shoulder of the cup is essential to prevent cup dislodgement if there is a break in the vacuum seal. The presenting part should descend with each pull and the cup should not dislodge more than once. If the baby is not delivered with three pulls and within 15 minutes from commencement of the procedure, then the procedure is abandoned and either forceps of caesarean section performed (Phillpott).

MATERNAL COMPLICATIONS

The vacuum extractor has the advantage of not occupying space in the pelvis (Malmstrom 1965, Plauche 1978, Kappy 1981). This, combined with less analgesia, in effecting delivery reduces the incidence of maternal trauma. The types of trauma incurred by the vacuum extractor include cervical and vaginal lacerations; episiotomy; perineal tears and extensions of episiotomies; postpartum haemorrhage and the need for blood transfusion; manual removal of placenta; and puerperal infectious morbidity.

Vaginal and cervical lacerations

There is wide agreement that the vacuum extractor is a safe method of delivery for the mother, provided that the cervix is fully dilated when the cup is applied (Sjostedt 1967, Ngan 1986, Malmstrom 1965, Chamberlain 1980, Schenker 1967). The risk of trauma is increased in the first-stage extraction, especially if the mother is nulliparous or the cervix unpliable or insufficiently dilated to permit the application of the vacuum cup. Cervical and vaginal injuries are preventable if appropriate attention is paid to application technique by ensuring that there is no entrapment of maternal tissue within the cup (Kappy 1981). In Sjostedt's series (1967) cervical lacerations occurred in 0.7% of vacuum extractions and were more common in multiparae than among primiparae. Significantly, more cervical and vaginal trauma occurred after forceps delivery—2.6% in this series. Most series support the concept that soft tissue injury is less frequent and less severe in vacuum extraction than it is in forceps delivery. Berggren recorded vaginal tears in 14.9% of his forceps series and 0% of his vacuum series (Berggren 1959). Brandstrup & Lange (1961) stated their figures of vaginal lacerations to be 3.7% in forceps deliveries and 0.9% in vacuum extraction deliveries. Plauche (1978), in examining 228 vacuum extraction deliveries, found maternal soft tissue injuries to be infrequent (1.7%), and no cervical lacerations required repair (Plauche 1978).

Correct application of the vacuum extractor cup should cause minimal cervical and vaginal trauma.

Episiotomy

Some may argue that listing episiotomy under maternal complications is inappropriate. It is, nevertheless, a traumatic procedure for the patient which may add morbidity to women recovering from their birthing experience. Most women who have an operative delivery also have an episiotomy (Hastie 1986). Among the reported vacuum extraction series, the frequency of episiotomy varies from 63% to 94.5% (Sjostedt 1967, Malmstrom 1965, Chamberlain 1980, Lillie 1960, Hammerstein 1962). Factors affecting the incidence of episiotomy include difficulty of delivery, size of the vacuum cup and the obstetrician's preference in performing such a procedure. Nyirjesy (1963) found that the frequency of episiotomy was not reduced by the use of the vacuum extractor, and in fact considers the procedure desirable for the majority of spontaneous deliveries.

Perineal tears

First- and second-degree tears are usually of minimal clinical importance. They are more common after forceps delivery, occurring in about 12.5% of recorded series compared with 10.9% in vacuum extraction series (Sjostedt 1967). The incidence of perineal tears is influenced by frequency of episiotomy. Minor perineal tears of first and second degree are more common if an episiotomy is not performed. Series of vacuum extractions reported by various investigators demonstrate a combined vulvovaginal laceration rate of between 10 and 19%. In these series the rates of episiotomy are between 45 and 85%. In the vacuum extraction series of Chalmers (1964), Brey (1962) and Karpathy (1965), they report a frequency of perineal tears of 4.3%, 14.6% and 9.7% respectively.

Major, or third-degree, perineal lacerations total 21% of Malmstrom's forceps series and 0.7% of the corresponding vacuum series. The higher frequency of third-degree tears with forceps delivery may be due to a higher frequency of pelvic contraction in the forceps group, but may also depend upon the pressure of the forceps blade on the perineum. It is also possible that in vacuum extractor deliveries, the timing of episiotomy is better judged and hence performed at the correct time, while in forceps delivery it is more difficult to gauge the stretching of the perineum and hence the higher incidence of the third-degree tears.

Among the reported vacuum extractor series, the incidence of third-degree tears is mostly less than 1%. A frequency of over 3% occurs only in the series by Tricomi (1961) and Pauly (1963). The rate of episiotomy reported by these authors is 76.3% and 72.1% respectively. But in the series of Chalmers (1964) in which perineal lacerations of third degree occurred in 0.5% of deliveries, the reported frequency of episiotomy is 63%, which is the lowest reported.

Postpartum haemorrhage

In producing significantly less maternal trauma, the vacuum extractor is less often associated with a primary postpartum blood loss in excess of 500 ml (Carter & Gudgeon 1987). Sjostedt (1967), in his extensive review, found the incidence of postpartum haemorrhage after forceps delivery to be 22%, which is four times the reported incidence of 5.2% in the vacuum extractor series. Brey (1962), Nyirjesy (1963) and Hammerstein (1962) have found the incidence of primary postpartum haemorrhage with the vacuum extractor to be 11.8%, 6.4% and 1.4% respectively.

Manual removal of placentae

Manual removal of placentae was down to 7.6% of patients after forceps delivery, four times the 1.9% incidence in vacuum extractor series (Sjostedt 1967, Schenker 1967). It may be that manual removal is done more readily with forceps delivery when the patient has had a conduction or general anaesthesia. The higher incidence of manual removal of placenta among forceps series must also contribute to the increased incidence of postpartum haemorrhage in this group.

Puerperal complications

Most authors agree that there are fewer puerperal complications following vacuum extraction than after forceps delivery (Malmstrom 1965, Schenker 1967, Lancet 1963). Schenker & Serr (1967), in their review of 600 cases of operative delivery, found that 5.6% of women after vacuum extraction had postpartum fever of genital tract origin in comparison with 15.3% following forceps delivery.

Two hundred patients, or 66.6% of women, after forceps delivery in Schenker's series received prophylactic antibiotics, as opposed to 146 or 48.6% after vacuum extraction deliveries.

Days of hospitalization after confinement has also been studied as an index of maternal morbidity. Sjostedt (1967) notes that the duration of treatment after delivery was over 10 days in 19.2% of forceps series. Obviously as a measure of morbidity, length of hospital stay is a crude index, for many variables may influence it, but it is still of interest that 80% of vacuum-delivered patients will be home within 10 days compared with 50% of forceps-delivered patients. Current hospital stay is about 50% less than in the review of Sjostedt. With less maternal trauma, patients delivered by the vacuum extractor are likely to be home earlier than patients delivered by forceps.

FETAL COMPLICATIONS

The reluctance to use the vacuum extractor by obstetricians has been mainly due to reports of fetal complications. The most serious have been the occurrence of subgaleal haematomas or intracranial haemorrhage (Malmstrom 1965, Earn 1967, Broekhuizen 1987, Fahmy 1971). Other fetal complications include artificial caput succedaneum formation, abrasions and lacerations, cephalhaematoma, cerebral irritation and asphyxia.

Subgaleal haemorrhage

The most serious fetal injury attributed to the vacuum extractor is that of subgaleal haemorrhage (synonymous with subaponeurotic haemorrhage). It probably occurs when emissary veins are ruptured beneath the galea aponeurotica. Malmstrom & Jansson (1965) believe that late subgaleal haemorrhage results from rupture of the interparietal synchondrosis, with bleeding from the saggital sinus into the subgaleal space. The subaponeurotic space is continuous across the cranium with no periosteal attachments. A haematoma in this space may dissect across the cranial vault, elevating a portion or all of the scalp. Subgaleal bleeding may thus be massive and life threatening. Subgaleal bleeding is often manifested late in the infant's nursery course, hours or even days after delivery (Ahuza 1969). Large reviews, one of which encompassed 2670 vacuum extraction deliveries, reported no subaponeurotic haemorrhages despite close attention to the status of the fetal scalp (Chalmers 1965, Fahmy 1971).

Ott believes that if the indications and techniques of vacuum extraction are followed, subaponeurotic haemorrhage should not be a complication associated with its use (Ott 1975). The cause and effect relationship between the vacuum extractor and subaponeurotic haemorrhage has not been really established, as they have been known to occur spontaneously, especially associated with prolonged labour.

Intracranial haemorrhage

Intracranial haemorrhage and evidence of cerebral irritation have also been associated with the use of the vacuum extractor (Malmstrom 1965, Plauche 1979, Aguero 1962). The incidence varies from less than 1% to approximately 8%, with an average of about 2.5%. Many of these cases too are associated with prolonged and difficult labours, and a cause–effect relationship with the vacuum extractor has not been definitely established. Malmstrom & Sjostedt both state that signs of cerebral irritation or intracranial haemorrhage are much less common in vacuum extraction deliveries than in forceps deliveries, although they are slightly more common in deliveries by vacuum extraction than in spontaneous deliveries (Sjostedt 1967).

Bird (1982) claims that the risk of the fetus suffering injury is directly related to the number of pulls (particularly negative or unrewarding ones), the number of times the cup lifts or becomes completely detached, and the duration of the cup's attachment to the scalp. Cerebral trauma occurs in less than 1% of infants when extraction is completed with less than five pulls, and in 5% when the number of pulls exceeds five.

The growing literature concerning intracerebral haemorrhage in infants of less than 33 weeks gestation (Cartwright 1979, Donat 1978) suggests an incidence of about 40%. Experience with term infants indicates a much lower occurrence, probably less than 1% (Cartwright 1979).

Cephalhaematoma

Cephalhaematoma is the most common fetal injury associated with the vacuum extractor (Carter & Gudgeon 1987). The reported frequency of this complication ranges from 0.7 to 39% (Sjostedt 1967). The ordinary subperiosteal cephalhaematoma is due to a tangential force on the fetal head, which causes recurrent displacement of the soft tissues of the scalp, and laceration of diploic veins. Periosteal attachments at the periphery of the bone prevent blood from disseminating. The parietal bone is most often involved, and may take many weeks to resolve. In Plauche's survey of 19 reports dealing with 8000 cases in which the vacuum extractor was used, the mean incidence was 6% (Plauche 1979). Fahmy (1971) studied factors predisposing to cephalhaematoma formation after vacuum extraction and found that high position of fetal head, slipping of the cup, large baby and traction for more than 10 minutes significantly increased the risk.

The majority of cephalhaematomata follow a benign course and cause no untoward effect on the fetus. Rarely they may increase in size and be so extensive as to cause fetal anaemia and require blood transfusion. Jaundice may further complicate such large cephalhaematomas. Linear fractures of the underlining bone have been found in as many as 25% of cases of cephalhaematoma, and bleeding from the fracture cranial bone may contribute to them (Fahmy 1971).

The incidence of cephalhaematoma can be reduced by care in selecting the cases, and experience which gives increased operative dexterity. Avoidance of prolonged traction or the use of the cup as a rotator and/or of sideways strain during extraction can minimize fetal scalp injury.

Cerebral irritation and asphyxia

Comparative clinical studies evaluating the effect of vacuum and forceps extraction on the Apgar score and neonatal outcome of the infants have yielded inconsistent results (Wider 1967, Schenker 1967, Munsat 1963). This may be due to the fact that the instruments have been used for a variety of maternal and fetal indications and in different obstetric conditions.

Phonocardiographic records were made by Snoeck (1960) at the time of cup application and found no changes in the fetal heart rate. Similarly, Lancet (1963) auscultated fetal heart sounds in all patients between contractions and could not detect any change in cardiac rhythm of the fetus.

Bird (1982) found that the vacuum extractor did not cause fetal hypoxia when it was used electively in uncomplicated cases for outlet delivery, or when extractions were smooth and easy and completed with no more than four pulls (Livnat 1978).

Saling & Hartung found that the risk of neonatal depression (Apgar score less than seven) was directly related to the extraction's force-time-integral (FTI), measured electronically in kilopound/second. Moreover, when depression occurred with extractions that were mildly difficult to difficult, it was always due to pre-existing hypoxia. Easy extractions (FTI less than 376 kp/s) did not result in depressed infants.

The incidence of postnatal asphyxia varies in different surveys, with a frequency between 2.6 and 12% (Malmstrom 1965). Livnat (1978) studied the acid–base balance of 63 neonates delivered either spontaneously or by vacuum extractor or forceps. He found that the outcome was similar in neonates delivered by vacuum extractor or forceps. When comparing pH and base deficit values between spontaneous deliveries and operative deliveries, no difference was apparent when the groups were corrected for length of second stage. Katz et al (1958), in a similar study on acid–base balance, found a significantly greater decrease in pH in the control compared with the vacuum group. They also found on analysis of CTG traces that mean total deceleration time amongst vacuum extraction fetuses was 22.8 minutes compared with 37.75 minutes amonst the control group ($P < 0.001$) Katz concluded that the application of the vacuum extractor during the second stage lessens fetal depression when compared with spontaneous delivery.

Scalp effects

The vacuum extractor places four types of force on to the fetal scalp: negative suction from the vacuum itself; downward traction from pulling; circular force if rotation occurs; and shearing force if the direction of traction is not perpendicular to the scalp surface. These forces either separately or together can cause damage to the fetal scalp. The most obvious of the injuries is the formation of the chignon or artificial caput. This is the oedematous, occasionally ecchymotic, area directly beneath the vacuum cup. It is the same as a normal caput succedaneum from spontaneous delivery. Although several observers have considered the artificial caput rather formidable at first sight, all agree upon the striking promptitude with which it disappears. In most babies the caput artificale 'chignon' disappears in a few hours, and what remains is a scalp mark with slight redness. In a few days it subsides, and in most cases when the baby leaves hospital the scalp is without any marks.

If the extraction time is too long and too high a vacuum pressure is used, the scalp membrane may present small ecchymosis, abrasions or tiny ulcers. Aguero et al (1962) commented on the high incidence of scalp lesions by saying that the vacuum extractor is a traumatic instrument, perhaps more so than any other. At the end of their report, however, they comment that 'its use is accompanied by the same risk common to other extraction instruments'. Plauche (1979) surveyed 12 independent studies for abrasions and lacerations. He showed a mean incidence of 12.6% in a total of 3543 cases.

Scalp necrosis followed by scalp scars has also been reported (Nyirjesy 1963, Brey 1962). These lesions can almost be eliminated by limiting extraction time to no more than 30 minutes. Their frequency among various investigators varies between 0.25 and 1.8% (Malmstrom 1965, Chalmers 1969, Plauche 1979).

Retinal haemorrhage

Retinal haemorrhage is a transient and subtle measurement of trauma and has been shown to be increased in Malmstrom vacuum extractor deliveries. Shenker reported 19.2% in spontaneous vaginal deliveries, 31% in forceps deliveries and 52% when the Malmstrom instrument is used (Schenker

1966). Although there is no correlation between retinal haemorrhage and intracerebral haemorrhage, there does appear to be an increase of these lesions with traumatic delivery. Fortunately, retinal haemorrhage has no influence on the subsequent function of the eye. Extraction with the new Silastic device does not increase the incidence of retinal haemorrhage compared with spontaneous vaginal delivery.

Neonatal jaundice

In recent years many investigators have studied the incidence of jaundice in the newborn after vacuum extraction. According to Munsat (1963), the degradation of large volumes of blood in cephalhaematomas may lead to hyperbilirubinaemia. However, he mentions that although the incidence of cephalhaematoma in his series was high (25.7%), he did not find an increased incidence of neonatal jaundice.

Other factors influence neonatal bilirubin levels, so a cause and effect relationship is difficult to establish. Premature neonates with immature hepatic enzymes are more likely to suffer neonatal jaundice. Prolonged labours, use of oxytocin and neonatal asphyxia have all been linked to increased neonatal jaundice.

Mild neonatal jaundice is probably increased after vacuum extraction delivery, but rarely does the serum bilirubin reach levels to cause significant problems for the neonate (Carter & Gudgeon 1987).

Fetal mortality

A comparison of fetal mortality in forceps and vacuum extraction studies most often shows lower mortality in cases delivered by the vacuum extractor. Bergman (1961), in his study of 29 Swedish obstetrical departments, found a perinatal mortality of 5.2% in 983 forceps deliveries and 1.9% in 1617 vacuum extractions. Lange (1964) had corresponding figures of 6.1% in forceps extractions and 3.8% in vacuum extractions.

Plauche (1979) reviewed the perinatal mortality for 8327 vacuum extractions that were reported in 24 papers from 10 countries. The uncorrected perinatal mortality rate was 25.8 per 1000, and when corrected for infants with absent heart sounds prior to delivery and those with anomalies incompatible with life, this fell to 15.5 per 1000 vacuum extractions. 30–40% of the extractions were done for fetal distress and another 20–30% for some other complication of labour.

Long-term effects

Recent reports on follow-up studies of children born by vacuum extraction have shown that this method of delivery appears to have little, if any, adverse effect on neurological, psychomotor, psychological or intellectual development (Bird 1982).

Evelbauer (1956) found all the children in his first vacuum extraction series of 100 cases well developed at the age of 5–6 years. Others have had the same experience (Berggren 1959).

Malmstrom has followed many of the infants delivered by vacuum extraction, year after year, and has found no reason to change his positive attitude toward this instrument (Malmstrom 1965).

Long-term outcome of infants delivered by vacuum extraction has also been analysed in a study by Bjerre & Dahlen (1974). Long-term follow-up of 101 infants delivered with vacuum extraction was carried out. A control group of 120 spontaneously delivered children was used. At 4 years of age, retarded development and/or neurological symptoms were seen in 5.9% of the controls and 5.3% of babies delivered with vacuum extraction. This difference was not statistically significant. They concluded that there should be no reluctance to use vacuum extraction for fear of late sequelae.

CONCLUSION

Over the past 30 years the vacuum extractor has gained wide use throughout Europe, with an associated decrease in perinatal mortality. Certain complications are associated with its use but in general these are minor and transitory. On analysis, most of the serious complications reported in the literature are considered to be due to other associated factors, or to misuse of the vacuum extractor.

The use of the vacuum extractor has not gained wide acceptance in many countries. I believe that the vacuum extractor is a useful addition to the obstetrician's armamentarium. With its ease of application, safety of the instrument and mechanism of 'autorotation' of the malpositioned fetal head, difficult forceps deliveries become easy vacuum extractions.

REFERENCES

Aguero O, Alvarez H 1962 Fetal injury due to the vacuum extractor. Obstetrics and Gynecology 19: 212–217
Ahuza G, Willoughby M, Kerr M, Hutchinson J 1969 Massive subaponeurotic haemorrhage in infants born by vacuum extraction. British Medical Journal 3: 743–745
Altaras M et al 1974 The use of the vacuum extractor in cases of cord prolapse during labour. American Journal of Obstetrics and Gynecology 118: 824–830
Berggren O G A Experience with Malmstrom's vacuum extractor. Clinical study of 100 cases. Acta Obstetricia et Gynecologica Scandinavica 38: 315
Bergman P, Malmstrom T, Schoon I 1961 Value of the vacuum extractor as judged from the use in elderly primipara. Acta Obstetricia et Gynecologica Scandinavica 42: 363–371
Berkus M D, Ramamurthy R S, O'Connor P S et al 1985 A cohort study of silastic obstetrical vacuum cup deliveries: safety of the instrument. Obstetrics and Gynecology 66: 503
Bird G C 1982 The use of the vacuum extractor. Clinical Obstetrics and Gynecology 9: 641–659
Bjerre I, Dahlin K 1974 The long term development of children delivered by vacuum extraction. Developmental Medicine and Child Neurology 16: 378–381
Bourne A W, Williams L H 1962 Recent advances in obstetrics and gynaecology, 10th edn. J and A Churchill London p 236

Brandstrup E, Lange P 1961 Clinical experience with vacuum extractor. Proceedings of the Third World Congress of the International Federation of Obstetricians and Gynaecologists, Vienna, vol 1, p 80

Brat T H 1965 Indications for and results of the use of the 'Ventouse obstetricale'—a ten year study. Journal of Obstetrics and Gynaecology of the British Commonwealth 72: 883–888

Brey J, Holtorff J, Kinzel W H, Schmidt G, Geburtsch V Frauenh 1962 The vacuum extractor. Geburtsch V Frauenheilk 22: 550–556

Broekhuizen F F, Washington J M, Johnson F, Hamilton P R 1987 Vacuum extraction versus forceps delivery: indications and complications, 1979–1984. Obstetrics and Gynecology 69: 338–342

Carter J R, Gudgeon C W 1987 Vacuum extraction and forceps delivery in a district hospital. Australian and New Zealand Journal of Obstetrics and Gynaecology 27: 117–119

Cartwright G W, Culbertson K, Schreiner R L 1979 Changes in clinical presentation of term infants with intracranial haemorrhage. Developmental Medicine and Child Neurology 21: 730

Chalmers J, Fothergill R 1960 Use of the vacuum extractor (ventouse) in obstetrics. British Medical Journal 1: 1684–1689

Chalmers J A 1964 Five years experience with the vacuum extractor. British Medical Journal 1: 1216–1220

Chalmers J A 1965 The vacuum extractor in difficult delivery. Journal of Obstetrics and Gynaecology of the British Commonwealth 72: 889

Chalmers J 1969 Complications of the vacuum extractor. British Medical Journal 4: 109

Chamberlain G 1980 Forceps and vacuum extraction. Clinical Obstetrics and Gynaecology 7: 511–527

Donat J F, Akazaki H, Kleinberg F 1978 Intraventricular haemorrhage in full term and premature infants. Mayo Clinic Proceedings 53: 437

Earn A A 1967 An appraisal of Malmstrom's vacuum-tractor (vacuum extractor). American Journal of Obstetrics and Gynecology 99: 732–743

Evelbauer K 1956 Vacuum extraction in obstetrics. Geburtsh V Frauenheilk 16: 223–227

Evelbauer K 1963 Side effect of the vacuum extractor. Archives of Gynecology 198: 523–529

Fahmy K 1971 Cephalohaematomata following vacuum extraction. Journal of Obstetrics and Gynaecology of the British Commonwealth 78: 369–372

Hammerstein J, Gromotke R 1962 Review of vacuum extractions. J Internat Coll Surg 37: 458

Hastie S J, MacLean A B 1986 Comparison of the use of the silastic obstetric vacuum extractor to Kiellands Forceps. Asia-Oceania Journal of Obstetrics and Gynaecology 12: 63–68

Holland E 1922 Cranial stress in the fetus during labour. Journal of Obstetrics and Gynaecology of the British Empire 29: 549

Kappy K A 1981 Vacuum extractor. Clinics in Perinatology 8: 79–86

Karpathy L 1965 Effects of Malmstrom's vacuum extractor. Gynecology 87: 501–509

Katz Z, Lancet M et al 1982 The beneficial effect of vacuum extraction on the fetus. Acta Obstetricia et Gynecologica Scandinavica 61: 337–340

Lancet M 1963 Use of the vacuum extractor. British Medical Journal 1: 165–169

Lange P 1964 The vacuum extractor ii. Value in relation to forceps and range of indications. Acta Obstetricia et Gynecologica Scandinavica 43: 53–56

Lillie E W 1960 The vacuum extractor. British Medical Journal 2: 602

Livnat E J, Felgin M, Scommegno A et al 1978 Neonatal acid base balance in spontaneous and instrumental vaginal deliveries. Obstetrics and Gynecology 52: 549–551

Malmstrom T, Janson I 1965 Use of the vacuum extractor. Clinical Obstetrics and Gynecology 8: 893–918

Maryniak G M, Frank J B 1984 Clinical assessment of the Kobayashi vacuum extraction. Obstetrics and Gynecology 64: 431

Matheson G W, Davajan V, Mishell D R 1968 The use of the vacuum extractor: a reappraisal. Acta Obstetricia et Gynecologica Scandinavica 47(2): 155–165

Mishell D, Kelly J V 1962 The obstetrical forceps and the vacuum extractor: an assessment of their compressive force. Obstetrics and Gynecology 19: 204–206

Munsat T L, Meerhout R, Nyirjesy I 1963 A comparative study of the vacuum extractor and forceps. Part ii. Evaluation of the newborn. American Journal of Obstetrics and Gynecology 85: 1083–1090

Ngan H Y S, Tang G W K, Ma H K 1986 Vacuum extractor: a safe instrument? Australian and New Zealand Journal of Obstetrics and Gynaecology 26: 177–181

Nyirjesy I, Hawks B L, Falls H C 1963 A comparative clinical study of the vacuum extractor and forceps—part 1 preliminary observations. American Journal of Obstetrics and Gynecology 85: 1071–1082

O'Neil A G B, Skull E, Michael C 1981 A new method of traction for the vacuum cup. Australian and New Zealand Journal of Obstetrics and Gynaecology 21: 24–25

Ott W J 1975 Vacuum extraction. Obstetrical and Gynecological Survey 30: 643–649

Paul R, Staisen K, Pine S 1973 The new vacuum extractor. Obstetrics and Gynecology 41: 800–802

Pauly J, Bepko F, Olson H 1963 Southern Medical Journal 56: 1219

Pelosi M A, Apuzzio J 1984 Use of the soft silicone obstetric vacuum cup for delivery of the fetal head at Caesarean section. Journal of Reproductive Medicine 79: 289

Phillpott H. Personal communication with editor

Plauche W C 1978 Vacuum extraction—use in a community hospital setting. Obstetrics and Gynecology 52: 289–293

Plauche W C 1979 Fetal cranial injuries related to delivery with the Malmstrom vacuum extractor. Obstetrics and Gynecology 53: 750–757

Roseman G 1969 Vacuum extraction of premature infants. South African Journal of Obstetrics and Gynecology 7: 10–12

Roszkowski I, Borkowski R, Kretowicz J 1963 Use of the vacuum extractor in fetal distress. American Journal of Obstetrics and Gynecology 87: 253–257

Rydberg E 1954 The mechanism of labour. Charles G Thomas, Springfield, Illinois

Schenker J B, Gombos G M 1966 Retinal lesions with vacuum extraction. Obstetrics and Gynecology 27: 521

Schenker J G, Serr D M 1967 Comparative study of delivery by vacuum extractor and forceps. American Journal of Obstetrics and Gynecology 98: 32–39

Sjostedt J E 1967 The vacuum extractor and forceps in obstetrics. A clinical study. Acta Obstetricia Gynecologica Scandinavica 46: 1–208

Tricomi V, Amorosi L, Gottschalk W 1961 A preliminary report on the use of Malmstrom's vacuum extractor. American Journal of Obstetrics and Gynecology 81: 681–687

Wider J A, Erez S, Steer C M 1967 An evaluation of the vacuum extractor in a series of 201 cases. American Journal of Obstetrics and Gynecology 98: 24–31

9. Appropriate technology in intrapartum fetal surveillance

S. Arulkumaran   I. Ingemarsson

INTRODUCTION

Intermittent auscultation of the fetal heart rate (FHR) and continuous electronic fetal heart rate monitoring (EFM) are the most popular methods of intrapartum fetal surveillance. Traditional teaching is that in the first stage of labour, auscultation every 15 minutes for a period of 1 minute immediately after a contraction, and auscultation after each contraction in the second stage may identify fetuses at risk. During auscultation the basal heart rate can be estimated; other qualities of the FHR such as baseline variability, accelerations and decelerations which better reflect fetal health are difficult to quantify. EFM has become popular because of the possible on-line documentation, easy application of the equipment, accuracy of picking up the fetal heart-rate signal and because of the additional information obtained about the FHR and uterine contractions. The development of technology which has reduced the cost of the equipment together with a shortage of experienced trained midwives has made continuous EFM a norm in many labour wards in western countries.

CONTROVERSY ABOUT EFM IN LABOUR

Despite its popularity controversy exists concerning the appropriate use of EFM. Randomized trials which showed no reduction in perinatal mortality and increased Caesarean section (CS) rate for fetal distress (Kelso et al 1978, Haverkamp et al 1979, Parsons et al 1981) lacked the numbers to derive meaningful conclusions. Two recent studies addressed the problem of EFM by recruiting adequate numbers. McDonald et al (1985) randomly allocated 13 000 patients to EFM or intermittent auscultation. There was no significant difference in perinatal mortality or long-term morbidity but the Caesarean section rate was marginally higher in those monitored electronically. Babies with neonatal seizures were significantly more common in those labours which lasted more than 5 hours and was 8.5% in the auscultation group compared with 2.4% in the electronically monitored group. Follow-up studies on these babies have shown no difference in terms of morbidity between the two groups.

The results of this study must be interpreted with caution. Only one-third (28/84) of the intrapartum and neonatal deaths during the study period were subjects of the clinical trial. The 56 deaths excluded were for rapid labour (10), gestation < 29 weeks (37) and meconium or absence of liquor (9). Only 80.7% in the EFM group were actually monitored in the first stage of labour and of these 11.0% had non-interpretable traces. Furthermore, those with thick meconium-stained liquor were monitored electronically and 2.3% of the women in the stethoscopic auscultation group were transferred to the EFM group due to abnormal stethoscopic findings. So in effect, the study compares intermittent auscultation with EFM in a low to moderate risk group where a little more than 70% of the women were monitored with acceptable tracings. This leaves us to conclude that although EFM is under scrutiny for routine use it is preferred in the high risk population. This is further strengthened by a recent study (Leveno et al 1986) involving 35 000 pregnancies comparing selective monitoring to universal monitoring. Universal monitoring was associated with a small but significant rise in Caesarean section for fetal distress but there was no difference in the perinatal mortality or morbidity between the two groups and the study recommended selective monitoring.

Despite such studies continuous EFM is practised as a routine in many labour wards because antenatal risk classification into high- and low-risk to select those who need monitoring is often considered insufficient to predict fetal compromise appearing in labour (Ingemarsson 1981). In addition, there is a tendency in the medical profession to use technology because it is available and not because it is necessary. This has aroused concern in consumer groups about the medicalization of child birth and has resulted in some women rejecting hospital confinement in favour of home confinement. In order to move away from this technological imperative and to use the technology of EFM appropriately, we should develop a reliable method of identifying those at risk. An admission test may be of value for this purpose.

Cases of litigation due to misinterpretation of the FHR trace or due to inadequate or inappropriate action taken in the presence of suspicious or abnormal FHR trace are becoming frequent. Fetal blood sampling (FBS) may help in some cases but facilities are not available in all institutions. In centres where facilities are available, over-enthusiasm and over-emphasis on performing FBS whilst ignoring the clinical picture has led to unnecessary fetal morbidity. The appropriate use of FBS, its misuse and possible alternatives should be considered.

ADMISSION TEST—A USEFUL TOOL TO SELECT PATIENTS FOR EFM?

Fetal morbidity and mortality occurs as a consequence of labour even in those categorized as low-risk based on various risk classifications (Hobel et

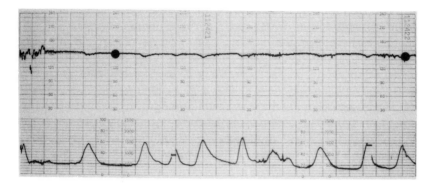

Fig. 9.1 Admission test FHR trace demonstrating the baseline rate, reduced baseline variability, absence of accelerations and some decelerations. Auscultation findings indicated by the dots reveal only the baseline FHR.

al 1973). A better way to screen patients admitted in labour would be to assess the ability of the fetus to withstand the functional stress of uterine contractions of early labour. A short recording of the FHR immediately after admission—the admission test (AT)—might select those fetuses with hypoxia present on admission or those who are likely to become hypoxic in the next few hours of labour (Fig. 9.1).

Results of a recent study (Ingemarsson et al 1986) which evaluated the admission test are given in Table 9.1. A *reactive* or *normal FHR trace* refers to a recording with normal baseline rate and variability, two accelerations of 15 beats above the baseline rate for 15 seconds, and no decelerations. A *suspicious* or *equivocal trace* refers to a trace with no FHR accelerations in addition to one abnormal feature such as reduced baseline variability (< 5 beats), presence of decelerations, baseline tachycardia or bradycardia. An *ominous trace* refers to more than one abnormal feature or repeated ominous variable or late decelerations. To evaluate the outcome, fetal distress was considered to be present when ominous FHR changes led to CS or forceps delivery or if the newborn had an Apgar score < 7 at 5 minutes after spontaneous delivery.

Table 9.1 Results of AT in relation to the incidence of fetal distress

Admission test		Fetal distress*
Reactive	$n = 982$ (94.3%)	13 (1.4%)
Equivocal	$n = 49$ (4.7%)	5 (10.0%)
Ominous	$n = 10$ (1.0%)	4 (40.0%)

*Fetal distress refers to those who had Caesarean section or forceps delivery for that indication or had a 5 minute Apgar score of less than 7 after normal delivery.

In those with ominous ATs, 4 out of 10 (40%) developed fetal distress compared with 13 out of 982 (1.4%) in those with a reactive AT. Closer scrutiny revealed that of the 13 who developed fetal distress after a reactive AT, 10 did so more than 5 hours after the AT. Of the other 3, one had cord prolapse and two fetuses at 35 weeks gestation showed signs of distress at birth 3 and 4 hours after the AT. This suggests that, excepting acute events, AT may be a good predictor of fetal condition during the next few hours in term fetuses. If labour continues beyond this period an electronic recording of the FHR for 20–30 minutes every 2–3 hours and complementary intermittent auscultation may help to pick up FHR changes suggestive of fetal compromise.

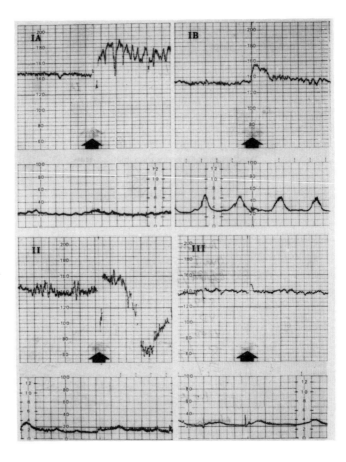

Fig. 9.2 Various responses to sound stimulation. Types Ia and Ib are normal and types II and III are abnormal. (With permission of the *American Journal of Obstetrics & Gynecology.*)

FETAL ACOUSTIC STIMULATION TEST (FAST) AND THE AT

The accuracy of the AT can be further enhanced and the number of suspicious traces reduced by using fetal acoustic stimulation test (FAST) at the time of the AT (Ingemarsson et al 1988). After a 15–20 minute AT we performed an acoustic stimulation test in all patients regardless of the outcome of the AT, and the FHR was recorded for another 5 minutes. A model 5C electronic artificial larynx (Western Electric, New York, NY) was applied to the maternal abdomen in the region of the fetal head and stimulus applied for 5 seconds. Sound pressure levels measured at 1 m in air averaged 82 dB and spectral analysis revealed a fundamental frequency of approximately 80 Hz and harmonics ranged from 20–9000 Hz.

Four different patterns of FHR response were observed (Fig. 9.2):
1. Type IA —a prolonged period of acceleration(s) > 15 beats lasting > 3 minutes.
2. Type IB —one acceleration lasting > 1 minute or two accelerations > 15 seconds each.
3. Type II —a biphasic response with accelerations followed by deceleration > 60 beats lasting > 60 seconds.
4. Type III —no acceleration or acceleration < 15 beats from baseline rate.

The prevalence of fetal distress in relation to the outcome of AT and FAST is given in Table 9.2. Based on these results one could conclude that those with a suspicious or an abnormal AT and FAST are at high risk of fetal distress compared with a low risk when both tests were normal. Thus AT in combination with FAST may be helpful in selecting those who would benefit by continuous monitoring.

USE OF FETAL SCALP BLOOD SAMPLING IN LABOUR

Difficulties are often encountered in interpreting FHR changes. Decelerations of the FHR are described as early, variable and late. Variable decelerations can be categorized as uncomplicated or complicated. The chance of acidosis is greater in the presence of repeated variable

Table 9.2 Incidence of fetal distress in relation to outcome of AT and FAST

AT (n = 766)	Normal		Suspicious and Abnormal	
	708		58	
FAST	Normal	Abnormal	Normal	Abnormal
Fetal distress	694 12(1.7%)	14 2(14.2%)	49 3(6.1%)	9 5(55.6%)

decelerations > 60 beats, lasts > 60 seconds, a late deceleration component, delayed recovery, rebound tachycardia or absence of variability between decelerations. Each of these descriptions can encompass different degrees of such changes, can overlap one another and it may be difficult to classify a given FHR tracing into a category of a described pattern. However, based on all the features of the trace, in most instances it is possible to classify them as suspicious or ominous requiring either observation or action which may be delivery or fetal scalp blood sampling (FBS). Differentiation of how ominous a trace may be difficult and opinion may differ between individuals. The clinical picture of the patient (age, parity, past obstetric history, intrauterine growth retardation, prolonged pregnancy, presence of meconium, stage and rate of progress of labour) should be taken into account when deciding on the action to be taken.

FHR changes of some form can be seen in 60% of all cases in an unselected population indicating that these changes are not specific to hypoxia (Ingemarsson et al 1980) and even if most of these changes were innocuous, they can cause anxiety. The risk of fetal acidosis is small when the trace is reactive (Beard et al 1971, Ingemarsson 1981). Alternatively, fetal acidosis is not a consistent finding when ominous FHR changes are seen (Beard et al 1971, Zalor & Quilligan 1979, Katz et al 1981). Understanding these difficulties, the National Institutes of Health in the USA considered EFM as a screening method to detect fetal hypoxia in labour and stressed the need for additional tests (which is usually a FBS) to confirm the fetal condition.

FBS for pH determination has been shown to be of value in selected cases when problems in interpretation of the FHR trace are encountered (Ingemarsson 1981, Katz et al 1981, Arulkumaran et al 1983). However, facilities and expertise are not widely available for performing FBS (Gillmer & Combe 1979) and alternatives to FBS are being studied.

There is also a move to de-emphasize the role of FBS in labour (Clarke & Paul 1985) because there is evidence to suggest that when properly interpreted, assessment of FHR patterns is in most cases equal to pH by FBS in the prediction of fetal outcome (Parer 1982). FHR assessment is superior to FBS in the prediction of a non-compromised fetus; the accuracy of prediction of infants with Apgar score > 7 is 99% with reactive FHR patterns (Schifrin & Dame 1972) compared with an 85–90% prediction with a scalp blood pH > 7.20 (Beard et al 1967, Bowe et al 1979, Tejani et al 1976). However, FHR pattern is poor in predicting a compromised fetus. When the FHR pattern is ominous only 50–65% of the newborns are depressed as judged by the Apgar score (Tejani et al 1976, Clark et al 1984) i.e. a 35–50% false prediction. The false prediction by a scalp blood pH < 7.20 is only 10–20% (Wood et al 1967, Tejani et al 1976). Contrary to these findings a series from UK reported that 73% of infants with cord

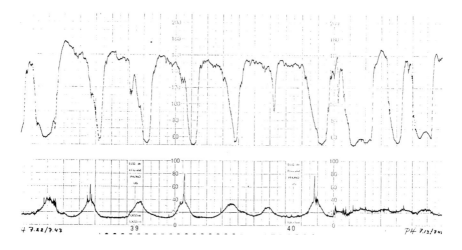

Fig. 9.3   An ominous FHR tracing where immediate delivery is better than performing a
FBS because of the possible rapid decline in pH.

arterial blood pH < 7.10 had a 1 minute Apgar score of > 7 and 86% had a
5 minute Apgar score > 7 (Sykes et al 1982). Such findings are usually due
to accumulation of carbon dioxide and its influence on the pH. Respiratory
acidosis is poorly correlated with fetal or neonatal condition.

Transitory low pH values of respiratory type with high Pco_2 and bi-
carbonate are not uncommon in low-risk labours (Ingemarsson &
Arulkumaran 1986). A pH value of 7.20 of respiratory type might revert to
7.27, 20 minutes later and hence the need to assess full acid base balance.
Alternatively, a normal pH value might rapidly deteriorate when an
ominous late or variable decelerations concomitant with silent pattern and
tachycardia are seen on the FHR trace (Fig. 9.3). Often a single pH value
may be misinterpreted. The pH value is an approximation even if correctly
sampled and analysed. The equipment for pH analysis may have a range of
error of 0.04. A value of 7.22 might be acidotic (7.18) or normal (7.26).
Useful information about fetal acid base balance in labour has been
presented by Willcourt (1989) in the previous volume of this series.

FHR CHANGES AND FETAL ACIDOSIS

Despite the shortcomings, acid base measurement plays an important role
because more than one pathophysiological mechanism gives rise to a
particular abnormal FHR pattern (Ingemarsson et al 1980), and because
fetal acidosis develops at various time intervals from the onset of a
suspicious or abnormal trace depending on the 'physiological reserve' of the
fetus and the type of abnormal FHR pattern observed (Fleischer et al 1982).

Pre-term, post-term, growth-retarded or fetuses with oligohydramnios or thick meconium-stained liquor are particularly at high risk of developing fetal acidosis early.

Baseline FHR variability and reactivity (spontaneous or provoked) give some indication of the physiological reserve of the fetus. If normal FHR variability was observed in the last 20 minutes prior to delivery the fetuses were found to be in a better condition at birth regardless of other features in the FHR trace (Paul et al 1975). Fetuses with loss of baseline variability were more prone to acidosis if there was tachycardia or late decelerations (Beard et al 1971, Schifrin & Dame 1972). Krebs et al (1979) considered those with normal baseline variability to be compensated and to have some reserve despite other abnormal features.

Some idea of the 'physiological reserve' of the fetus should help in managing patients with abnormal but transient changes in FHR patterns in the form of prolonged bradycardia of less than 80 beats/min for more than 2 minutes or less than 100 beats/min for more than 3 minutes. These are not uncommon findings in any labour ward. In the majority of cases signs of spontaneous recovery can be expected within 5–10 minutes if the episode is preceded by a reassuring trace. A bolus injection of a beta receptor agonist (e.g. terbutaline 0.25 mg IV) for relaxation of uterus may be helpful when excessive uterine activity due to oxytocin overstimulation is causing the prolonged bradycardia (Ingemarsson et al 1985). Other common causes are maternal hypotension after epidural block or fetal vagal response to vaginal examination. Cord prolapse, abruptio placentae and scar dehiscence should be ruled out as possible causes of prolonged bradycardia. When intrauterine growth retardation, prematurity, prolonged pregnancy with thick meconium-stained liquor or an abnormal FHR pattern prior to the episode

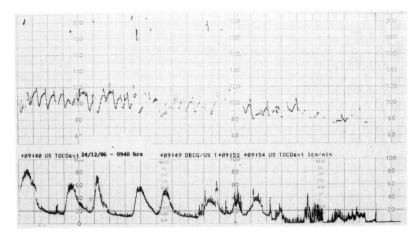

Fig. 9.4   FHR trace showing terminal bradycardia.

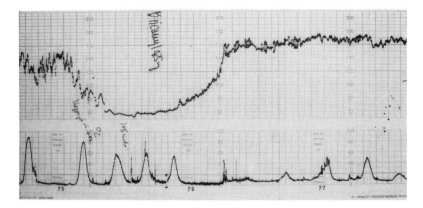

Fig. 9.5   A case with prolonged fetal bradycardia showing recovery. Terbutaline 0.25 mg IV abolishes uterine contractions for 7 to 25 minutes.

of bradycardia are part of the scenario, the option of early delivery should be considered to pre-empt terminal bradycardia (Fig. 9.4). Absence of baseline variability over 4 minutes during the episode of bradycardia may be suggestive of diminished physiological reserve as these fetuses have low scalp blood pH (Ingemarsson et al 1985). During the episode of bradycardia there is reduction in fetal perfusion, essential blood flow being maintained. Reduced perfusion leads to anaerobic metabolism as well as less clearance of CO_2. Hence the results of an FBS at the time of bradycardia or soon after the event often show a low pH. The return of FHR to normal values re-establishes normal perfusion and the acidosis is spontaneously corrected by a fetus with good physiological reserve (Figs 9.5 and 9.6).

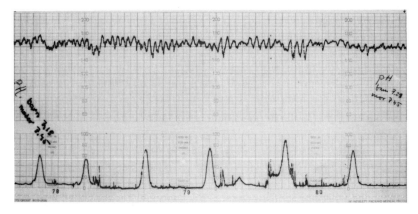

Fig. 9.6   Low scalp blood pH soon after the bradycardia and normal scalp blood pH value in the same fetus 40 minutes later.

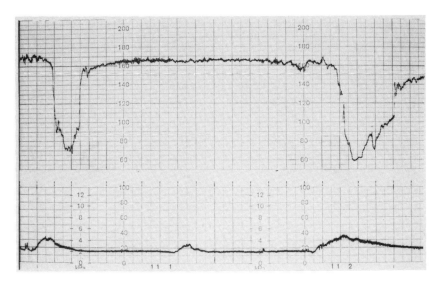

Fig. 9.7   FHR trace (tachycardia, absence of accelerations, reduced baseline variability and ominous declerations) at 3 cm dilatation with infrequent contractions and thick meconium-stained liquor in a patient at 41 weeks.

WHEN NOT TO PERFORM FETAL BLOOD SAMPLING

FHR changes may be iatrogenic and may follow administration of epidural anaesthesia, sedation or analgesia, hyperstimulation with oxytocics, dehydration by restriction of fluids or maternal postural changes causing supine hypotension. These can be corrected by taking appropriate action. After having excluded such causes and those due to head compression in the late first stage of labour, FBS is the rational choice to exclude fetal acidosis if the abnormal FHR patterns persist, especially when there is loss of reactivity and baseline variability. The clinical picture should be always considered before embarking on FBS. Often there is failure to progress, in addition to a suspicious or an abnormal trace for some hours. Such a patient may need long hours of labour and oxytocics to achieve vaginal delivery which is likely to worsen the condition of the fetus. In such situations it is better to deliver the fetus than to waste time with FBS. Similar situations where it might be better to deliver the fetus than to perform an FBS are summarized below:

1. When the clinical picture demands early delivery (Fig. 9.7);
2. When an ominous FHR trace prompts immediate delivery (Figs 9.3 and 9.4);
3. When the FHR trace is reassuring (Fig. 9.8);
4. When the changes are due to oxytocic overstimulation;
5. When there is associated failure to progress in labour;

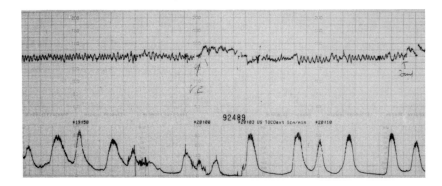

Fig. 9.8 Sinusoidal-like pattern but the presence of spontaneous or provoked FHR accelerations reassures fetal health.

6. During or soon after an episode of prolonged bradycardia (Figs 9.5 and 9.6);
7. If spontaneous vaginal delivery is imminent or easy instrumental vaginal delivery is possible.

Often one FBS may not be adequate, as the FHR changes might persist or may become more ominous. When a declining trend in pH is observed, and certainly when the pH falls into the acidotic range, it may be wise to opt for operative delivery unless spontaneous delivery is imminent. A sense of security after one FBS and failure to repeat the procedure within 30 minutes, allowing labour despite abnormal FHR pattern, and poor progress are common problems that have led to fetal morbidity and litigation.

ALTERNATIVES TO FETAL SCALP BLOOD SAMPLING

It may not be possible to perform an FBS at times because the cervix may not be dilated sufficiently or the head might be too high to obtain a satisfactory sample. In these situations a painful stimulus to the fetal scalp or vibroacoustic stimulation of the fetus may be an alternative (Clarke et al 1984, Arulkumaran et al 1987, Edersheim et al 1987). FHR accelerations to these stimuli have been uniformly associated with non-acidotic scalp blood pH values. Although promising, and many reports have appeared supporting this concept, it is difficult to understand how an arbitrary cut-off point of pH 7.20 and above invariably should be associated with FHR accelerations. In a recent study (Ingemarsson & Arulkumaran 1989) it was observed that although the presence of accelerations was strongly associated with a normal pH, two fetuses with low scalp blood pH (7.16 and 7.18) demonstrated a reactive response (Fig. 9.9). They responded with acceleration at the time of scalp blood sampling as well and were found to have respiratory acidosis. It is also notable that nearly 50% of those who

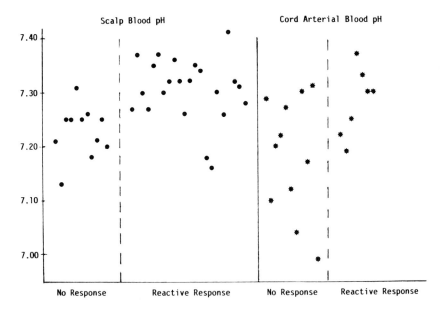

Fig. 9.9 Scalp blood and cord arterial blood pH values in relation to reactive or nonreactive responses to vibroacostic stimulation. (With permission from the *British Journal of Obstetrics & Gynaecology*.)

did not react with accelerations were found to have non-acidotic pH values.

Due consideration has to be given to fetal behavioural states prior to the action of FBS or manoeuvres such as vibroacoustic stimulation. Periods of non-reactive FHR pattern with reduced baseline variability up to periods of 25–40 minutes alternate with reactive periods in labour (Spencer & Johnson 1986). Failure to recognize this by inspecting the preceding trace results in unnecessary interference. At times, this period may last longer, especially after the administration of analgesic drugs.

CONCLUSION

The routine use of technology does not appeal to the consumer or to the scientific world. Selective EFM with an AT, followed by intermittent electronic monitoring every 2–3 hours and auscultation in between, may be adequate and appropriate in low-risk pregnancies. High-risk pregnancies would benefit by continuous EFM.

Determination of fetal scalp blood pH is helpful in assessing the fetal well-being in a few percent of all labours when interpretation of the FHR trace causes problems. However, the value of a single pH is limited and the type of acidosis will not be established unless a full acid base status is obtained. Imprudent use of the method may in fact delay delivery and must be avoided. Stimulation of the fetus may in selected cases replace sampling of fetal scalp blood. The time spent on learning the proper interpretation of

FHR patterns compared with time spent on learning other subjects in obstetrics is disproportionate in our training programmes. Until reliable alternative methods of fetal surveillance in labour become available, obstetricians in training should have weekly meetings reviewing the FHR traces of interest and educational courses in EFM.

REFERENCES

Arulkumaran S, Gibb D M F, Ratnam S S 1983 Experience with a selective intrapartum fetal monitoring policy. Singapore Journal of Obstetrics and Gynaecology 14: 47–51
Arulkumaran S, Ingemarsson I, Ratnam S S 1987 Fetal heart rate response to scalp stimulation as a test of fetal well-being in labour. Asia Oceania Journal of Obstetrics and Gynaecology 13: 131–135
Beard R W, Morris E D, Clayton S G 1967 pH of fetal capillary blood as an indicator of the condition of the fetus. Journal of Obstetrics and Gynaecology of the British Commonwealth 74: 812–817
Beard R W, Filshie G M, Knight C A, Roberts G M 1971 The significance of the changes in the continuous fetal heart rate in the first stage of labour. Journal of Obstetrics and Gynaecology of the British Commonwealth 78: 865–881
Bowe E T, Beard R W, Finster M, et al 1979 Reliability of fetal blood sampling. American Journal of Obstetrics and Gynecology 133: 762–768
Clarke S L, Gimovsky M L, Miller F C 1984 The scalp stimulation test: a clinical alternative to fetal scalp blood sampling. American Journal of Obstetrics and Gynecology 148: 274–277
Clarke S L, Paul R H 1985 Intrapartum fetal surveillance: the role of fetal scalp blood sampling. American Journal of Obstetrics and Gynecology 153: 717–720
Edersheim T G, Hutson J M, Druzin M L, Kogut E A 1987 Fetal heart rate response to vibratory acoustic stimulation predicts fetal pH in labor. American Journal of Obstetrics and Gynecology 157: 1557–1560
Fleischer A, Schulman H, Jagani N, Mitchell J, Randolph G 1982 The development of fetal acidosis in the presence of an abnormal fetal heart rate tracing. I. The average for gestational age fetus. American Journal of Obstetrics and Gynecology 144: 55–60
Gillmer M D G, Combe D 1979 Intrapartum fetal monitoring practice in the United Kingdom. British Journal of Obstetrics and Gynaecology 86: 753–758
Haverkamp A D, Orlean M, Langerdoerfer S, et al 1979 A controlled trial of the differential effects of intrapartum fetal monitoring. American Journal of Obstetrics and Gynecology 134: 399–408
Hobel C J, Hyvarinen M A, Okada D M, Oh W 1973 Prenatal and intrapartum high-risk screening. I. Prediction of the high-risk neonate. American Journal of Obstetrics and Gynecology 117: 1–9
Ingemarsson E 1981 Routine electronic fetal monitoring during labor. Acta Obstetrica Gynaecologica Scandinavica (suppl) 99: 1–29
Ingemarsson E, Ingemarsson I, Solum T, Westgren M 1980 A one-year study of routine fetal heart rate monitoring during the first stage of labour. Acta Obstetrica Gynecologica Scandinavica 59: 297–300
Ingemarsson E, Ingemarsson I, Solum T, Westgren M 1980 Influence of occiput posterior position on the fetal heart rate pattern. Obstetrics and Gynecology 155: 301–305
Ingemarsson I, Arulkumaran S, Ratnam S S 1985 Bolus injection of terbutaline in term labour. 1. Effect on fetal pH in cases with prolonged bradycardia. American Journal of Obstetrics and Gynecology 153: 859–865
Ingemarsson I, Arulkumaran S 1986 Fetal acid-base balance in low-risk patients in labour. American Journal of Obstetrics and Gynecology 155: 66–69
Ingemarsson I, Arulkumaran S 1989 Reactive FHR response to sound stimulation in fetuses with low scalp blood pH. British Journal of Obstetrics and Gynaecology 96: 562–565
Ingemarsson I, Arulkumaran S, Ingemarsson E, Tambyraja R L, Ratnam S S 1986 Admission test: a screening test for fetal distress in labour. Obstetrics and Gynecology 68: 800–806

Ingemarsson I, Arulkumaran S, Paul R H, Ingemarsson E, Tambyraja R L, Ratnam S S 1988
Fetal acoustic stimulation in early labour in patients screened with the admission test.
American Journal of Obstetrics and Gynecology 158: 70–74

Katz M, Mazor M, Insler V 1981 Fetal heart rate patterns and scalp pH as predictors of fetal
distress. Israel Journal of Medical Sciences 17: 260–265

Kelso J, Parsons R, Lawrence G F, Arora S S, Edmonds D K, Cooke I D 1978 An
assessment of continuous fetal heart rate monitoring in labour—a randomized trial.
American Journal of Obstetrics and Gynecology 131: 526–532

Krebs H B, Petres R E, Dunn L J, Jordann H V F, Segreti A 1979 Intrapartum fetal heart
rate monitoring. I. Classification and progress of fetal heart rate patterns. American
Journal of Obstetrics and Gynecology 133: 762–772

Leveno K J, Cunningham F G, Nelson S et al 1986 A prospective comparison of selective and
universal electronic fetal monitoring in 34,995 pregnancies. New England Journal of
Medicine 315: 615–619

MacDonald D, Grant A, Sheridan-Pereira M, Boylan P, Chalmers I 1985 The Dublin
randomised controlled trial of intrapartum fetal heart rate monitoring. American Journal of
Obstetrics and Gynecology 152: 524–539

Parer J T 1982 In defense of FHR monitoring's specificity. Contemporary Obstetrics and
Gynecology 19: 228–234

Parsons R J, Brown V A, Cooke I D 1981 Second thoughts on routine monitoring in labour.
In: Studd J W W (ed) Progress in Obstetrics and Gynaecology vol I. Churchill
Livingstone, London, pp 139–150

Paul R H, Suidan A K, Yeh S-Y, Schifrin B S, Hon E H 1975 Clinical fetal monitoring. VII.
The evaluation and significance of intrapartum baseline variability. American Journal of
Obstetrics and Gynecology 123: 206–210

Schifrin B S, Dame L 1972 Fetal heart rate patterns: prediction of Apgar score. Journal of the
American Medical Association 219: 1322–1325

Sykes G S, Johnson P, Ashworth F, et al 1982 Do Apgar scores indicate asphyxia? Lancet i:
494–496

Spencer J A D, Johnson P 1986 Fetal heart rate variability changes and fetal behavioural
cycles during labour. British Journal of Obstetrics and Gynaecology 93: 314–321

Tejani N, Mann L I, Bhakthavathsalan A, Weiss R R 1975 Correlation of fetal heart rate
uterine contraction patterns and fetal scalp blood pH. Obstetrics and Gynecology 46:
392–396

Tejani N, Mann L I, Bhakthavathsalan A 1976 Correlation of fetal heart rate patterns and
fetal pH with neonatal outcome. Obstetrics and Gynecology 48: 460–463

Willcourt R J 1989 Fetal blood gases and pH: current application. In: Studd J W W (ed)
Progress in Obstetrics and Gynaecology vol 7. Churchill Livingstone, London, pp 155–174

Wood C, Ferguson R, Leeton J et al 1967 Fetal heart rate and acid base status in the
assessment of fetal hypoxia. American Journal of Obstetrics and Gynecology 98: 62–68

Zalor R W, Quilligan E J 1979 The influence of scalp sampling on the Caesarean section rate
for fetal distress. American Journal of Obstetrics and Gynecology 135: 239–246

10. Early amniocentesis

James C. Dornan   David Sim

The basis of all medicine is the search for, and the securing of, a diagnosis. The duty of all those workers associated with the prenatal diagnosis area is to use methods which are reliable, safe and as non-invasive as possible. These should provide timely information which will allow appropriate counselling so that the best management possible can be planned for the fetus and its parents. The whole concept of prenatal diagnosis must not be seen as one of 'search and destroy', but rather to 'search carefully and counsel wisely'.

Improvements in ultrasound technology mean that the vast majority of fetal *structural* anomalies may now be observed antenatally. This assessment must be carried out at the correct time and by appropriately trained personnel looking for the right markers with the best machines.

Most *chromosomal* abnormalities are detected antenatally because of a planned action by those involved in the care of the pregnancy. The mother may have attended the genetic clinic because she is in a 'high risk' group, i.e. raised maternal age, relevant past obstetric or family history, or an antenatally detected structural anomaly may have triggered a search for a genetic cause.

Prenatal diagnosis of genetic anomalies will require one of three invasive procedures:

1. Amniocentesis
2. Chorionic villus sampling (CVS)
3. Cordocentesis

In each case the aim is to obtain fetal cells which can be cultured and karyotyped in order to diagnose chromosomal, metabolic and blood disorders of the fetus.

Needles were first intentionally inserted into the uterus nearly 60 years ago (Menees et al 1930) with the purpose of injecting dye and thus diagnosing fetal structural anomalies and the placental site. In the past two decades, amniocentesis (the removal of liquor from the amniotic cavity) has played a major role in prenatal diagnosis of chromosomal and other birth defects.

Advantages of various methods

Amniocentesis

The procedure is traditionally carried out between 15 and 16 weeks gestation, liquor invariably being obtained at this time. Ideally the procedure should be carried out under ultrasonic control but this is not absolutely necessary and the level of expertise required is lower than that needed for the other two procedures. Fetal cells are invariably cultured from the liquor, and unless maternal cell contamination has occurred, which is uncommon, the result should produce no false positives or false negatives. The integrity of the feto placental unit is not intentionally insulted. There is a low abortion rate associated with the procedure and post-procedure vaginal loss is rare. The results obtained allow termination of pregnancy well before the 28th week which is, at the present time, the legally held gestation of viability.

Chorionic villus sampling

Using this method, mesenchymal cells of the chorionic villi are obtained for chromosomal and DNA analysis by inserting a needle, under ultrasonic control, into the placenta along the chorionic plate and aspirating villi. Nowadays the transabdominal approach is generally preferred to the transcervical approach because of the reduced risk of introducing infection (Lilford 1985). The advantages of the technique are that the procedure can be carried out in early pregnancy from the ninth menstrual week onwards and the amniotic cavity is left intact. Direct cytotrophoblastic preparation allows a diagnosis to be obtained 24 hours after the procedure and so termination of the pregnancy, if desired, may be carried out as a one-stage procedure under anaesthetic.

Cordocentesis

Under ultrasound control a needle is passed into the umbilical artery or vein where the cord is inserted into the placental chorionic plate. A transplacental route is used when the placenta is anterior and a transamniotic route when posterior. This technique has the main advantage that it can be used in pregnancy after 18 weeks gestation to produce fetal cells which can be karyotyped within 24 hours, and therefore offer a swift diagnosis. This is of special use when a major obstetrical complication is diagnosed late in pregnancy, e.g. intrauterine fetal growth retardation with oligohydramnios, when a genetic cause is strongly suspected and confirmation is likely to alter obstetric management. The sample obtained may also be used in the diagnosis of blood disorders such as haemoglobinopathies, immuno deficiencies, viral infections and metabolic disorders, or when the fetal acid base status is desired.

Disadvantage of various methods

Amniocentesis

Traditionally amniocentesis was not performed until the 16th week as there were thought to be insufficient viable fetal cells, insufficient amniotic fluid and a higher fetal loss rate if the procedure was carried out prior to this gestation (Crane 1983). Results of culture, however, are not obtained until three or four weeks after the procedure and the pregnancy will then be around the 19th week. Quickening will have been experienced by the mother and the fetus is beginning to enter the realms of 'viability'. In Britain there have been recent attempts to make termination of pregnancy after 18 weeks' gestation illegal. As yet these efforts have been unsuccessful, but it is likely in the future that the present limit of 28 weeks' gestation will be reduced, perhaps to 22 or 24 weeks.

A late diagnosis of chromosomal abnormality necessitating termination may involve the mother going through a lengthy process which is not only potentially dangerous and painful, but may be associated with severe emotional problems.

In their review of amniocenteses, Ager and Oliver (1986) showed an overall fetal loss rate of 2.1%. Most centres attribute only one-quarter of this figure to the procedure of amniocentesis, although many units, including our own in Belfast, would quote a rate of 0.5% for loss associated with the procedure itself. The NICHD collaborative study of 1976 suggested that the frequency of spontaneous abortion was not significantly higher among patients undergoing mid-trimester amniocentesis against a matched control group not having the procedure.

Chromosomal analysis as a result of amniocentesis is known to be highly accurate, though some diagnostic errors have been reported. The major source of error is due to maternal self-contamination, which can be minimized by using laboratory techniques such as multiple primary cultures and maternal amniotic fluid quinacrine chromosome polymorphisms. However, this complication is unlikely to arise if the needle is inserted into the amniotic sac under ultrasound control, the stillete not removed until the position is confirmed and the first few drops of liquor allowed to spill free before a sample is taken.

Chorionic villus sampling

There are concerns that chorionic villus sampling carries a higher risk of fetal loss than amniocentesis, although this has not been borne out by the Canadian Multicentre randomized trial (Canadian Collaborative CVS, 1989). Undoubtedly the fetal loss rate will decrease with the increasing experience of the operator (Jackson & Wagner 1987). The fetal loss rate may also be less if the transabdominal route rather than the transcervical route is used (Lilford 1985). Of course, since the procedure is commonly performed at earlier gestations than amniocentesis it is clear that there is an increased 'background' abortion incidence. Trials of CVS show variable fetal loss rates until 28 weeks' gestation. Brambati et al (1985) quotes an abortion rate of 4% with CVS whereas Elias et al (1986) and Jackson et al (1986) quote 2.3%. The Canadian Multicentre randomized clinical trial of CVS and amniocentesis showed 7.6% total losses (spontaneous and induced abortions and late losses) in the CVS group and 7.0% in the amniocentesis group. However, perinatal mortality was greater in the CVS group for no obviously recognizable reason. Although maternal morbidity was similar in each group, 9.9% of women eligible for CVS had a further amniocentesis and almost 27% of the CVS group had bleeding or spotting following the procedure. The possible higher risk of CVS is attributed to the higher risk of the procedure, although Jackson & Wagner (1987) disagree with this. Protagonists of one procedure or another obviously tend to be slightly biased. Complication rates are probably more influenced by operator skill, instrumentation, ultrasound resolution and suitability of the patient, rather than the procedure itself.

CVS may also provide erroneous results. Maternal cell contamination is not a problem with direct preparations, as the villi themselves are examined, but may be a problem in long-term cultures. Discrepancies have been reported between chorionic villus (placental) and fetal cell analysis especially in first trimester fetal diagnosis (Simoni et al 1985). Most are due to placental mosaics and it is suggested that all mosaics identified should have amniocentesis in order to confirm the diagnosis prior to deciding on ultimate management.

False positives—the chances of an abnormal CVS with a normal follow-up amniocentesis is quoted as 4.6% in the Canadian study—are disturbingly high. Confined mosaicism of chorionic villi can occur during rapid cell proliferation in the early embryo and lead to cell lines which may be found in only some tissue of the pregnancy. Therefore if only extraembryonic tissue is analysed false positives will occur. Culture preparations are composed of three cells that make up the inner cell mass and give rise to the embryo proper (Markert and Petters 1978). Discrepancies between karyotypes in cells of trophoblast, mesenchyme and fetus therefore become possible.

There have also been cases reported of normal karyotype chorionic cells with mosaic fetal cells (Martin et al 1986, Linton & Lilford 1986). These findings were not revealed on direct examination but were found on long-term culture. If results of karyotyping from CVS are to be 100% accurate then all samples would need to be subjected to long-term culture and this makes the procedure much more time-consuming and expensive.

Cordocentesis

The major problem with cordocentesis is that it requires a high degree of skill in order to obtain a sample in every case. Documented complications include cord haematomata formation, fetal haemorrhage and vagal stimulation producing fetal bradycardia. When haemorrhage is noted from the point of entry in the cord, haemostasis usually occurs within a short period of time, but unfortunately not always, and these very real complications must be considered. Again, the complication rate must be balanced against the need for a diagnosis. This procedure should only be carried out by highly skilled operators with a wide experience of ultrasound-guided biopsy.

EARLY AMNIOCENTESIS

To combine the advantages of the accuracy and reduced complications of amniocentesis and the benefits of early diagnosis provided by chorionic villus sampling, the efficacy of early amniocentesis has been assessed and reported by several centres (Godmilow et al 1988, Elejalde & Elejalde 1988). The procedures were carried out between 12 and 14 weeks and would suggest that early amniocentesis is a simple, safe and accurate method of prenatal diagnosis.

Since January 1987, we in Belfast have been offering early genetic amniocentesis at our Regional Obstetric Clinic as early as 9.5 weeks from the last menstrual period. Amniocenteses have been performed on 222 patients prior to 14 completed weeks. Eight millilitres of amniotic fluid was obtained following the ultrasound-guided procedure. Amniocytes were successfully cultured and harvested according to routine procedure in all but one case, which required a repeat amniocentesis.

The average time to harvest was 10 days and the number and quality of metaphases were comparable to those from 16-week gestation samples.

There were seven abnormal karyotypes (3.2%), including four trisomy 21, two trisomy 18 and one with a metacentric chromosome. One fetus had spina bifida and one had Meckel's syndrome. No fetal loss has been observed to date and a careful follow-up study is in progress.

Patient selection

Patients selected for early amniocentesis are, in the main, the same group of patients who would be appropriate for CVS or routine amniocentesis at 16–18 weeks (Crane 1983). As usual, the patient will have had the exact risks of fetal abnormality, the possible means of diagnosis and the relevant risks of the procedure discussed with her. An ultrasonic scan is carried out to confirm viability, gestation, number of fetuses, possible growth abnormalities and placental site.

It is wise to tailor the method to the patient herself. During the learning days of early amniocentesis it is best to avoid the patient who is grossly obese, has a retroverted uterus, fibroids or presents a history of a heavy threatened abortion.

The patient is asked to have a full bladder at the time of procedure and, if required, she can then empty her bladder appropriately.

The procedure

The procedure should not be carried out blindly but rather under ultrasound control (Fig. 10.1). This is best carried out with a sector or curved linear array probe. An attempt should be made to avoid placental tissue, but at the 12-week stage this can be difficult. It is better to insert the needle cleanly and atraumatically through a placenta than to poke and push the uterus and its contents around and perhaps miss the whole point of the exercise which is to obtain clear liquor.

An appropriate site of entry on the abdominal wall having been located, the skin, deeper structures and the peritoneum are infiltrated with approximately 5 ml of local anaesthetic. A 20 gauge spinal needle is then introduced under ultrasound guidance into the amniotic sac; 8 ml of amniotic fluid is removed; 2 ml is required for alpha fetoprotein estimation, and the remainder is used to obtain fetal cells for culture and analysis.

Previous reports (Crane 1983, McNay & Whitfield 1984) recommended that 15–20 ml of amniotic fluid is required for analysis. This represents 10% of the average volume of fluid at 16 weeks (Fig. 10.2). In our own unit 8 ml is all that is required and at 12 weeks represents 10% of the average volume of liquor for that gestation. Using this technique and suitably selected patients there have been no difficulties in obtaining liquor.

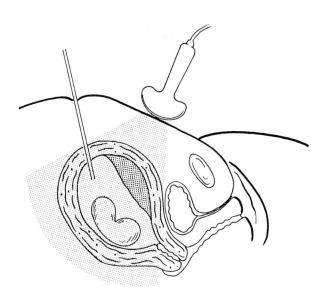

Fig. 10.1 Early amniocentesis.

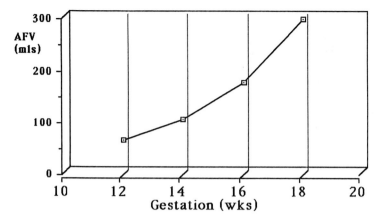

Fig. 10.2   Amniotic fluid volume v. gestation.

Occasionally the membranes appear to occlude the needle tip but if this occurs, a short sharp pierce of the membranes will suffice in order to enter the amniotic sac. The first few drops of liquor are allowed to flow freely.

Following removal of the needle, observation is made for intra-uterine haemorrhage or fetal bradycardia. If either are noted the duration of the event is recorded. Rhesus negative mothers are given 500 i.u. of anti-D immunoglobulin.

Since we introduced this new technique of early amniocentesis into our unit we now carry out over 90% of amniocenteses at gestations of less than 14 weeks. As the Canadian group admit, in deciding to undergo prenatal diagnosis, women consider more than just fetal loss rates. Factors such as the likely success of the procedure on the first attempt, the accuracy of the results obtained and the risk of vaginal bleeding are all likely to influence their choice.

Culture failure occurs due to either insufficient fetal cells or bacterial or fungal contamination. Failure rates of one in 200 are quoted at 16 weeks (Crane 1983). Traditionally, of course, amniocentesis at 16 weeks was considered to be the correct gestation because there would be sufficient cells present, less risk of abortion and the procedure could be carried out before cornification of the fetal skin. It would now appear that at the earlier gestations the risks of abortion are slight, and there are in fact more than adequate numbers of fetal cells in the small volume of liquor required.

In carrying out early amniocentesis one cannot always avoid the placenta, but merely try to traverse the thinnest portion of it and so avoid trauma from forcing the needle laterally. Crane (1983) reports no increase in abortion rates in his series where 37% of amniocenteses were transplacental. McNay & Whitfield (1984) reports that fetomaternal haemorrhage occurs in only 1% of cases as detected by Kleihauer testing before and after amniocentesis.

CONCLUSION

Ideally, antenatal diagnosis should involve only non-invasive procedures. It is theoretically possible in the future that a sample of maternal blood taken at the time of the first missed period could be processed by cell separation and that the fetal cells present in the maternal circulation could be replicated, cultured and analysed in order to determine the total genetic make up of the fetus. Until such times as this is possible, we must continue to try to find invasive methods that are safe and reliable. No procedure fills all the criteria, but early amniocentesis seems to have the advantages of an early diagnosis, a reduced operator expertise requirement, a low complication rate, reliability and acceptability.

REFERENCES

Ager R P, Oliver R W A 1986 The risks of midtrimester amniocentesis. Harboro Publications, Bramhall

Brambati B, Simoni G, Danesine C et al 1985 First trimester fetal diagnosis of genetic disorders. Clinical evaluation of 250 cases. Journal of Medical Genetics 22: 92–99

Canadian Collaborative CVS-Amniocentesis Clinical Trial Group 1989 Multicentre randomised clinical trial of chorion villus sampling and amniocentesis. Lancet i: 1–6

Crane J P 1983 Genetic amniocentesis. In: Studd J (ed) Progress in Obstetrics and Gynaecology, Vol. 3. Churchill Livingstone, Edinburgh

Elejalde B R, Elejalde M M de 1988 Early genetic amniocentesis, safety complications time to obtain results and contradictions (Abstract). American Journal of Human Genetics 43(3): A232

Elias S, Simpson J L, Martin A O et al 1986 Chorionic villus sampling in continuing pregnancies. I. Low fetal loss rates in initial 109 cases. American Journal of Obstetrics and Gynecology 154: 1349–1352

Godmilow L, Weiner S, Dunn L K 1988 Early genetic amniocentesis: experience with 600 consecutive procedures and comparison with chorionic villus sampling (Abstract). American Journal of Human Genetics 43(3): A234

Jackson L G, Wapner R A, Barr M A 1986 Safety of chorionic villus biopsy. Lancet i: 674–675

Jackson L G, Wapner R J 1987 Risks of chorionic villus sampling. In: Rodeck C H (ed) Clinics in Obstetrics and Gynaecology, Vol. 1, No. 3, Baillière Tindall, London

Lilford R J 1985 Chorionic villus biopsy. Editorial. Archives of Diseases in Childhood 60: 897–899

Linton G, Lilford R J 1986 False negative finding on chorionic villus sampling. Lancet ii: 630

Markert C H, Petters P M 1978 Manufactured hexaparental mice show that adults are derived from three embryonic cells. Science 202: 56–58

Martin A O, Elias S, Roskinsky B, Bombard A T, Simpson T L 1986 False negative finding on chorionic villus sampling. Lancet ii: 391–392

Menees T O, Miller S D, Holly L E 1930 Amniography. Preliminary Report. American Journal of Roentgenology 24: 363–366

McNay M B, Whitfield C R 1984 Prenatal diagnosis. Amniocentesis. British Journal of Hospital Medicine 31(6): 406–416

NICHD National Registry for Amniocentesis Study Group. 1976 Midtrimester amniocentesis for prenatal diagnosis—safety and accuracy. JAMA 236: 1471–1476

Simoni G, Gimelli G, Cuoco C et al 1985 Discordance between prenatal cytogenetic diagnosis after chorionic villi sampling and chromosomal constitution of the fetus. In: Fraccaro M, Simoni G, Brambati B (eds) First Trimester Fetal Diagnosis. Springer, Berlin, pp 137–143

11. The therapeutic roles of prostaglandins in obstetrics

I. Z. MacKenzie

INTRODUCTION

In 1968 the first reports of the use of prostaglandin E2 (PGE2) and prostaglandin F2α (PGF2α) appeared in the medical literature (Karim et al 1968, Embrey 1969). In each instance they were given by intravenous infusion and appeared an exciting new development. Following many subsequent controlled and uncontrolled trials over the following 8 years, it was concluded that when given by intravenous infusion, these powerful oxytocics offered no advantage over titrated infusions of oxytocin for most labour inductions; gastrointestinal side-effects were frequently experienced and intravenous infusions of PGE2 and PGF2α were largely abandoned. However, by the mid-1970s, evidence was starting to accumulate of the value of PGE2 when used to induce labour when the cervix was unripe and as a result of further research during the latter years of the 1970s, a renewed enthusiasm for prostaglandins for labour induction occurred. Over the past

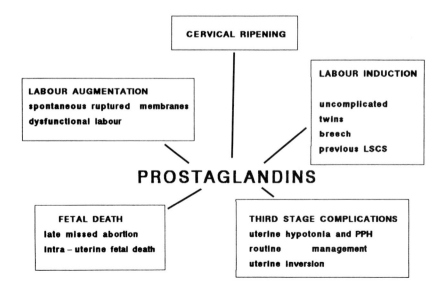

Fig. 11.1 Roles of prostaglandins in relation to labour induction.

149

10 years more precise roles for the prostaglandins in relation to labour induction have been identified (Fig. 11.1).

Prostaglandin chemistry

It is now realized that the prostaglandins, members of the group of prostanoids which include the leukotrienes and thromboxanes, are ubiquitous and are probably involved in most organ functions. Their place in reproductive medicine was the first to be explored and a considerable effort has been made to elucidate their possible roles. They are a family of highly active, structurally similar, modified unsaturated hydroxy fatty acids. A number have now been identified in tissues and biological fluids and each is derived from the basic, but not itself active, prostanoic acid, a cyclopentane fatty acid consisting of a five-carbon ring with two hydrocarbon side chains attached to neighbouring carbon atoms. Depending upon the configuration of the five-carbon ring, each belongs to one of four groups (A, B, E or F) while for each group a suffix numeral (1, 2 or 3) describes the degree of unsaturation of the side chain, thus denoting the number of double bonds each molecule contains. The group of primary prostaglandins consists of six which are formed by conversion of three precursor essential unsaturated fatty acids. In reproduction PGE2 and PGF2α appear to be of major significance and are formed from 5, 8, 11, 14-eicosatetraenoic acid (arachidonic acid) via the cycloendoperoxides PGG2 and PGH2 following the influence of the cyclo-oxygenase enzyme system. They are locally produced and immediately active since they are rapidly metabolized via 15-hydroxy prostaglandin dehydrogenase and ^13 reductase enzymes which are widely dispersed in the body.

Prostaglandins and parturition

Although the precise function of prostaglandins in the evolution of spontaneous parturition remains uncertain, there is convincing evidence that they are essential for the initiation and normal progress of labour (Thorburn & Challis 1979, Bleasdale & Johnstone 1984). Whether the prostaglandins are the primary stimulator of uterine contractions or act through second messengers to sensitize the myometrium to oxytocin still needs to be determined. However, increases in the prostaglandins and their metabolites have been demonstrated both in late pregnancy and during cervical dilatation in advanced labour (Husslein 1985, Sellers 1985). The use of prostaglandins to induce cervical ripening and labour may thus be considered appropriate, by striving to foreshorten a normal physiological process using physiological substances in physiological amounts.

USES IN LABOUR INDUCTION

In considering the role of prostaglandins for labour induction, attention needs to be paid to any pregnancy complication that exists either precipitating or complicating the delivery, and also the state of the uterine cervix at the time the delivery is indicated. There has been a much greater awareness of the importance of cervical condition over the past 15 years.

Induction with an unripe cervix

Cervical state can have a profound influence on the outcome of induced labour as demonstrated by Friedman et al (1966) and Calder et al (1974). When delivery is indicated for maternal and/or fetal reasons and the cervix is unripe, the prospects for a successful outcome to labour are reduced: this rarely represents a problem for induction in multiparae except for those previously delivered by Caesarean section. In such cases, the decision to deliver needs to be reaffirmed and an accurate assessment of cervical state should be made. As long ago as 1969, Embrey (1969) noted the benefits of PGE2 compared with PGF2α in successfully inducing labour in this situation.

There have now been numerous studies, many involving control groups, demonstrating the benefits of using prostaglandins as part of the induction process when the cervix is unripe, most noticeable by the reduction in the

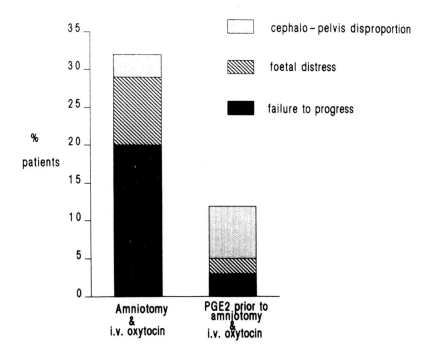

Fig. 11.2   The effect of the use of PGE2 for induction upon the need for Caesarean section. (Derived from Calder et al 1977 and MacKenzie & Embrey 1977).

need for Caesarean section for failure to progress in labour (Fig. 11.2). Of the prostaglandin administration routes that have been explored for induction, oral and intravenous have been abandoned and local administration by extra-amniotic injection, endocervical instillation, and intravaginal placement are favoured; a technique of direct injection into cervical tissue has been described (Boemi et al 1982) but has not been widely adopted. For extra-amniotic and endocervical treatment, PGE2 250–500 μg in a viscous gel is used, in general usually with one instillation, although protocols are described with repeated treatment after 6–8 hours (Calder et al 1977, Thiery et al 1977, Ulmsten et al 1982). For vaginal therapy, PGE2 2–10 mg incorporated into a variety of vehicles have been used including viscous gels (MacKenzie & Embrey 1977), dry tablets (Wilson 1978), lipid pessaries (Shepherd et al 1979), and non-biodegradable pessaries (Embrey et al 1980, Brundin et al 1983). Table 11.1 illustrates doses and protocols commonly used. Opinions vary on optimum regimes between single-prostaglandin treatment followed by oxytocin titration and low amniotomy after 15–20 hours, and repeated treatments several hours later if significant improvement in cervical state has not been achieved. In general, the results are similar with the different protocols although dry tablets are generally much less effective, probably due to poor absorption of the prostaglandins (Sellers & MacKenzie 1985).

The prostaglandins characteristically induce frequent low-amplitude contractions, often not felt by the patient, which may continue for 3–4 hours and then wane. In 30–50% labour will gradually establish and if treatment is given in the evening this results in a disturbed night for the woman and added demands upon the delivery unit when staffing levels are generally reduced. To try and reduce the incidence of labour occurring overnight, the concomitant administration of a tocolytic agent has been used which reduces the frequency of labour ensuing without apparently affecting the cervical ripening impact of the prostaglandins and subsequent improved labour outcome (Goeschen et al 1985, Insull et al 1989).

From most reports, up to 12% will require delivery by Caesarean section, of which 2–5% will be because of a failure to establish progressive labour, the induction attempt having been unsuccessful. Explanations for these failed inductions may be manifold, but in many instances it is possibly due either to the uterus and cervix not being sensitive to the prostaglandins and consequently unresponsive to oxytocin, or due to an inadequate transfer of the administered prostaglandins from the vagina to the target organs. In support of the former hypothesis is the finding of low-circulating oestradiol concentrations in those women with a failed induction compared with the levels in successfully induced women (MacKenzie et al 1979a) and this may not facilitate the rise in PGF metabolite in the circulation which appears to be necessary for progressive labour to occur (Husslein et al 1981). Kinetic studies to explore the second explanation are at present inconclusive (Sellers & MacKenzie 1985). What does seem clear however is

Table 11.1 Cervical ripening with PGE2 in primiparae: results of selected series

Reference	Protocol	N	Max Cx score	L.O.L. (h)	Failed inductions
Calder et al 1977	240–480 µg extra-amniotically — induced next day	121	3	10.7	0.8%
Thiery et al 1977	250–500 µg extra-amniotically — repeat in 8 hours	68	4	N.S.	4.4%
Ekman et al 1983	500 µg endocervically — induced the next day	27	5	N.S.	3.7%
Ulmsten et al 1982	500 µg endocervically — induced the next day	35	5	N.S.	6.3%
MacKenzie & Embrey 1977	2 mg vaginal gel — induced the next day	102	3	10.5	3.0%
O'Herlihy & MacDonald 1979	2 mg vaginal gel — induced the next day	54	3	8.5	1.5%
Shepherd et al 1979	3 mg vaginal pessary — repeated in 12 hours	110	4	16.0	5.5%
Wilson 1978	2 mg vaginal tablets — induced the next day	15	3	N.S.	13.3%

L.O.L.: length of labour.

that the results are not dose-related within the dose ranges quoted earlier (MacKenzie 1981, Reed & Mattock 1982, Graves et al 1985).

The vast majority of studies on labour induction with an unripe cervix have explored the value of PGE2. PGF2α has been used but objective comparisons (MacKenzie & Embrey 1979, Neilson et al 1983) strongly suggest that PGE2 has greater collagenolytic properties, which has been supported by in vitro studies (Hillier & Wallis 1981). Some of the prostaglandin analogues may be more effective in inducing cervical ripening and labour, but stringent toxicology studies are necessary before they can be used clinically with reassurance.

Conclusions

When induction is necessary in a primipara with an unfavourable cervix, locally administered PGE2 as part of the induction procedure will produce a more favourable outcome than is achieved with intravenous oxytocin and low amniotomy alone. A variety of vehicles incorporating the prostaglandins and different regimens have been described and there is probably little to choose between them. When administered extra-amniotically or endocervically, PGE2 0.5 mg appears to be the appropriate dose and with vaginal treatment PGE2 2–3 mg in most vehicles is required; for some patients at least 12–18 hours should be allowed for the prostaglandins to produce the necessary cervical changes either directly or through mediators. PGF2α appears to be much less effective. The precise mechanism responsible for cervical ripening and initiation of labour with local prostaglandins still remains uncertain and at present up to 5% of primiparae will end as a failed induction. More study is necessary to determine the optimum release rate of prostaglandins from administration vehicles and further developments of sustained-release preparations incorporating the prostaglandins or a prostaglandin analogue may provide improved results.

Routine induction

In the late 1970s in the UK, there were growing demands for less invasive, more 'natural' methods of labour induction. The demands added impetus to the searches already in progress by the profession to develop better, simpler procedures to improve the outcome for all concerned. Most of this effort was directed towards exploring the roles of prostaglandins. While the early studies of intravenous, oral and vaginal administration all indicated that gastrointestinal side-effects were a problem, side-effects could be largely avoided if doses were kept down with oral and vaginal use.

Oral protocols are seen as non-invasive, simple and attractive by patients generally. Repeated ingestion of PGE2 0.5 mg to 2 mg 1–4 hourly in the form of dry tablets have been found to induce progressive labour in

Table 11.2 PGE2 and labour induction: results from selected series

Reference	Protocol	Cx score	N	L.O.L. (h)	Augmented labour	L.S.C.S.
Primiparae						
Matthews et al 1976	0.5–2.0 mg orally 2–4 hourly	favourable	25	6.25	25%	0%
Mundow 1977	0.5–1.5 mg orally 1–2 hourly	6+	18	8.62	0%	0%
MacKenzie et al 1981	5 mg vaginal pessary	5+	96	8.1	37%	N.S.
Khoo et al 1981	5 mg vaginal tablet	5.9 mean	25	N.S.	42%	16%
Shepherd et al 1981	3 mg vaginal pessary 4–6 hourly	5+	226	8.7	34%	7%
Multiparae						
Matthews et al 1976	0.5–2.0 mg orally 2–4 hourly	favourable	25	6.01	12%	4%
Mundow 1977	0.5–1.5 mg orally 1–2 hourly	6+	82	6.81	0%	0%
MacKenzie et al 1981	2.5 mg vaginal pessary	5+	167	4.8	19%	N.S.
Khoo et al 1981	3 mg vaginal tablet	6.5 mean	22	N.S.	23%	0%
Shepherd et al 1981	3 mg vaginal pessary 4–6 hourly	5+	253	5.1	10%	2%

L.O.L.: length of labour.
L.S.C.S.: lower segment Caesarean section.
N.S.: Not stated.

virtually all multiparae with a favourable cervix. Nausea, vomiting and diarrhoea occur occasionally, but the method is otherwise acceptable. For most primiparae and multiparae with a less-favourable cervix, the results are less impressive. The alternative vaginal approach is equally attractive and results are very satisfactory for all groups; gastrointestinal side-effects are virtually eliminated although some vaginal burning may be experienced for 15–30 minutes after treatment. With this route, much less agreement exists as to optimum treatment regimens, both regarding prostaglandin dose and subsequent management. Most reports of vaginal administration have assessed the use of hospital pharmacy-produced gels and pessaries since a commercial product has not been available until recent years. Lipid-based pessaries, a variety of viscous gels of cellulose and dextran, as well as tablets marketed for oral and vaginal use have all been used vaginally, each producing similar results (Table 11.2). PGE2 dosages have mostly been in the same range as that used for cervical ripening, 2–5 mg.

Since part of the drive to use vaginal instillation has been the desire to avoid intravenous infusions, many workers have devised protocols using repeated vaginal treatments at 4–6 hour intervals with low amniotomy performed once labour is established. Where observations have been controlled, the outcome compared with conventional induction by low amniotomy and immediate oxytocin titration is of a generally longer induction-delivery interval with prostaglandins, but similar duration of labour and neonatal condition for both groups; analgesia requirements and postpartum haemorrhage are usually reduced in prostaglandin-treated patients. While there is little doubt that PGF2α can be used for inducing labour when the cervix is ripe most work has involved intravenous infusions; there have been only a few reports of local administration of PGF2α 40–50 mg (MacLennan & Green 1979) and it is thus difficult to comment on its value compared with PGE2.

Although labour can be reliably induced in most cases, there remains a degree of unpredictability about the speed with which the myometrium responds to the administered prostaglandins. Of particular concern are those patients who respond quickly, resulting in very painful labours with an increased risk of fetal distress. Uterine overstimulation occurs in approximately 1% of cases and a sustained tetanic contraction, or hypertonus, occurs about once in 500 cases, an incidence similar to that observed in spontaneous labour and labour induced with oxytocin. When it occurs, acute fetal distress is a likely consequence and immediate action is required. Delivery by Caesarean section may be appropriate, while the alternative is urgent administration of a tocolytic, either by infusion or inhalation to reverse the hypertonia; after an hour, normal labour can usually be allowed to continue (Khoo et al 1982, Shepherd et al 1981). Experience has led most workers to recommend either very cautious use in highly parous patients in whom the cervix is effaced and partly dilated, or avoiding prostaglandins in these patients altogether since they are more likely to be overstimulated. The sustained-release pessary could have distinct advantages in these patients (Embrey & MacKenzie 1985, Embrey et al 1986).

Conclusions

Prostaglandins given orally by repeated doses at hourly intervals will induce labour with few side-effects in almost all multiparae if the cervix is moderately favourable. Vaginal administration is effective in both primiparae and multiparae and causes virtually no side-effects. Hyper-stimulation occurs in less than 1% and facilities should be readily available for these rare cases either for rapid delivery or for the administration of a tocolytic agent: an inhalant or syringe loaded with a β-sympathomimetic agent should be ready for emergency use in all obstetric units using prostaglandins. Women with a very favourable cervix are best not treated with prostaglandins since a rapid uncontrolled labour may be provoked. Caution must be exercised since vaginal administration is simple and attractive and could lead to wanton labour induction without good clinical indication.

Role in previous Caesarean section

There is an increasing incidence of multiparae presenting in pregnancy with a history of delivery by lower segment Caesarean section in most countries as a result of the rising rates of Caesarean section (Chalmers 1985). In consequence there is a greater need to consider how best to manage subsequent confinements, and the use of prostaglandins to induce labour in these women has not been explored in any logical objective manner: coincidental reference to such cases has been made in analyses of labour inductions using prostaglandins. Since the prostaglandins usually provoke frequent low-pressure contractions (MacKenzie & Embrey 1977, Steiner et al 1979), their use in cases with a lower-segment scar could well be an advantage. There have, however, been occasional reports in the literature of cases of scar rupture (Bennett & Laurence 1981, Fay & Fraser 1983).

One large prospective study of 143 consecutive patients whose labours were induced using vaginal PGE2 has been reported: 68% patients with an unfavourable cervix delivered vaginally, the incidence increasing to 83% with an intermediate cervix, and 89% with a favourable cervix (MacKenzie et al 1984). In none did the lower-segment scar rupture. It was concluded that the use of local prostaglandins in this situation is safe and offers patients with an unfavourable cervix a high chance of vaginal delivery, since many obstetricians might otherwise have advised delivery by elective section without any attempt at labour. A recent extension of the series above to 439 patients has been reported (MacKenzie 1988). Overall the results were very similar but four cases of scar dehiscence and one of rupture were found at repeat section when labour was abandoned: in all five cases, oxytocin augmentation was required, compared with 62% for the total study group. This incidence of scar damage is similar to that reported following oxytocin-induced labour and spontaneous labour (Case et al 1971, Molloy et al 1987, Phelan et al 1987). Objective evidence of a definite advantage over oxytocin in such cases, however, has not been presented although a prospective randomized study of the two treatment modalities has shown a reduction in subsequent failed inductions or failure to progress in labour when PGE2 is used compared with oxytocin (Sellers et al 1988).

Conclusion

The prostaglandins may be used to induce labour in women who have previously been delivered by lower-segment Caesarean section and provides a high chance of a safe vaginal delivery but there is approximately a 1% risk of scar damage. Due care and attention should therefore be maintained throughout such labours, especially if oxytocin augmentation is necessary. It is inappropriate if cephalopelvic disproportion is anticipated. Whether there are any definite advantages over the use of intravenous infusions of oxytocin however has not yet been adequately demonstrated, but there is probably a greater chance of a vaginal delivery in cases with an unfavourable cervix.

Induction in twin pregnancies

Apart from occasional anecdotal cases in series of prostaglandin inductions reported in the literature, there is virtually nothing written concerning the use of prostaglandins in multiple pregnancies. Personal experience suggests that the prostaglandins are as effective in multiple pregnancies as in singletons. However, since primary post-partum haemorrhage due to uterine hypotonia occurs in approximately 10–15% of twin labours, it could be argued that the use of prostaglandins as part of the induction procedure would seem to be more than justified. An analysis of 144 twin-pregnancy labours managed in the unit in Oxford is illustrated in Figure 11.3; primary postpartum haemorrhage was lower following labour induced with prostaglandins (2.5%) compared with oxytocin-induced labour (11.5%) and spontaneous-onset labour (14.1%). The numbers are small and the differences do not reach statistical significance, but it suggests there may be some advantage from the use of PGE2; no obvious dis-advantages were detected.

Conclusion

Prostaglandins may be used in the induction of labour in twin pregnancies

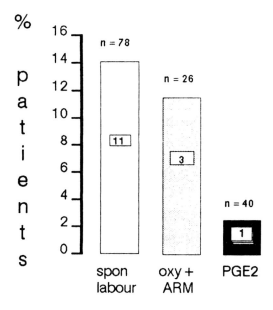

Fig. 11.3   Incidence of primary post-partum haemorrhage following vaginal delivery of twins according to mode of labour onset in 144 patients (MacKenzie & McKinlay 1988, unpublished data).

and this might reduce the incidence of postpartum haemorrhage from uterine hypotonia. There is presently little reported use of prostaglandins for twin labours and more studies are required before any firm conclusions can be drawn.

Fetal breech presentation

There remains some controversy over delivery management when the fetus presents by the breech. Only one study has specifically assessed the value of prostaglandins for inducing labour in this situation (O'Herlihy 1981): of 13 primigravidae with an unripe cervix given PGE2 2 mg vaginally as a viscous gel, 9 delivered vaginally and 4 required Caesarean section because of poor progress in labour. Similar results were reported in a large series of vaginally-treated patients of mixed parity which included 54 with a breech presentation when 13% were ultimately delivered by section, most in the second stage of labour (Shepherd et al 1981). A personal series (MacKenzie 1987) of 177 patients of mixed parity with all degrees of cervical favourability resulted in a Caesarean section rate of 22%, of which almost half were in the second stage of labour. No obvious detriment to mother or baby was recorded.

Conclusions

An objective assessment of the use of prostaglandins in breech presentation has not been made. The probable advantage compared with intravenous oxytocin titration and low amniotomy is the delay in rupturing the fore-waters until the breech has descended well into the maternal pelvis. The high rate of Caesarean section during the second stage of labour is a matter of some concern; whether this is a consequence of the use of prostaglandins or merely a reflection of current attitudes to breech management remains speculative at present.

Ruptured membranes without ensuing labour

When the fetal membranes rupture spontaneously around term, labour generally establishes within a few hours. When there is a delay in labour starting, there are concerns of intrauterine infection developing and many obstetricians favour stimulating contractions with an oxytocic. Prostaglandins have been used for this purpose in a variety of ways. Thiery et al (1982) treated 38 patients of mixed parity with cervical score of 5 or less with low-dose intravenous infusions of PGE2 0.1 mg/hr increasing the rate until labour was stimulated; 37 delivered vaginally with a low rate of gastrointestinal side-effects. Oral administration has been used and compared with intravenous (i.v.) oxytocin by Hauth et al (1977) and Lange et al (1981). Both conducted randomized prospective trials and found that oral PGE2 0.5–1.5 mg/hr was safe and efficient compared with i.v. oxytocin, although oxytocin tended to result in shorter treatment to delivery intervals according to Lange et al (1981). The design used by Hauth et al (1977) unfortunately does not allow any worthwhile comparison since PGE2 was instilled 3 hours after membranes ruptured while oxytocin was given after 12 hours. Vaginal administration as a PGE2 4 mg gel (Ekman-Ordeberg et al 1985) or as a PGE2 3 mg pessary (Magos et al 1983, Chapman et al 1984) has been used generally with favourable conclusions. Further augmentation with prostaglandins or i.v. oxytocin appears necessary in about 40% of primiparae and 20% multiparae treated with vaginal prostaglandins.

Conclusions

Despite the fact that these series and others have been reported there remains uncertainty over the place for prostaglandins in this situation. Apart from the different routes explored and different protocols used, there are large discrepancies over the recommended interval before trying to stimulate labour after the membranes have ruptured and how long treatment should continue before resorting to other augmentation methods. Appropriate attention has often not been paid to the influence of parity and cervical state upon results and worthwhile conclusions comparing prostaglandins with intravenous oxytocin are not possible. It is evident, however, that the prostaglandins are effective in stimulating labour when the membranes have ruptured and appear to be safe whichever administration route is used. Large, well-designed prospective trials are still required before it will be possible to be sure of any advantage or disadvantage when compared with i.v. oxytocin or even awaiting the spontaneous onset of labour.

Augmentation of dysfunctional labour

One area where the prostaglandins might have a particularly important role is to improve the outcome in cases of incoordinate uterine activity or cervical dystocia. In such cases when intravenous oxytocin infusions fail to produce progressive labour, delivery by Caesarean section is necessary. The exposure of the uterus to a small dose of prostaglandins could well enhance the prospects of a vaginal delivery. This potential use of the prostaglandins has not yet been explored.

Conclusions

This aspect of labour warrants studying with randomized prospective controlled trials.

FETAL AND NEONATAL CONSEQUENCES

Any method of labour induction requires not only a careful appraisal of the risks and benefit of the method over alternatives with regard to the various indices of labour outcome, but also critical assessment of possible fetal benefits and morbidity. The low-amplitude contractions characteristically stimulated by the prostaglandins should theoretically cause little disturbance to placental bed blood flow with a consequent small risk of fetal distress developing. However, the possibility of fetal distress occurring once labour is established is presumably similar to that following induction with oxytocin. Observations on cord blood gas values at delivery following extra-amniotic prostaglandin-induced labour have indicated that fetal and neonatal acidosis and asphyxia is no more common than during labour induced with oxytocin or following spontaneous onset (Thiery et al 1978, Steiner et al 1979). Whether continuous electronic fetal monitoring should be instituted before and following prostaglandin treatment remains controversial; the place for routine continuous monitoring of the fetal heart in labour, induced or spontaneous, has still to be proven with virtually all controlled studies showing no advantage.

Since the development of vaginal prostaglandin treatment was in part the consequence of a desire to move away from invasive mechanized labour management, the case for continuous electronic fetal monitoring needs to be proven before being widely recommended. Continuous monitoring for the first 4 hours following treatment would seem appropriate in women in whom placental function is thought to be reduced but there is as yet no evidence that such management improves the outcome. One retrospective analysis of 53 patients (MacKenzie & Embrey 1981) comparing continuous electronic monitoring with intermittent auscultation found no obvious benefits for fetal wellbeing from continuous monitoring but the diagnosis of suspected fetal distress was made in 48% of the monitored cases, of which all were delivered by Caesarean section, compared with 4% in the intermittent auscultation group; neonatal outcome was similar for both groups. It would seem wise for all patients to be carefully watched for the first 4–5 hours after prostaglandin treatment by intermittent fetal auscultation at 15–30 minute intervals as a minimum to ensure that fetal distress does not occur from an unexpected response to the exogenous prostaglandins. Isolated cases of acute fetal distress and death following prostaglandin treatment for ripening or labour induction have appeared in the press at intervals over the past 12 years (Felmingham et al 1976, Quinn & Murphy 1981, Stewart & Calder 1981). These cases however are not a justification for continuously monitoring all patients. There has been one report suggesting placental abruption may be a consequence of prostaglandin induction (Leung et al 1987). This appears to be an isolated report to date, the significance of which is at present uncertain.

Since the prostaglandins are implicated in numerous physiological processes, the possible consequences for the fetus and neonate of maternal treatment with prostaglandins needs to be considered. Concentrations of PGE are raised in cord blood following vaginal PGE2 treatment compared with values found following oxytocin-induced labour, spontaneous labour and at elective Caesarean section, while there is no difference in PGF concentrations (MacKenzie et al 1980). This implies that the exogenous prostaglandins reach the fetus, a conclusion substantiated by the finding of higher PGE metabolite levels in cord plasma in babies delivered after short PGE treatment-delivery intervals compared with those delivered after longer intervals as shown in Figure 11.4 (Sellers & MacKenzie 1985). Despite these findings, there has been no evidence of any adverse effects upon neonatal cardiovascular physiology such as prolonged patency or premature closure of the ductus arteriosis with PGE2 or PGF2α administration to the mother. There have however been few reports of follow-up studies of babies delivered after prostaglandin-induced labours, although Van Pelt et al (1984) found no ill-effects in 20 babies assessed up to 12 months of age. A follow-up analysis of 300 babies up to 3 years after various types of labour onset including prostaglandins inductions has failed to observe any deleterious effects attributable to these oxytocics (MacKenzie & McKinlay 1988, unpublished data).

One proven advantage of prostaglandins over oxytocin for labour

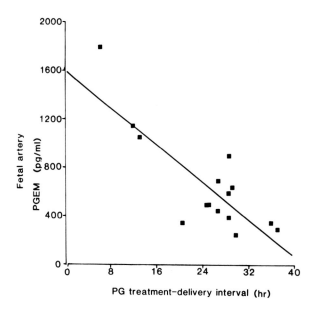

Fig. 11.4   PGEM concentrations in umbilical artery at delivery related to the time from PGE2 administration to delivery in 15 patients ($P = 0.0002$). (Reproduced with permission from Sellers & MacKenzie 1985.)

induction is a reduced incidence of neonatal hyperbilirubinaemia (Beazley et al 1976, Conway et al 1976, Chew 1977); the incidence following PGE2-induced labour is similar to that for spontaneous-onset labour. This could be explained by the apparent steroidogenic properties of prostaglandins (Saruta & Kaplan 1972, Flack & Ramwell 1972). Thus there may be particular benefits for the fetus if very preterm induction is planned.

Maternal water intoxication due to hyponatraemia is a rare hazard of oxytocin-induced labour and is generally the result of high-dose infusion over a long period (Schwartz & Jones 1978). In such instances, electrolyte imbalance of the neonate has also been reported and the use of prostaglandins in such cases should avoid such a potentially dangerous condition.

Conclusions

Prostaglandins administered to the mother result in increased plasma concentrations of the prostaglandin and its metabolite in the fetal and neonatal circulation. However, no direct ill-effects have been reported as yet, although fetal distress is a potential hazard of any therapy that stimulates uterine contractions. Reduced frequencies of neonatal hyper-bilirubinaemia and hyponatraemia are definite advantages of the prostaglandins compared with oxytocin, especially in preterm inductions and if a prolonged labour may result. Further studies of the long term consequences for the baby are still required.

USES DURING THE THIRD STAGE OF LABOUR

Induced labours have been shown to be associated with a greater incidence of primary post-partum haemorrhage than occurs with spontaneous-onset labour (Brinsden & Clark 1978). The incidence however appears to be reduced if prostaglandins are used as part of the induction procedure rather than oxytocin alone (MacKenzie 1979, Kennedy et al 1982). The potent oxytocic properties of prostaglandins make them of value in the management of post-partum haemorrhage.

Routine third-stage management

There has been very little attention paid to the possible role of prostaglandins in routine third-stage management. Kerekes and Domokos (1979) in a prospective randomized trial found that PGF2α 1–2 mg intra-myometrially resulted in less blood loss than occurred with intramuscular ergometrine. Further consideration of this possible role for the prostaglandins is warranted, although intramyometrial injections would probably prove unacceptable as a routine.

Primary post-partum haemorrhage

Primary post-partum haemorrhage due to uterine atonia that does not respond to other oxytocics may be staunched by the timely administration of prostaglandins avoiding the need for laparotomy and ligation of the internal iliac arteries or hysterectomy. Various regimens have been described as shown in Figure 11.5. Vaginal administration would seem to be an inappropriate route and direct administration transabdominally or transvaginally into the myometrium may well be the ideal route.

Uterine inversion

The intramuscular injection of 15mePGF2α 250 µg has been advocated in combination with intrauterine packing as treatment for recurrent uterine inversion (Heyl et al 1984). Thiery and Delbeke (1985) have used intra-myometrial injections of either PGE2 or 15mePGF2α after an i.v. injection of a tocolytic to permit replacement of the uterus. Further studies are necessary to support the use of prostaglandins for this potentially lethal condition.

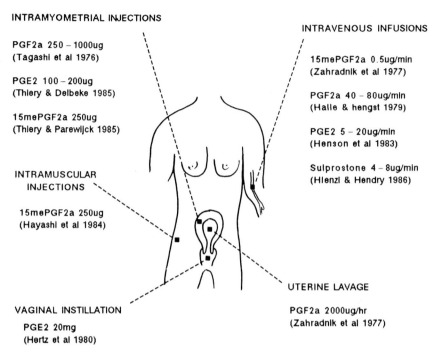

INTRAMYOMETRIAL INJECTIONS

PGF2a 250 – 1000ug
(Tagashi et al 1976)

PGE2 100 – 200ug
(Thiery & Delbeke 1985)

15mePGF2a 250ug
(Thiery & Parewijck 1985)

INTRAMUSCULAR
INJECTIONS

15mePGF2a 250ug
(Hayashi et al 1984)

VAGINAL INSTILLATION

PGE2 20mg
(Hertz et al 1980)

INTRAVENOUS INFUSIONS

15mePGF2a 0.5ug/min
(Zahradnik et al 1977)

PGF2a 40 – 80ug/min
(Halle & hengst 1979)

PGE2 5 – 20ug/min
(Henson et al 1983)

Sulprostone 4 – 8ug/min
(Hienzl & Hendry 1986)

UTERINE LAVAGE

PGF2a 2000ug/hr
(Zahradnik et al 1977)

Fig. 11.5 Administration of prostaglandins for the management of intractable haemorrhage from uterine hypotonia following the third stage of labour.

Secondary post-partum haemorrhage

Prostaglandins have been used in the management of secondary post-partum haemorrhage by one group (Andrinopoulos & Mendenhall 1983); PGF2α was injected transvaginally and transabdominally into the myometrium 21 days after delivery with benefit although marked side-effects occurred for a few minutes. The precise mechanism whereby the prostaglandins have a beneficial effect in this situation, however, is not clear. Further evidence of the value of prostaglandins in the treatment of this condition is needed before widespread advocacy can be made.

Conclusions

It is evident from the number of reports in the literature that the control of massive haemorrhage due to third-stage uterine hypotonia, can be obtained using the natural prostaglandins or an analogue. It is therefore suggested that all obstetric units should have supplies of a prostaglandin available for this potentially very serious emergency. The best regimen however has not been established and indeed each may have some advantages. The intra-myometrial route has the benefit of speed of action with injection into the dysfunctioning organ. Although no randomized trials have been conducted into their use for this purpose, the present evidence is compelling. Their place in the management of uterine inversion and secondary post-partum haemorrhage is less clear and further studies on routine use for third-stage management are warranted with the current climate against routine ergometrine administration despite good evidence of its impact in reducing post-partum haemorrhage and transfusion rates (Prendiville et al 1988).

MANAGEMENT OF FETAL DEATH IN UTERO

Provoking abortion or delivery when fetal death has been diagnosed, is one of the major advances of recent years in obstetric practice provided by the prostaglandins. The primary objective in the management of such cases is to succeed in expelling the pregnancy as safely and as quickly as possible with minimal disturbance and distress to the patient. Expulsion within 24 hours has generally been the goal.

Late missed abortions

When the uterus is less than 16 weeks' gestational size, evacuation using prostaglandins alone is often unsuccessful and surgical aspiration or curettage should be used. At sizes equivalent to 16–28 weeks' pregnancy, intravenous infusions can be used with success but result in frequent gastrointestinal side-effects. Local application is thus to be preferred. Extra-amniotic instillation as a single injection of PGE2 1–2 mg or PGF2α 10 mg in viscous gel, or as a continuous infusion of PGE2 200 µg/2-hourly or PGF2α 60 µg/2-hourly results in abortion within 24 hours in the vast majority of patients; gastrointestinal side-effects are rarely encountered (Calder et al 1976).

Vaginal instillation using a viscous gel or lipid pessary has also been advocated. PGE2 15–25 mg as a single treatment with intravenous oxytocin augmentation after 15–20 hours results in abortion in up to 95% within 24 hours with vomiting or diarrhoea in 15%; lower doses are generally less effective (MacKenzie et al 1979b). Alternatively, PGE2 20 mg repeated at 3–6 hourly intervals avoids the need for oxytocin augmentation in most, but causes 60–80% to suffer gastrointestinal side-effects (Rutland & Ballard 1977, El-Demarawy et al 1977). Recent experience with 16-16dimethyl-PGE1 1–2 mg either as a single treatment with oxytocin augmentation after 16–18 hours when necessary, or as repeated insertions at 3-hour intervals has produced similar results, but with many fewer side-effects. Protocols using intramuscular injections of the PGE2 analogue, sulprostone 0.5 mg at 6-hour intervals (Karim et al 1979) or 15mePGF2α 0.125–0.250 mg at 2-hour intervals (Wallenburg et al 1980) are effective but offer no advantage over local applications of the natural compounds and tend to result in frequent side-effects (Table 11.3).

Table 11.3 Management of missed abortion and late fetal death using prostaglandins: selected series

Reference	Protocol	N	Mean Treatment Time (h)	Expulsion in 24 hours	Side-effects vomit.	diarrh
Calder et al 1976	{ PGE2 0.2–3.9 mg extra-amniotically { PGF2α 3.9–5.7 mg extra-amniotically	50	7.8–17.2	N.S.	40%	0%
Lippert & Luthi 1978	PGE2 0.5–1.0 mg extra-amniotic gel 3 hourly	20	12.0	90%	N.S.	
Toppozada et al 1979	16 phenoxy PGE2 500 µg i.m. 4–6 hourly	27	12.4	93%	48%	
Karim et al 1979	16 phenoxy PGE2 500 µg i.m. 6 hourly	49	9.5	97%	21%	
Wallenburg et al 1980	15mePGF2α 125–250 µg i.m. 2 hourly	97	8.6	93%	52%	59%
Rutland & Ballard 1977	PGE2 20 mg pessaries 3 hourly	50	11.3	86%	60%	60%
El-Demarawy et al 1977	PGE2 20 mg pessaries 3–6 hourly	31	14.6	80%	87%	70%
MacKenzie et al 1979b	PGE2 5–15 mg pessary	50	15.0	74%	15%	

vomit.: vomiting.
diarrh.: diarrhoea.

Third trimester intra-uterine fetal death

For fetal death in later pregnancy, the local administration of prostaglandins provides the ideal method for the management of these cases. Similar treatment protocols to those used for late missed abortions are appropriate, although lower doses of prostaglandins should be used. PGE2 10 mg in viscous gel or lipid pessary as a single instillation with intravenous oxytocin augmentation when required is generally very effective with less than 5% remaining undelivered for more than 24 hours (MacKenzie et al 1979b). Repeated administration of PGE2 20 mg pessaries at 3–6 hour intervals have been advocated, particularly by units in the USA (Rutland & Ballard 1977, Southern et al 1978), but this is almost certainly overdosing the patient and leads to an unacceptable incidence of gastro-intestinal side-effects. Cases of uterine rupture have been reported by a number of workers (MacKenzie 1988) and have usually been associated with prolonged attempts to achieve delivery by overstimulating the uterus. Occasionally, difficulty is experienced in establishing progressive labour and in such cases the attempt should be deferred for 2 or 3 days. This situation is very rare having occurred on only three occasions among more than 200 cases of missed abortion and late fetal death managed in the unit in Oxford.

Conclusions

Local prostaglandins, especially if given intravaginally, are very effective in terminating pregnancy when the fetus is dead. The procedure causes minimal disturbance to an already-distressed patient and does not commit the obstetrician to delivery since the fetal membranes can be kept intact until abortion or delivery is imminent.

WHAT COULD THE FUTURE HOLD?

It is evident that the introduction of prostaglandins into clinical obstetric practice has improved the management and outcome of many aspects of labour. There can be little doubt that the chances of a vaginal delivery being achieved for women with an unfavourable cervix are increased compared with 15 years ago, although the improvement is masked by a greater willingness to resort to Caesarean section for suspected fetal distress, fetal growth retardation, breech presentation and other reasons. For those requiring induction when the cervix is riper, the approach using vaginal administration of prostaglandins is seen by many to represent a less invasive, more natural event than the alternative of a continuous intra-venous infusion of oxytocin. Similarly management of fetal death and severe uterine atonia leading to haemorrhage have been revolutionized by the use of prostaglandins, a supply of which should be available in all obstetric units.

The popularity of the idea of vaginal administration of prostaglandins has at last led to the introduction of commercial preparations for clinical use, thus enabling obstetricians and hospital pharmacies to discontinue using hospital-made, potentially unstable and unsafe gels and pessaries. The introduction of a pessary with a more predictable release profile should be hailed as a major advance although more experience with it is required. The recent approach of concomitant tocolytic therapy to prevent or reduce uterine contractions during cervical ripening, especially in cases of suspected placental insufficiency and the possible at-risk fetus, looks promising and further studies are needed. The introduction of the anti-progestogens shortening mid-trimester prostaglandin-induced abortion times with lower prostaglandin doses (Selinger et al 1987) could have similar benefits, particularly if they can be shown not to have any adverse effects upon the fetus or newborn since it is conceivable that cervical effacement and dilatation might be produced with reduced uterine contractions and thus less potential insult to the baby during labour. When the antiprogestins are explored for labour induction, the same objective assessments using prospective controlled trials that have been a feature of many of the studies investigating prostaglandins will be required.

REFERENCES

Andrinopoulos G C, Mendenhall H W 1983 Prostaglandin F2α in the management of delayed postpartum haemorrhage. American Journal of Obstetrics and Gynecology 146: 217–218

Beazley J M, Weekes A R L 1976 Neonatal hyper-bilirubinaemia following the use of prostaglandin E2 in labour. British Journal of Obstetrics and Gynaecology 83: 62–67

Bennett M J, Laurence D T 1981 Induction of labour with prostaglandin E2 vaginal pessaries in high-risk pregnancies. Journal of Obstetrics and Gynaecology 2: 71–73

Bleasdale J E, Johnstone J M 1984 Prostaglandins and human parturition: regulation of arachidonic acid mobilization. Reviews of Perinatal Medicine 5: 151–191

Boemi P, Reitano S, Cianci S 1982 A new cervical perfusion method for induction of labour with prostaglandins. American Journal of Obstetrics and Gynecology 144: 476–479

Brinsden P R S, Clark A D 1978 Postpartum haemorrhage after induced and spontaneous labour. British Medical Journal ii: 855–856

Brundin J, Christensen N J, Fuchs T, Larsson M 1983 The A-rod—a new possibility for cervical dilatation and/or induction of uterine contractions for abortion or delivery by combined pharmacological and mechanical action. Acta Obstetrica et Gynecologica Scandinavica (suppl) 113: 159–162

Calder A A, Embrey M P, Hillier K 1974 Extra-amniotic prostaglandin E2 for induction of labour at term. British Journal of Obstetrics and Gynaecology 81: 39–46

Calder A A, MacKenzie I Z, Embrey M P 1976 Intrauterine (extra-amniotic) prostaglandins in the management of unsuccessful pregnancy. Journal of Reproductive Medicine 16: 271–275

Calder A A, Embrey M P, Tait T 1977 Ripening of the cervix with extra-amniotic prostaglandin E2 in viscous gel before induction of labour. British Journal of Obstetrics and Gynaecology 84: 264–268

Case B D, Corcoran R, Jeffcoate N, Randle G H 1971 Caesarean section and its place in modern obstetric practice. Journal of Obstetrics and Gynaecology of the British Commonwealth 78: 203–214

Chalmers I 1985 Trends and variations in the use of Caesarean section. In: Clinch J, Matthews T (eds) Perinatal Medicine. M.T.P. Press, Lancaster, pp 145–149

Chapman M, Lawrence D, Sims C, Bennett M 1984 Induction of labour by prostaglandin pessaries or oxytocin infusion after spontaneous rupture of membranes. Journal of Obstetrics and Gynaecology 4: 185–187

Chew W C 1977 Neonatal hyperbilirubinaemia: a comparison between prostaglandin E2 and oxytocin inductions. British Medical Journal 2: 679–680

Conway D I, Read M D, Baver C, Martin R H 1976 Neonatal jaundice—a comparison between intravenous oxytocin and oral prostaglandin E2. Journal of International Medical Research 4: 241–246

Corson S L, Bolognese R J 1977 Postpartum uterine atony treated with prostaglandins. American Journal of Obstetrics and Gynecology 129: 918–919

Ekman-Ordeberg G, Persson P H, Ulmsten U, Wingerup L 1983 The impact on labour induction of intracervically applied PGE2 gel related to gestational age in patients with an unripe cervix. Acta Obstetricia et Gynecologica Scandinavica (suppl) 113: 173–175

Ekman-Ordeberg G, Uldbjerg N, Ulmsten U 1985 Comparison of intravenous oxytocin and vaginal prostaglandin E2 gel in women with unripe cervices and premature rupture of the membranes. Obstetrics and Gynecology 66: 307–310

El-Demarawy H, El-Sahwi S, Toppozada M 1977 Management of missed abortion and fetal death in utero. Prostaglandins 14: 583–590

Embrey M P 1969 The effect of prostaglandins on the human pregnant uterus. Journal of Obstetrics and Gynaecology of the British Commonwealth 76: 783–789

Embrey M P, MacKenzie I Z 1985 Labour induction with a sustained release prostaglandin E2 polymer vaginal pessary. Journal of Obstetrics and Gynaecology 6: 38–41

Embrey M P, Graham N B, McNeill M E 1980 Induction of labour with a sustained release prostaglandin E2 vaginal pessary. British Medical Journal 281: 901–902

Embrey M P, Graham N B, McNeil M E, Hillier K 1986 In vitro release characteristics and long-term stability of polyethylene oxide hydrogel vaginal pessaries containing prostaglandin E2. Journal of Controlled Release 3: 39–45

Fay R A, Fraser I S 1983 Vaginal prostaglandins and scar rupture. Journal of Obstetrics and Gynaecology 4: 139–140

Felmingham J E, Oakley M C, Atlay R D 1976 Uterine hypertonus after induction of labour with prostaglandin E2 tablets. British Medical Journal i: 586

Flack J D, Ramwell P W 1972 A comparison of the effects of ACTH, cyclic AMP, Dibutyryl cyclic AMP, and PGE2 on corticosteroidogenesis in vitro. Endocrinology 90: 371–377

Friedman E A, Niswander K R, Bayonet-Rivera N P, Sachtleben M R 1966 Relation of prelabour evaluation in inducibility and the course of labour. Obstetrics and Gynecology 28: 495–501

Goeschen K, Fuchs F, Rasmussen A B, Rehnstrom J V, Salinge E 1985 Effect of β mimetic tocolysis in cervical ripening and plasma prostaglandin F2α metabolite after endocervical application of prostaglandin E2. Obstetrics and Gynecology 65: 166–171

Graves G R, Baskett T F, Gray J H, Luther E R 1985 The effect of vaginal administration of various doses of prostaglandin E2 gel on cervical ripening and induction of labour. American Journal of Obstetrics and Gynecology 151: 178–181

Halle H, Hengst P 1979 Der einsatz von prostaglandin F2α in der nachgeburtsperiode. Zentralblatt für Gynäkologie 101: 916–917

Hauth J C, Cunningham F G, Whalley P J 1977 Early labour initiation with oral PGE2 after premature rupture of the membranes at term. Obstetrics and Gynecology 49: 523–526

Hayashi R H, Castillo M S, Noah M L 1984 Management of severe postpartum haemorrhage with a PGF2α analogue. Obstetrics and Gynecology 63: 806–808

Heinzl S, Hendry M 1986 Die Behandlung der postpartalen Atonie mit Prostaglandinen. Zeitschrifte für Geburtshilfe und Perinatologie 190: 92–94

Henson G, Gough J D, Gillmer M D 1983 Control of persistent primary postpartum haemorrhage due to uterine atony with intravenous prostaglandin E2: case report. British Journal of Obstetrics and Gynaecology 90: 280–282

Hertz R H, Sokol R J, Dierker L J 1980 Treatment of postpartum uterine atony with prostaglandin E2 vaginal suppositories. Obstetrics and Gynecology 56: 129–139

Heyl P S, Stubblefield P G, Phillippe M 1984 Recurrent inversion of the puerperal uterus managed with 15(s)15methyl prostaglandin F2α and uterine packing. Obstetrics and Gynecology 63: 263–264

Hillier K, Wallis R M 1981 Prostaglandins, steroids and the human cervix. In Ellwood D A, Anderson A B M (eds) The cervix in pregnancy and labour. Churchill Livingstone, London, pp 144–162

Hunter I W E, Cato E, Ritchie J 1984 Induction of labor using high dose or low dose prostaglandin vaginal pessaries. Obstetrics and Gynecology 63: 418–420

Husslein P, Fuchs A R, Fuchs F 1981 Oxytocin and the initiation of human labor. I. Prostaglandin release during induction of labor by oxytocin. American Journal of Obstetrics and Gynecology 141: 688–697

Husslein P 1985 Mode of action of oxytocin and the role of its receptors in the production of prostaglandins. In: Wood C (ed) The role of prostaglandins in labour. Royal Society of Medicine Symposium No 92, pp 15–24

Insull G M, Cooke I, MacKenzie I Z 1989 Tocolysis during cervical ripening with vaginal PGE2. British Journal of Obstetrics and Gynaecology 96: 179–182

Karim S M M, Trussell R R, Patel R C, Hillier K 1968 Response of pregnant human uterus to prostaglandin F2α—induction of labour. British Medical Journal 4: 621–623

Karim S M M, Lim A L, Prasad R N V et al 1979 Termination of abnormal intrauterine pregnancy with intramuscular administration of sulprostone. Singapore Journal of Obstetrics and Gynecology 10: 33–37

Kennedy J H, Stewart P, Barlow D H, Hillan E, Calder A A 1982 Induction of labour: a comparison of a single prostaglandin E2 vaginal tablet with amniotomy and intravenous oxytocin. British Journal of Obstetrics and Gynaecology 89: 704–707

Kerekes L, Domokos N 1979 The effects of prostaglandin F2α on the third stage of labour. Prostaglandins 18: 161–166

Khoo P P T, Kalshekar M, Jogee M, Elder M G 1981 Induction of labour with prostaglandin E2 vaginal tablets. European Journal of Obstetrics and Gynecology and Reproductive Biology 11: 313–318

Lange A P, Secher N J, Nielsen F H, Pederson G T 1981 Stimulation of labor in cases of premature rupture of the membranes at or near term: a consecutive randomised study of prostaglandin E2 tablets and intravenous oxytocin. Acta Obstetrica et Gynecologica Scandinavica 70: 207–210

Leung A, Kwok P, Chang A 1987 Association between prostaglandin E2 and placental abruption. British Journal of Obstetrics and Gynaecology 94: 1001–1002

Lippert T H, Luthi A 1978 Induction of labour with prostaglandin E2 gel in cases of intrauterine fetal death. Prostaglandins 15: 533–542

MacKenzie I Z 1981 Clinical studies on cervical ripening. In: Ellwood D A, Anderson A B M (eds) The cervix in pregnancy and labour. Churchill Livingstone, London, pp 161–186

MacKenzie I Z 1987 The clinical use of prostaglandins for cervical ripening and induction of labour. In: Hillier K (ed) Eicosanoids and reproduction. M.T.P. Press, Lancaster, pp 195–224

MacKenzie I Z 1988 Previous Caesarean section and labour induction with PGE2. In: Egarter C, Husslein P (eds) Prostaglandins for cervical ripening and/or induction of labour. Facultas Universitätsverlag, Vienna, pp 53–57

MacKenzie I Z, Embrey M P 1977 Cervical ripening with intravaginal prostaglandin E2 gel. British Medical Journal 2: 1381–1384

MacKenzie I Z, Embrey M P 1979 A comparison of PGE2 and PGF2α vaginal gel for ripening the cervix before induction of labour. British Journal of Obstetrics and Gynaecology 85: 657–661

MacKenzie I Z, Embrey M P 1981 Prostaglandins in obstetrics. British Medical Journal 283: 142

MacKenzie I Z, Bradley S, Embrey M P 1981 A simpler approach to labour induction using a lipid-based prostaglandin E2 vaginal suppository. American Journal of Obstetrics and Gynecology 141: 158–162

MacKenzie I Z, Jenkin G, Bradley S G 1979a The relation between plasma oestrogen, progesterone and prolactin concentrations and the efficacy of vaginal prostaglandin E2 gel in initiating labour. British Journal of Obstetrics and Gynaecology 86: 171–174

MacKenzie I Z, Davies A J, Embrey M P 1979b Fetal death in utero managed with vaginal prostaglandin E2 gel. British Medical Journal ii: 1764–1765

MacKenzie I Z, Bradley S, Mitchell M D 1980 Prostaglandin levels in cord venous plasma at delivery or related to labour. In: Samuelsson B, Ramwell P W, Paoletti R (eds) Advances in Prostaglandin and Thromboxane Research, Vol. 8, Raven Press, New York, pp 1401–1405

MacKenzie I Z, Bradley S, Embrey M P 1984 Vaginal prostaglandins and labour induction for patients previously delivered by Caesarean section. British Journal of Obstetrics and Gynaecology 91: 7–10

MacLennan A, Green R 1979 Cervical ripening and induction of labour with intravaginal PGF2α. Lancet *i*: 117–119

Magos A L, Noble M C B, Wong Ten Yuen A, Rodeck C H 1983 Controlled study comparing vaginal prostaglandin E2 pessaries with intravenous oxytocin for the stimulation of labour after spontaneous rupture of membranes. British Journal of Obstetrics and Gynaecology 90: 726–731

Matthews D D, Hossain H, Bhargava S, D'Souza F 1976 A randomised controlled trial of an oral solution of prostaglandin E2 and oral oxytocin used immediately after low amniotomy for induction of labour in the presence of favourable cervix. Current Medical Research and Opinion 4: 233–240

Molloy B G, Sheil O, Duignan N M 1987 Delivery after Caesarean section: review of 2176 consecutive cases. British Medical Journal 294: 1645–1647

Mundow L S 1977 The induction of labour with prostaglandin E2 tablets. Journal of the Irish Medical Association 70: 74–75

Neilson D R, Prins R P, Bolton R N, Mark C, Watson P 1983 A comparison of prostaglandin E2 gel and prostaglandin F2α gel for pre-induction cervical ripening. American Journal of Obstetrics and Gynecology 146: 526–530

O'Herlihy C 1981 Vaginal prostaglandin E2 gel and breech presentation. European Journal of Obstetrics Gynecology and Reproductive Biology 11: 299–303

O'Herlihy C, MacDonald H N 1979 Influence of pre-induction prostaglandin E2 gel on cervical ripening and labour induction. Obstetrics and Gynecology 54: 708–710

Phelan J P, Clark S L, Diaz F, Paul R H 1987 Vaginal birth after Caesarean section. American Journal of Obstetrics and Gynecology 157: 1510–1515

Prendiville W J, Harding J E, Elbourne D R, Stirrat G M 1988 The Bristol third stage trial: active versus physiological management of third stage of labour. British Medical Journal 297: 1295–1300

Quinn M A, Murphy A J 1981 Fetal death following extra-amniotic prostaglandin gel: report of two cases. British Journal of Obstetrics and Gynaecology 88: 650–651

Reed M D, Mattock E J 1982 Cervical ripening with prostaglandin E2 pessaries—a question of dose. Journal of Obstetrics and Gynaecology 3: 71–74

Rutland A, Ballard C 1977 Vaginal prostaglandin E2 for missed abortion and intrauterine fetal death. American Journal of Obstetrics and Gynecology 128: 503–505

Saruta T, Kaplan N M 1972 Adrenocortical steroidogenesis: the effects of prostaglandins. Journal of Clinical Investigation 51: 2246–2251

Schwartz R H, Jones R W A 1978 Transplacental hyponatraemia due to oxytocin. British Medical Journal i: 152–153

Selinger M, MacKenzie I Z, Gillmer M D, Phipps S, Ferguson J 1987 Progesterone inhibition in midtrimester termination of pregnancy: physiological and clinical effects. British Journal of Obstetrics and Gynaecology 94: 1218–1222

Sellers S M 1985 Plasma concentrations of prostaglandins and oxytocin in labour. In: Wood C (ed) The role of prostaglandins in labour. Royal Society of Medicine Services Symposium No. 92, pp 45–50

Sellers S M, Ah-Moy M, MacKenzie I Z 1988 Randomised controlled trial of vaginal PGE2 versus intravenous oxytocin for labour induction in cases of previous Caesarean section. Abstracts for First European Congress on Prostaglandins in Reproduction, Vienna

Sellers S M, MacKenzie I Z 1985 Prostaglandin release following vaginal prostaglandin treatment for labour induction. In: Wood C (ed) The role of prostaglandins in labour. Royal Society of Medicine Services Symposium No. 92, pp 77–84

Shepherd J H, Pearce J M F, Sims C 1979 Induction of labour using prostaglandin E2 pessaries. British Medical Journal ii: 108–110

Shepherd J H, Bennett M, Laurence D, Moore F, Sims C D 1981 Prostaglandin vaginal suppositories: a simple and safe approach to the induction of labour. Obstetrics and Gynecology 58: 596–600

Southern E M, Gutnecht G D, Mohberg N R, Edelman D A 1978 Vaginal prostaglandin E 2 in the management of fetal intrauterine death. British Journal of Obstetrics and Gynaecology 85: 437–441

Steiner H, Zahradnik H P, Beckwoldt M, Robrecht D, Hillemanns H G 1979 Cervical ripening prior to induction of labour (intracervical application of PGE2 viscous gel). Prostaglandins 17: 125–133

Stewart P, Calder A A 1981 Cervical ripening. British Journal of Obstetrics and Gynaecology 88: 1071–1072

Takagi S, Yoshida T, Togo T, et al 1976 The effects of intramyometrial injection of PGF2α on severe postpartum haemorrhage. Prostaglandins 12: 565–579

Thiery M, Delbeke L 1985 Acute puerperal uterine inversion: two-step management with a β-mimetic and a prostaglandin. American Journal of Obstetrics and Gynecology 153: 891–892

Thiery M, Parewijck W 1985 Local administration of 15(s)-15methyl PGF2α for management of hypotonic postpartum haemorrhage. Zeitschrifte für Geburtshilfe Perinatologie 189: 179–180

Thiery M, Parewijck W, de Grezelle H et al 1977 Pre-induction ripening of the cervix with extra-amniotic prostaglandin E2 gel. Zeitschrifte für Geburtshilfe und Perinatologie 182: 251–357

Thiery M, Parewijck W, Martens G 1982 Intravenous infusion of prostaglandin E2 for management of premature rupture of membranes. Zeitschrifte für Geburtshilfe und Perinatolgie 186: 87–88

Thorburn G D, Challis J R G 1979 Endocrine control of parturition. Physiological Reviews 59: 863–918

Toppozada M, Warda A, Ramada M 1979 Intramuscular 16-phenoxy-PGE2 ester for pregnancy termination. Prostaglandins 17: 461–467

Ulmsten U, Wingerup L, Belfrage P, Ekman G, Wiqvist N 1982 Intracervical application of prostaglandin gel for induction of term labor. Obstetrics and Gynecology 59: 336–339

Van Pelt C, De Coster W, Thiery M et al 1984 Preinduction cervical ripening with prostaglandin E2: influence on psychomotor evolution in the first year. European Journal of Obstetrics, Gynecology and Reproductive Biology 18: 299–301

Wallenburg H C S, Keirse M J N C, Freie H M P, Blacquiere J F 1980 Intramuscular administration of 15(s)-15methyl Prostaglandin F2α for induction of labour in patients with fetal death. British Journal of Obstetrics and Gynaecology 87: 203–209

Wilson P D 1978 A comparison of four methods of ripening the unfavourable cervix. British Journal of Obstetrics and Gynaecology 85: 941–944

Zahradnik H P, Steiner H, Hillemans H G, Breckwoldt M, Ardelt W 1977 Prostaglandin PF2α und 15 methyl-prostaglandin F2α-anwendung bei massiven uterinen blutungen. Geburtshilfe Frauenheilk 37: 493–495

12. Human immunodeficiency virus infection

Alison Webster   Margaret Johnson

INTRODUCTION

The acquired immune deficiency syndrome (AIDS) was first recognized in male homosexuals in 1981 (Morbidity and Mortality Weekly Report 1981). This group still forms the largest group of HIV-infected individuals in the developed world, and also accounts for the majority of AIDS patients. Consequently, most of the data gathered concerning the natural history of HIV infection has been amassed by follow-up of this patient group.

Natural history of HIV infection

Initial infection with HIV may be asymptomatic, or may produce an acute glandular fever-like seroconversion illness, and antibodies are detectable in serum usually within 6 weeks. Subsequently, the HIV infection may remain clinically silent for a variable period of time, and this may correspond to the virus establishing a latent infection within various cell types (reviewed by Fauci 1988). The mean incubation period for AIDS is estimated to be about 8–10 years from the time of seroconversion (Moss et al 1988, Lui et al 1988). It has been suggested that as yet unidentified factors may precipitate the onset of AIDS in HIV-infected individuals. Persistent generalized lymphadenopathy (PGL) may be present for many years before AIDS develops, and does not adversely affect the prognosis in otherwise asymptomatic patients.

With the development of AIDS there is a progressive loss of CD4-positive lymphocytes leading to loss of immune surveillance, and hence the appearance of opportunistic infections and tumours. Typically, p24 Ag, a protein present in the core of the virus, is detectable in serum at the time of seroconversion, but then becomes undetectable, only to reappear late in the course of disease when it indicates a poor prognosis (Allain et al 1987). Antibodies to this viral protein show a reverse trend, and are therefore inversely related to disease progression; there is, however, wide individual variation.

Serum beta-2 microglobulin, a component of the class I histocompatibility complex, is found in the serum of HIV-infected individuals, presumably as a result of lymphocyte turnover, and levels rise during the course of the disease (Zolla-Pazner et al 1984). Neopterin is produced by stimulated macrophages, and elevated levels have been found in the urine and serum of patients with AIDS; again levels tend to rise as disease progresses (Fuchs et al 1988). Measurement of both of these substances has been shown to be useful in determining the prognosis of HIV-infected individuals. Unfortunately, these assays are not widely available outside research laboratories.

Sequential measurement of all the above parameters is likely to provide the most information on disease progression in an individual patient. There has been much speculation as to whether all HIV-infected individuals will eventually develop AIDS; there is as yet no conclusive evidence that this is not the case, although a few asymptomatic individuals have been documented to lose anti-HIV antibodies.

A second human immunodeficiency virus, HIV2, has been identified, and is prevalent mainly in West Africa (reviewed in Editorial, Lancet 1988). It has been suggested that this virus may be less virulent than HIV1, with a longer incubation period to AIDS; in other respects the natural history of HIV2 infection is as described above for HIV1. Most assays currently in routine use for the detection of HIV antibodies will not however detect antibodies to HIV2, and specific tests must therefore be performed. At present, infection with HIV2 is very infrequent in the UK.

Zidovudine (azidothymidine, AZT) is the only drug so far shown to be of proven benefit in AIDS, in that it decreases the frequency of opportunistic infections, and increases patient survival (Fischl et al 1987a). Unfortunately, it is associated with significant toxicity in these patients, the most limiting of which are anaemia, which can be treated by regular blood transfusions, and a reversible neutropenia which must be managed by dose modification. Multicentre trials are currently being conducted in the USA and in the UK and France to assess the safety and efficacy of zidovudine in halting disease progression in asymptomatic HIV-infected patients. The expectation is that inhibition of viral replication will arrest the disease at an early stage, and that these patients, being in a much better state of general health than AIDS patients, will suffer fewer serious side-effects. However, these patients may find minor side-effects, such as nausea and headache, to be less acceptable than do more severely ill patients with AIDS.

Many other agents with documented in vitro activity against HIV are currently being assessed as possible therapies for HIV disease and alternative approaches, such as using CD4 molecules to block HIV attachment to lymphocytes (Capon et al 1989), offer new prospects for HIV therapy.

There is as yet no evidence that the natural history of HIV infection in women, or its response to treatment, differs from that described above, with the exception being that Kaposi's sarcoma is less frequent in women with AIDS, being found in only 1% of females, as opposed to 3% of heterosexual and 23% of homosexual males (Saltzman et al 1988). Two additional areas must be considered which are relevant to women with HIV: pregnancy and childbearing, dealt with in detail below, and cervical dysplasia. Immunocompromised women following renal transplantation are at increased risk of cervical dysplasia (Halpert et al 1986); there is some evidence that this is also the case for HIV-infected women. An increased incidence of cervical dysplasia has been reported in HIV-infected as opposed to uninfected prostitutes (Muggiasca et al 1989). Women who have acquired HIV infection as a result of sexual promiscuity may be especially at risk of this complication. All HIV-infected women should thus have regular cervical smear examinations. There is no information about HIV infection and the incidence of vulval dystrophies in young women, and this clearly needs further study.

Heterosexual transmission

The first women identified as having AIDS were intravenous drug abusers (IVDA) in the United States. This group still forms the majority of HIV-infected women, and women with AIDS, in Europe, North America and Australia. Blood transfusion-acquired AIDS was also recognized in women, but as a result of screening of blood donors, this mode of transmission has now been virtually eliminated.

It subsequently became clear that AIDS could be acquired by heterosexual contact; a ratio of HIV-infected males:females approaching 1:1 confirms this as the major means of transmission in sub-Saharan Africa, and consequently, by extrapolation, the major means of transmission worldwide. The contribution of heterosexually-acquired HIV infection in this country appears to be rising. HIV has been isolated from blood, semen, saliva, female genital tract secretions, and breast milk, and transmission could therefore theoretically occur via exchange of any of these body fluids. Heterosexual transmission has been documented to occur from both male to female, and vice versa, but it is not clear whether the efficiency of transmission is increased in one or other direction. Studies of this phenomenon are confounded by the fact that, unless seroconversion is demonstrated, it is impossible to prove which partner was infected first.

Widely differing rates of HIV seropositivity amongst spouses of AIDS patients have been reported (Kim et al 1988, Fischl et al 1987b, Padian et al 1987, Mann et al 1986, Peterman et al 1988). Predictably, the risk of heterosexually acquired HIV infection shows a correlation with the number of sexual partners. In addition, several factors have recently been associated with HIV seropositivity, including various sexually transmitted diseases, receptive anal intercourse, and intercourse during menses. Since these factors may simply be markers of sexual promiscuity, it is necessary to control for the number of sexual exposures.

There is good evidence for an association of HIV transmission with anal intercourse (Padian et al 1987, Zorilla et al 1989), herpes simplex virus type 2 (Holmberg et al 1988), and for *Haemophilus ducreyi* (chancroid) among patients in Africa (Kreiss et al 1986, Holmberg et al 1988, Piot et al 1989). There is also evidence of an association with syphilis (Quinn et al 1988), *Chlamydia trachomatis* (Plummer et al 1988) and gonorrhoea (Fischl et al 1988). Breaching of the mucosal barrier as a result of genital ulceration, or due to trauma associated with anal intercourse, presumably increases the efficiency of exchange of infected blood or body fluids. In addition, the recruitment of inflammatory cells during a genital-tract infection may also increase the likelihood of transmission of virus. Genital ulcer disease is more prevalent in Africa than in Europe and North America, and is therefore likely to be a more frequent risk factor for HIV transmission in African patients.

The stage of HIV disease, as judged by the CD4-cell count or presence of symptoms of AIDS, has not been conclusively shown to influence transmission of HIV. Several conflicting reports have been published but it is clear that completely asymptomatic individuals may transmit virus. Within a monogamous relationship, there appears to be no correlation between the number of acts of sexual intercourse and the risk of acquiring HIV, although recently it has been suggested that the risk of HIV transmission increases with number of exposures, but in a non-linear fashion (Padian & Shiboski 1989). The role that these factors play in transmission cannot be elucidated by prospective study, since partners of HIV-infected individuals are advised to refrain from unprotected sexual intercourse as soon as the infection is recognized. Other, as yet unidentified factors may affect transmission, such as the viral strain involved, or the individual's susceptibility to infection. Despite the theoretical risk, there is no evidence that activities such as kissing or biting are involved in transmission of HIV.

Epidemiology

Although intravenous drug abusers account for the majority of HIV-infected women in the United Kingdom identified so far, this is not the case in other parts of the world where heterosexual transmission plays the major role. High rates of HIV seropositivity have been reported among prostitutes in many cities in Central and East Africa, and these rates appear to have risen rapidly in recent years. More than 80% of Nairobi prostitutes are now reported to be infected (Plummer et al 1987). Use of prostitutes is strongly influenced by cultural factors, and there is evidence that this behaviour is more frequent in Africa than in Europe. We would conclude that female prostitution play a major role in the progression of the AIDS epidemic in Central and East Africa.

In Europe and North America, prostitution is linked with IVDA, and widely differing rates of HIV seropositivity are reported for this group, depending on whether or not they admit to IVDA. For example, HIV-seroprevalence in Italy has been reported to vary from less than 2% of non-IVDA prostitutes to 36% of IVDA prostitutes (Tirelli et al 1989). Intravenous drug abusers are likely to have sexual partners who are also IVDA, and possibly HIV-infected, thus some cases of heterosexually acquired HIV may have been misclassified as IVDA-acquired. A number of recent reports suggest a change to safer sexual practices by prostitutes with clients, but they may continue to have unsafe sex with private partners (Hooykaas et al 1989).

In the United States, AIDS and HIV infection appear to be more frequent amongst Black and Hispanic women than Whites, and it appears that these individuals are concentrated within major cities. This observation could be related to the fact that male intravenous drug abusers from these ethnic groups within the same cities also have a high incidence of HIV infection (Haverkos & Endelman 1988).

Various studies have attempted to assess the prevalence of HIV infection in the general population. HIV seroprevalence amongst female applicants for military service in the United States during 1985/86 was 0.061% (Burke et al 1987). This may be an underestimate of the prevalence, since women with risk factors for HIV infection may be under-represented among military service applicants. Similarly, the rate of HIV infection among blood donors may underestimate the prevalence in the population as a whole. Conversely, women attending clinics for sexually transmitted diseases are likely to have more risk factors for HIV disease. Recent surveys have revealed that less than 0.1–3.0% of women attending STD clinics in Europe and the USA are HIV infected (Table 12.1).

Table 12.1   HIV seroprevalence among female STD clinic attenders in the United States and Britain

Study population	Year	Number	HIV pos (%)	Ref.
San Francisco	1988	N/S	(0.7%)	1
Washington state	1988	528	4 (0.8%)	2
Los Angeles County	1988	782	8 (1%)	3
North Carolina	1988	N/S	(0.5%)	4
Baltimore	1987	1310	4 (3%)	5
USA multicentre	1988/9	N/S	(3%)	6
London	1987	412	4 (1%)	7
	1987	1115	3 (0.3%)	8
	1988	2025	3 (0.1%)	9
South-East Thames region	1986	233	3 (1.3%)	10
	1987	949	7 (0.7%)	10
Other regions in England and Wales	1986	752	3 (0.4%)	10
	1987	4778	1 (0.02%)	10

1. Wilson et al 1989; 2. Handsfield et al 1989; 3. Ford et al 1989; 4. Landis et al 1989; 5. Quinn et al 1988; 6. McCray et al 1989; 7. Loveday et al 1989; 8. Evans et al 1988; 9. Barlow et al 1989; 10. Collaborative study group 1989.

In order to obtain a more representative sample of sexually active women, investigators have turned their attention to women attending for obstetric services, although women who are infertile, or elect not to become pregnant, would not be included by such an approach. Samples for antibody testing have either been collected antenatally, or at the time of delivery from mother or infant. Infant heel-prick samples, collected on filter paper for determination of metabolic disease, have been used in some seroepidemiologic surveys. Some studies have been conducted anonymously on samples from which all identifying information has been removed, whilst others have sought the woman's consent before testing. Unfortunately, the results of these studies are not comparable as there is evidence that women who refuse HIV testing have a higher incidence of HIV infection than those who consent (O'Sullivan et al 1989).

Surveys undertaken at the time of delivery will exclude those women who undergo elective termination of pregnancy, or spontaneous abortion; they may provide useful information on the number of predicted paediatric AIDS cases, but not the incidence of HIV infection in the female population.

Anonymous testing may provide useful epidemiological data but unfortunately, individual infected women cannot be identified and appropriately managed. Testing with consent has the advantage of being able to identify seropositive women, but may exclude many who decline to be tested. Information useful to both the epidemiologist and the individual patient will be derived by employing the two testing systems in parallel. The alternative strategy, compulsory testing, is unlikely to be ethically acceptable.

Results of recent anonymous surveys have revealed that from 0.02% (London) to 4.4% (Newark, New Jersey) of women in Europe and the United States are infected (Table 12.2). However, these figures may mask wide variations in seropositivity within individual hospitals, depending on the risk factors of the population that they serve. HIV seropositivity rates among similar patients in Africa are likely to be far higher; surveys of antenatal clinic patients in Africa over the past few years have revealed that between 4% and 13.5% of women are infected (Table 12.2).

PREGNANCY WITH HIV INFECTION

There are conflicting reports as to the effect of pregnancy on the course of HIV disease. CD4-cell counts fall during pregnancy, and recover during the post-partum period. These changes are paralleled, but at a lower level, in HIV infected women, although there is some evidence that counts may not recover to their pre-pregnancy levels in these patients (Delfraissy et al 1989a). Although a number of studies have suggested that pregnancy is not associated with progression of HIV disease (Berebbi et al 1989a, Selwyn et al 1989, MacCallum et al 1989), there have been two recent case-

Table 12.2   HIV seroprevalence among antenatal patients or newborns in Africa, the United States, and Europe

Study population	Year	Infants (I) Mothers (M)	Number	HIV pos	Ref
Lusaka, Zambia	1985	M	184	8.7%	1
Kinshasa, Zaire	1986/7	M, I	8108	5.8%	2
Ivory Coast	1987	M	1000	4%	3
Malawi	1987	M	290	6.5%	4
Uganda	1987	M	1011	13.5%	5
State of Massachusetts	1986/7	I	30 708	2.1%	6
State of New York	1987/8	I	276 609	0.66%	7
State of New Jersey	1988	I	29 309	0.49%	8
Newark, New Jersey	1987/8	I	2205	4.4%	9
Miami, Florida	1988	I*	7400	2.3%	10
Los Angeles County	1988	I	7186	0.04%	11
New York City	1987/8	I	224	2.7%	12
London	1988	I	46 600	0.02%	13
Italy	1988	I	20 683	0.09%	14
Paris	N/S	M*	30 525	0.9%	15

* Only those mothers/infants giving consent were screened.
1. Melbye et al 1986; 2. Ryder et al 1989b; 3. Leonard et al 1988; 4. Ntaba et al 1988; 5. Giraldo et al 1988; 6. Hoff et al 1988; 7. Novick et al 1989; 8. Altman et al 1989; 9. Connor et al 1989; 10. O'Sullivan et al 1989; 11. Hill et al 1989; 12. Sperling et al 1989; 13. Tedder et al 1989; 14. Ippolito et al 1989; 15. Goudeau et al 1989.

controlled studies, in Haiti (Deschamps et al 1989) and France (Delfraissy et al 1989b) which have reported that pregnancy adversely affects the course of HIV disease, although in the French study this association was observed only in women who carried their pregnancies to term, not among those whose pregnancies were aborted. The weight of evidence appears to be in favour of pregnancy per se having no effect on disease progression in HIV positive women when compared with nonpregnant controls. Transient p24 antigenaemia has been described during pregnancy, but seems to have no particular significance in terms of maternal or fetal HIV disease. There is no evidence from European studies that maternal HIV infection is associated with intrauterine growth retardation (IUGR) or prematurity when their infants are compared with those born to uninfected women with similar behavioural factors, such as drug abuse and smoking (Johnstone et al 1988, Berrebi et al 1989b). However, a higher incidence of prematurity, IUGR and perinatal mortality has been recently reported among infants born to HIV-seropositive mothers when compared with those born to seronegative mothers in Zaire (Ryder et al 1989b).

Perinatal infection

Infants born to HIV-infected women are at risk of HIV infection in utero, at the time of birth, or postnatally. Virus has been isolated from fetuses obtained at therapeutic abortion, and viral antigen has been demonstrated in fetal tissues, confirming that in utero transmission may occur. The presence of p24 antigen in cord blood in the absence of maternal anti-genaemia is highly suggestive of in utero transmission of virus. A recent study, using the polymerase chain reaction, reports that 22 out of 33 spleens obtained from fetuses aborted at 16–24 weeks were found to be positive for the HIV genome (Courgnaud et al 1989). An HIV embryopathy has been described as an infrequent complication of in utero transmission (Marion et al 1986). However, the existence of a specific HIV embryopathy has been disputed since many of the facial abnormalities described are susceptible to observer bias, or may be related to other maternal behavioural factors (Cordero 1988, Garn 1988). HIV is present in blood and genital tract secretions of infected women, and theoretically the infant may be exposed to infected body fluids at the time of delivery, whichever mode of delivery is employed. There is as yet no good evidence that the mode of delivery affects the risk of HIV transmission, and therefore there are at present no grounds on which to recommend delivery by Caesarian section if this is not otherwise indicated.

Recently, postnatal transmission of HIV via breast feeding has been documented (Colebunders et al 1988). Only a small number of infants have been identified who have been infected via this route. These were babies born to women infected with HIV post-partum as a result of blood transfusion, or (in one case) a seroconverting intravenous drug-abusing woman. However, HIV infection of women in the immediate post-partum period is likely to be a rare event with the advent of screening of blood donors, and infectivity of breast milk at the time of maternal primary infection may not be representative of the more usual situation where maternal infection precedes pregnancy. The additional risk that breast feeding represents in the transmission of HIV has yet to be determined.

Determining the rate of ante- or perinatal transmission of HIV is beset by several problems. All infants born to HIV seropositive mothers will have passively acquired IgG, and therefore conventional serological testing cannot confirm or refute infection in the neonate. This antibody may be detectable for many months; currently, persistence of antibody beyond the age of 15 months is regarded as indicative of infection in the child. Unfortunately, IgM estimations are unhelpful in this situation; presence or absence of this immunoglobulin class has been shown not to correlate with other evidence of infection (Ryder et al 1989a).

In order to confirm infection within the first 15 months of life, it is necessary to demonstrate viraemia, or p24 antigenaemia, although p24 Ag may be present in the neonatal period as a result of passive transfer from antigenaemic mothers. Virus isolation is a laborious technique, requiring lymphocyte cultivation, and is therefore usually undertaken only in reference laboratories. A recent report suggests that in vitro synthesis of

HIV-specific antibody by lymphocytes obtained from neonates may also be a useful way of determining their HIV status (Amadori et al 1988). Detection of viral genomes, using the polymerase chain reaction (PCR) is an extremely sensitive technique, which can be undertaken using minute quantities of tissue. This method has been reported to detect evidence of HIV infection in adult contacts of HIV-infected individuals several months before seroconversion was documented. The technique however is prone to laboratory contamination, and hence false positive results, and it has not been evaluated in a routine diagnostic setting. The high rate of HIV infection detected by PCR in fetal spleens described above does not correlate with the rates of HIV infection reported by follow-up of infants (see below), although the two types of study are not directly comparable. A recent study among infants has reported a good correlation between a positive result for the HIV genome by PCR, and eventual development of AIDS (Rogers et al 1989).

At present, in the absence of a positive viral isolate or p24 antigenaemia, infants must be followed up for at least 15 months in order to determine their HIV status. A large number of infants are labelled as being of 'indeterminate' HIV status until they reach this age, and this must be very distressing to the mothers. The situation is further complicated by the fact that AIDS has recently been described in children who were previously antibody-negative (Aiuti et al 1987).

It has recently been suggested by mathematical modelling that the incubation period of paediatric AIDS may have two distributions, one with a median of 4.1 months, and the other with a median of 6.1 years (Auger et al 1988). It is tempting to surmise that these differing incubation periods may result from differing modes of transmission of HIV, i.e. in utero as opposed to perinatal.

The results of several large studies have now been reported, where infants have been followed until at least 15 months of age, or until death from AIDS or AIDS-related complex (Table 12.3). Most of the mothers in

Table 12.3   Perinatal transmission of HIV to infants followed for at least 15 months

Study population	Number	Mother with AIDS (%)	Infants infected (%)	Ref
Europe	100	5%	24 (24%)	1
Italy	89	N/S	29 (33%)	2
France	117	3%	32 (27%)	3
Zaire	92	18%	36 (39%)	4
Uganda	87	N/S	29 (33%)	5

1. European Collaborative Study 1988; 2. Italian Multicentre Study 1988; 3. Blanche et al 1989; 4. Ryder et al 1989b; 5. Mworozi et al 1989.

the European studies were IVDA, and so may not be representative of all HIV-infected women. Transmission rates of between 24% and 39% were reported by these groups. These figures, although showing reasonable agreement, may be an underestimate of the true transmission rate, for the reasons outlined above. Stage of maternal disease did not appear to affect HIV transmission, although very few of the women in the European studies had symptoms of HIV disease, whereas 18% of the African women in one study had AIDS. It is quite clear however that women with good immunological function can transmit virus to their offspring (Rehmet et al 1989). However, Davachi and Kabena (1989) have reported a very high perinatal mortality (90%) among children born to women with AIDS in Africa; the quality of care that these women are able to provide may be responsible for this depressing statistic.

At present, there is no available therapy which has been shown to interrupt transmission of virus from mother to infant. Antiviral agents such as zidovudine may have a role to play in this setting, and the pharmacokinetics of this drug are currently being investigated in pregnant women (Watts et al 1989). However, it will be some time before the safety and efficacy of zidovudine are established in this situation. If a beneficial effect of this drug is demonstrated in ongoing trials in asymptomatic, non-pregnant patients, it will be important to establish whether this therapy can be safely continued through pregnancy.

MANAGEMENT

In the UK, reports of HIV infection in women are rare outside those groups acknowledged to be at high risk, principally intravenous drug abusers, and sexual contacts of bisexual or African men. Heterosexual transmission is, however, becoming increasingly important in the United Kingdom (Gill et al 1989). Women at risk of HIV infection may decline testing for a variety of reasons. However, women should be made aware of the benefits of knowing their HIV status so that they may receive optimal medical care and appropriate advice. It is important that medical and nursing staff in general practice family-planning clinics receive adequate training so that they can identify and counsel women at risk. Unfortunately, these women may have infrequent contact with medical services, and unless they positively seek HIV testing, the opportunity to discuss this matter will not arise. Diagnosing HIV infection at an antenatal clinic visit is not wholly satisfactory in that this deprives the woman of her choice of whether to conceive in full knowledge of her HIV status.

HIV is a progressive immunological disease, and for this reason all HIV-infected individuals should be regularly reviewed so that onset of HIV disease may be anticipated, and appropriate therapy instituted at the earliest possible opportunity, as this will improve survival. Monitoring of CD4 lymphocyte counts and p24 antigen will provide important information on the stage of HIV disease, and regular clinical examination may detect early signs of opportunistic infection. Examination should also include regular cervical cytological screening. Women who fulfill the criteria for diagnosis of AIDS should be offered zidovudine therapy and also prophylaxis to prevent *Pneumocystis carinii* pneumonia. They should be monitored closely for signs of toxicity and development of opportunistic infections or tumours. HIV-infected women should be counselled as to the risks of transmission to their sexual partners and how to reduce these risks, and should be encouraged to bring forward their partners for counselling and HIV testing.

The male condom is the only widely available method for protection of sexual partners from acquiring HIV, and its efficacy in preventing transmission is likely to be increased by concomitant use of a spermicide such as nonoxynol-9, which has antiviral activity. Unfortunately, faults may occur during manufacture of condoms, and they may rupture or slip off during use, so reducing their effectiveness. The recently developed female condom, a flexible polyurethane membrane which covers the cervix, vagina and external genitalia, is claimed to be less susceptible to these faults. The reader should refer to Chapter 26 on barrier methods of contraception for further details.

Asymptomatic women attending for monitoring of HIV infection may also be offered the opportunity of participating in trials of therapy.

Women with AIDS should be advised not to become pregnant, since their long-term prognosis is currently poor, and the risks to the fetus are significant. These facts should be explained, and termination recommended should pregnancy arise.

Pregnancy in asymptomatic HIV-infected women is a vexed issue. The long-term prognosis for these women is unclear, but there is no evidence as yet that pregnancy adversely affects the course of HIV disease. However, there are clearly significant risks of transmission of HIV to the infant. There is no evidence to support the theory that the risks of transmission from mother to infant increase progressively with time, and so we can see no reason to advise women who are determined to conceive to do so earlier rather than later, except for reasons of the individual woman's life expectancy. At present, we would advise any HIV-infected woman not to conceive, since a minimum of about one-quarter to one-third of infants born will be HIV-infected, and the future for such infected infants remains depressing. However, many women conceive despite advice to the contrary (Kaplan et al 1989). The currently available information on the risks of HIV transmission should be explained to them, and termination offered.

It is also clear that many women choose to carry their pregnancies to term (Barbacci et al 1989b), perhaps because of our present inability to diagnose infection in the infant antenatally. In view of the possible risks of transmission via breast milk, women in developed countries should be discouraged from breast feeding as suitable alternative formula feeds are available, and HIV-infected women should not contribute to milk banks. Transmission of HIV on the labour or post-natal ward could theoretically occur via contact of blood or other body fluids with broken skin or mucous membranes. However, if current practices on the ward adhere to those recommended for the prevention of transmission of hepatitis B, then additional measures need not be taken. Thus staff will be protected against transmission of HIV from patients whose HIV infection is not suspected at the time of delivery, and identified HIV-infected women will not be subjected to the stigma of excessive isolation procedures.

Infants should be monitored from birth for the presence of signs and symptoms of AIDS, and serum samples for determination of antibody status and p24 antigenaemia should be obtained at regular intervals, together with lymphocytes for virus isolation or genome detection. It is unfortunate that many mothers must remain in doubt as to their infant's HIV status for many months, and that the development of AIDS remains a possibility, even in infants previously thought to be uninfected due to loss of HIV antibody.

REFERENCES

Aiuti F, Luzi G, Mezzaroma I, Scano G, Papetti C 1987 Delayed appearance of HIV infection in children. Lancet ii: 858
Allain J P, Laurian Y, Paul D A et al 1987 Long term evaluation of p24 antigen and antibodies to p24 and gp41 in patients with haemophilia. Potential clinical importance. New England Journal of Medicine 317: 1114–1121
Altman R, Grant C M, Brandon D et al 1989 Statewide HIV1 serologic survey of newborns with resultant changes in screening and delivery system policy. 5th International Conference on AIDS, Montreal, Abstract WA07
Amadori A, de Rossi A, Giaquinto C, Faulkner-Valle G, Zacchello F, Chieci-Bianchi L 1988 In vitro production of HIV-specific antibody in children at risk of AIDS. Lancet i: 852–854
Auger I, Thomas P, De Gruttola V et al 1988 Incubation period for paediatric AIDS cases. Nature 336: 575–577
Barbacci M, Chaisson R, Anderson J, Horn J 1989 Knowledge of HIV serostatus and pregnancy decisions. 5th International Conference on AIDS, Montreal, Abstract MBP10
Barlow D, Bradbeer C, Thin R N, Christie I, Palmer S, Banatvala J E 1989 Heterosexual transmission of HIV is rare among attenders at an STD clinic in London. 5th International Conference on AIDS, Montreal, Abstract MAP58
Berrebi A, Puel J, Tricoire J, Herne H, Pontonnier G 1989a Influence of gestation on HIV infection. 5th International Conference on AIDS, Montreal, Abstract MBP25
Berrebi A, Kobuch W E, Puel J, Tricoire J, Herne P, Fournie A 1989b Effects of HIV infection on pregnancy. 5th International Conference on AIDS, Montreal, Abstract MBP26
Blanche S, Rouzioux C, Moscato M G et al 1989 A prospective study of infants born to women seropositive for human immunodeficiency virus type 1. New England Journal of Medicine 320: 1643–1648
Burke D S, Brundage J F, Herbold J R et al 1987 Human immunodeficiency virus infections among civilian applicants for United States military service, October 1985 to March 1986. New England Journal of Medicine 317: 131–136
Capon D J, Chamow S M, Mordenti J et al 1989 Designing CD4 immunoadhesins for AIDS therapy. Nature 337: 525–531
Colebunders R L, Kapita B, Nekwei W, Bahwe Y, Baenda F, Ryder R 1988 Breast feeding and transmission of HIV. 4th International Conference on AIDS, Stockholm, Abstract 5103

Collaborative Study Group 1989 HIV infection in patients attending clinics for sexually transmitted diseases in England and Wales. British Medical Journal 298: 415–418

Connor E, Thomas D, Goode L et al 1989 Seroprevalence of HIV1 and HTLV1 among pregnant women in Newark, NJ. 5th International Conference on AIDS, Montreal, Abstract MBP19

Cordero J F 1988 Issues concerning AIDS embryopathy. American Journal of Diseases of Childhood 142: 9

Courgnaud V, Laure F, Barin F, Goudaeu A, Brossard A, Brechot C 1989 In utero HIV1 transmission identified through PCR. 5th International Conference on AIDS, Montreal, Abstract MBP1

Davachi F, Kabena M 1989 Outcome of advanced maternal AIDS in offspring. 5th International Conference on AIDS, Montreal, Abstract B646

Delfraissy J, Sereni D, Pons J C, et al 1989a Antigenaemia p24 and CD4 cell counts in HIV pregnant women. 5th International Conference on AIDS, Montreal, Abstract MBP2

Delfraissy J F, Pons J C, Sereni D et al 1989b Does pregnancy influence disease progression in HIV positive women? 5th International Conference on AIDS, Montreal, Abstract MBP34

Deschamps M, Pape J W, Madhavan S, Johnson W D 1989 Pregnancy and acceleration of HIV disease. 5th International Conference on AIDS, Montreal, Abstract MBP6

Editorial 1988 HIV-2 in perspective. Lancet i: 1027–1028

European Collaborative Study 1988 Mother to child transmission of HIV infection. Lancet ii: 1039–1043

Evans B A, McCormack S M, Bond R A, MacCrae K D, Thorp R W 1988 Human immunodeficiency virus infection, hepatitis B virus infection and sexual behaviour of women attending a genitourinary medicine clinic. British Medical Journal 296: 473–475

Fauci A S 1988 The human immunodeficiency virus: infectivity and mechanisms of pathogenesis. Science 239: 617–622

Fischl M A, Richman D D, Grieco M H, et al 1987a The efficacy of azidothymidine (AZT) in the treatment of patients with AIDS and AIDS-related complex. New England Journal of Medicine 317: 185–191

Fischl M A, Dickinson G M, Scott G B, Klimas N, Fletcher M A, Parks W 1987b Evaluation of heterosexual partners, children and household contacts of adults with AIDS. Journal of the American Medical Association 257: 640–644

Fischl M, Fayne T, Flanagan S et al 1988 Seroprevalence and risks of HIV infections in spouses of persons infected with HIV. 4th International Conference on AIDS, Stockholm, Abstract 4060

Ford W L, Rose T, Kerdt P, Onorato L, Waterman S 1989 HIV seroprevalence in sexually transmitted disease clinics in Los Angeles County. 5th International Conference on AIDS, Montreal, Abstract MAP74

Fuchs D, Hausen A, Reibnegger G et al 1988 Neopterin as a marker for activated cell-mediated immunity. Immunology Today 9: 150–155

Garn S M 1988 HIV-related dysmorphogenesis. American Journal of Diseases of Childhood 142: 10

Gill N O, Porter J D H, Ellam G A et al 1989 The extent of heterosexual transmission in England and Wales: evidence from surveillance data. 5th International Conference on AIDS, Montreal, Abstract TAP4

Giraldo G, Serwadda D, Mugerwa R et al 1988 Seroepidemiologic analyses on populations from Uganda and Tunisia—high- and low-risk African regions for HIV. 4th International Conference on AIDS, Stockholm, Abstract 5036

Goudeau A, Brossard Y, Larsen M et al 1989 A prospective sero-epidemiological study of HIV in 30525 pregnant women screened in the Paris metropolitan area between February 1987 and July 1988. 5th International Conference on AIDS, Montreal, Abstract MAP15

Halpert R, Fruchter R G, Sedlis A, Butt K, Boyce J G, Sillman F H 1986 Human papillomavirus and lower genital neoplasia in renal transplant patients. Obstetrics and Gynecology 68: 251–258

Handsfield H H, Sohlberg E, Hopkins S, Swenson P D, Harris N 1989 Trends in HIV seroprevalence in an urban sexually transmitted disease clinic 1986–1989. 5th International Conference on AIDS, Montreal, Abstract MAP61

Haverkos H W, Endelman R 1988 The epidemiology of acquired immunodeficiency syndrome among heterosexuals. Journal of the American Medical Association 260: 1922–1929.

Hill D, Kerndt P, Frenkel L M et al 1989 HIV seroprevalence among parturients in Los Angeles County, 1988. 5th International Conference on AIDS, Montreal, Abstract MAP12

Hoff R, Berardi V P, Weiblen B J, Mahoney-Trout L, Mitchell M L, Grady G F 1988 Seroprevalence of human immunodeficiency virus among childbearing women. New England Journal of Medicine 318: 525–530

Holmberg S D, Stewart J A, Gerber A R et al 1988 Prior herpes simplex virus type 2 infection as a risk factor for HIV infection. Journal of the American Medical Association 259: 1048–1050

Hooykaas C, Van der Pligt J, Van Doornum G J J, Van der Linden M M P, Coutinho R A 1989 High-risk heterosexuals: differences between private and commercial partners in sexual behaviour and condom use. 5th International Conference on AIDS, Montreal, Abstract TAP14

Ippolito G, Angeloni P, Stegagno M et al 1989 Anonymous HIV testing of newborns in 63 Italian hospitals: as estimate of prevalence of HIV infection among women of reproductive age. 5th International Conference on AIDS, Montreal, Abstract MAP8

Italian Multicentre Study 1988 Epidemiology, clinical features and prognostic factors of pediatric HIV infection. Lancet *ii*: 1043–1046

Johnstone F D, MacCallum L, Brettle M, Inglis J M, Peutherer J F 1988 Does infection with the human immunodeficiency virus affect the outcome of pregnancy? British Medical Journal 296: 467

Kaplan M H, Farber B, Hall W H, Mallow C, O'Keefe C, Harper R G 1989 Pregnancy arising in HIV-infected women while being repetitively counselled about 'safe sex'. 5th International Conference on AIDS, Montreal, Abstract MBP4

Kim H C, Raska K, Clemow L et al 1988 Human immunodeficiency virus infection in sexually-active wives of infected hemophilic men. American Journal of Medicine 85 472–476

Kreiss J K, Koech D, Plummer F A et al 1986 AIDS infections in Nairobi prostitutes: spread of the epidemic to East Africa. New England Journal of Medicine 314: 414–418

Landis S, Schoenbach V, Weber D, Mittal M, Koch G, Levine P 1989 HIV1 seroprevalence in sexually transmitted disease clinics in central North Carolina. 5th International Conference on AIDS, Montreal, Abstract MAO23

Leonard G, Mournier M, Verdier M et al 1988 Seroepidemiological study of sexually transmitted pathogenic agents (HIV1, HIV2, *T. pallidum*, *C. trachomatis*) in Ivory Coast. 4th International Conference on AIDS, Stockholm, Abstract 5014

Loveday C, Pomeroy L, Weller I V D et al 1989 Human immunodeficiency viruses in patients attending a sexually transmitted disease clinic in London, 1982–87. British Medical Journal 298: 419–421

Lui K J, Darrow W W, Rutherford W 1988 A model based estimate of the mean incubation period for AIDS in homosexual men. Science 240: 1333–1335

MacCallum L R, Cowan F M, Whitelaw J, Burns S M, Brettle R P 1989 Disease progression following pregnancy in HIV seropositive women. 5th International Conference on AIDS, Montreal, Abstract MBP3

McCray E, Onorat I M, Sweeney P A 1989 Seroprevalence of HIV among clients attending sexually transmitted diseases clinics in the US. 5th International Conference on AIDS, Montreal, Abstract MAO20

Mann J M, Quinn T C, Francis H et al 1986 Prevalence of HTLVIII/LAV in household contacts of patients with AIDS and controls in Kinshasa, Zaire. Journal of the American Medical Association 256: 721–724

Marion R W, Wiznia A A, Hutcheon G et al 1986 Human T-cell lymphotropic virus type III (HTLVIII) embryopathy: a new dysmorphic syndrome associated wth intrauterine HTLVIII infection. American Journal of Diseases of Childhood 140: 638–640

Melbye M, Njelesani E K, Bayley A et al 1986 Evidence for heterosexual transmission and clinical manifestations of human immunodeficiency virus infection and related conditions in Lusaka, Zambia. Lancet *ii*: 1113–1115

Morbidity and Mortality Weekly Report 1981 Pneumocystis pneumonia—Los Angeles. 30: 250–252

Moss A R, Bachetti P, Osmond D et al 1988 Seropositivity for HIV and the development of AIDS or AIDS related condition: three-year follow up of the San Francisco General Hospital cohort. British Medical Journal 296: 745–750

Muggiasca M L, Conti E, Ravasi L, Imperiale D, Agarossi A, Conti M 1989 Human immunodeficiency virus and human papilloma virus in the cervical intraepithelial neoplasia (CIN) in development of past intravenous drug abusers women. 5th International Conference on AIDS, Montreal, Abstract MBP56

Mworozi E A, Ndugwa C M, Kataaha P K, Kiguli S 1989 Perinatal transmission of HIV infection in Uganda 0–34 months follow-up. 5th International Conference on AIDS, Montreal, Abstract TBP 189

Novick L, Glebatis D, Stricof R, Berns D 1989 HIV infection in adolescent childbearing women. 5th International Conference on AIDS, Montreal, Abstract WAO8

Ntaba H M, Liomba G N, Schmidt J H, Schonhals C, Gurtler L, Deinhardt F 1988 HIV prevalence in hospital patients and pregnant women in Malawi. 4th International Conference on AIDS, Stockholm, Abstract 5036

O'Sullivan M J, Fajardo A, Ferron P, Efantis J, Senk C, Duthely M 1989 Seroprevalence in a pregnant multiethnic population. 5th International Conference on AIDS, Montreal, Abstract MBP23

Padian N, Marquis L, Francis D P et al 1987 Male to female transmission of human immunodeficiency virus. Journal of the American Medical Association 258: 788–791

Padian N, Shiboski S 1989 Heterogeneous male to female transmission of human immunodeficiency virus. 5th International Conference on AIDS, Montreal, Abstract TAO16

Peterman T A, Stoneburner R L, Allen J R, Jaffe H W, Curran J W 1988 Risk of human immunodeficiency virus transmission from heterosexual adults with transfusion-associated infections. Journal of the American Medical Association 259: 55–58

Piot P, Van Dyck E, Ryder R W et al 1989 Serum antibody to *Haemophilus ducreyi* as a risk factor for HIV infection in Africa, but not in Europe. 5th International Conference on AIDS, Montreal, Abstract MAO32

Plummer F A, Simonsen J N, Ngugi E N, Cameron D W, Piot P, Ndinya-Achola J O 1987 Incidence of human immunodeficiency virus (HIV) infection and related disease in a cohort of Nairobi prostitutes. 3rd International Conference on AIDS, Washington, Abstract M8.4

Plummer F, Cameron W, Simonsen N et al 1988 Cofactors in male–female transmission of HIV. 4th International Conference on AIDS, Stockholm, Abstract 4554

Quinn T C, Glasser D, Cannon R O et al 1988 Human immunodeficiency virus infection among patients attending clinics for sexually transmitted diseases. New England Journal of Medicine 318: 197–203

Rehmet S, Staszewski S, Wegerich B, Kreuz W, Stille W 1989 Perinatal and heterosexual transmission through HIV-positive women. 5th International Conference on AIDS, Montreal, Abstract MBP200

Rogers M F, Ou C, Rayfield M et al 1989 Use of the polymerase-chain reaction for early detection of the proviral sequences of human immunodeficiency virus in infants born to seropositive mothers. New England Journal of Medicine 302: 1649–1654

Ryder R, Nsa W, Francis H et al 1989a HIV IgG antibody at the age of 12 or 18 months but not HIV IgM antibody at birth or age 3 months correlates with clinical evidence of perinatally acquired HIV infection. 5th International Conference on AIDS, Montreal, Abstract B625

Ryder R W, Nsa W, Hassig S E et al 1989b Perinatal transmission of human immunodeficiency virus type 1 to infants of seropositive women in Zaire. New England Journal of Medicine 320: 1637–1642

Saltzman B R, Friedland G H, Klein R S, Villeno J, Freeman K, Gutelle P 1988 Comparison of AIDS clinical manifestations between men and women in a primarily homosexual population. 4th International Conference on AIDS, Stockholm, Abstract 4001

Selwyn P A, Schoenbaum E E, Davenny K et al 1989 Prospective study of human immunodeficiency virus infection and pregnancy outcomes in intravenous drug users. Journal of the American Medical Association 261: 1289–1294

Sperling R S, Sacks H S, Mayer L, Joyner M, Berkowitz R L 1989 Umbilical cord blood serosurvey for human immunodeficiency virus in parturient women in New York City. Obstetrics and Gynecology 73: 179–181

Tedder R, Briggs M, Parra N, Helm M, Peckham C 1989 Measurement of HIV seroprevalence in childbearing women in London. 5th International Conference on AIDS, Montreal, Abstract WAO9

Tirelli U, De Mercato R, Caprilli F, Guliani M, Saracco A, Rezza G 1989 HIV seropositivity and risk behaviour of Italian prostitutes. 5th International Conference on AIDS, Montreal, Abstract MAP48

Watts H, Brown Z, Tartaglione T et al 1989 Pharmacokinetics of zidovudine in HIV-positive pregnant women. 5th International Conference on AIDS, Montreal, Abstract MBP56

Wilson M J, Greenhalgh J B, Lemp G F, Perkins C I 1989 HIV seroprevalence in the San Francisco Bay area. 5th International Conference on AIDS, Montreal, Abstract MAP64

Zolla-Pazner S, William D, El-Sadr W, Marmor M, Stahl R 1984 Quantitation of B2 microglobulin and other immune characteristics in a prospective study of men at risk for the acquired immune deficiency syndrome. Journal of the American Medical Association 251: 2951–2955

Zorrilla C, Romaguera J, Torres J, Morales L, Adamson K 1989 Effect of lifestyles and high-risk sexual behaviour between HIV seropositive HIV seronegative pregnant women. 5th International Conference on AIDS, Montreal, Abstract MBP28

PART THREE

Gynaecology

13. Urodynamics

Eboo Versi   Linda Cardozo

INTRODUCTION

Urodynamics, as the name suggests, is the study of urine flow but in broader terms it encompasses all the investigations used for assessing lower urinary tract function. The bladder has a dual role; on the one hand to act as a storage organ and on the other, to expel the urine contained therein when it is appropriate to do so. Consequently, lower urinary tract disorders can be divided into incontinence (and related problems) and voiding difficulties.

The traditional approach to the management of bladder dysfunction relied upon localization of anatomical abnormalities which were thought to be the cause of symptoms (Jeffcoate & Roberts 1952, Green 1962). Thus the presence of anterior vaginal wall prolapse was thought to be the prime cause of incontinence and effective repair of the defect was expected to lead to a permanent cure. Unfortunately, it became evident that such a naïve policy was not always effective; objective cure rates for stress incontinence treated by anterior colporrhaphy are about 50% (Stanton 1975, Stanton & Cardozo 1979, Weil et al 1984) so it became important to develop accurate investigations to increase the clinician's diagnostic acumen. Urodynamics also serves to provide a rational set of criteria for patient selection when operative treatment is contemplated.

BACKGROUND

Cystometry, which is the measurement of the pressure/volume relationship of the bladder, was the first urodynamic test to be described and remains the most useful. The first cystometer was designed by Mosso and Pellacani in 1882. It utilized a water manometer to measure the intravesical pressure at different volumes and recorded the pressure on a smoked drum. The same principle can be used today in the very simplest form of cystometry by filling the bladder, via a urethral catheter attached to a central venous pressure line (see Vol. 1, p. 159). The water manometer cystometer is subject to several errors, one of which is the inability to measure pressure during bladder filling, so incremental filling must be employed. This problem was overcome by Lewis (1939) who measured bladder pressure by means of an aneroid barometer and recorded the results on a paper drum. His cystometer was accurate with regard to the intravesical pressure, but did not account for the effect that changes in intra-abdominal pressure can have on the intravesical pressure recording.

The advent of pressure transducers allowed for accurate measurement of both intravesical (bladder) and intra-abdominal (rectal or vaginal) pressures via independent fluid-filled catheters. The intra-abdominal pressure can be electronically subtracted from the intravesical pressure to give a measurement of detrusor pressure changes. All these parameters can be recorded onto a computer disk or printed out by a multichannel chart recorder to provide a permanent record. This type of subtracted cystometry is widely used today in urodynamic units throughout Europe.

The measurement of urethral closure pressure was first described by Bonney (1923) who termed it 'sphincterometry' and tried to quantify the pressure required to force fluid from the external meatus into the bladder. This was grossly unphysiological and urethral pressure profilometry was not recognized as a clinically useful test until 1969 when Brown and Wickham described a fluid-perfused catheter withdrawal technique designed to measure urethral resistance. Since then various methods of urethral pressure profilometry have been described but the accuracy of the test for the diagnosis of female urinary incontinence is limited (Versi et al, 1986b).

The first flow meter was not described until 1956 (von Garrelts), but uroflowmetry has rapidly gained popularity as it is simple, non-invasive and very informative, especially in men.

Micturition cystography has also been used since the 1950s. Jeffcoate and Roberts (1952) described loss of the posterior urethrovesical angle on coughing or straining, which they thought was diagnostic of urethral sphincter incompetence. It has since become evident that the posterior urethrovesical angle is absent in some continent women, may be present in some incontinent women and is lost when normal micturition occurs and when the detrusor contracts. So although urine loss may be demonstrated by micturition cystography, it does not shed much light on the underlying pathology.

Thus the major urodynamic investigations were developed independently and it was not until 1964 that Enhorning and colleagues first described simultaneous cystometry and radiological screening of the bladder and urethra, both of which were recorded by individual television cameras, the images being fused to give a composite picture of bladder function. The investigation was refined by Bates et al (1970), whose technique of 'synchronous cine/pressure flow cystography' is virtually the same as videocystourethrography which is the routine method of urodynamic assessment currently employed in many tertiary referral centres.

SYMPTOMS

Precise and uniform terminology is an essential prerequisite for progress in any scientific field and urodynamics is no exception. In 1970 a multi-disciplinary group including urologists, gynaecologists, physiotherapists, nurses, physiologists and biomedical engineers founded the International Continence Society, whose membership and influence continue to grow. This society has a standardization committee (see Abrams et al 1988) which has drawn up a list of clearly defined terms to avoid misunderstanding, and wherever possible, clinicians should use these terms for the sake of uniformity, and to ensure that we all speak the same language.

Stress incontinence

Stress incontinence is a symptom: the patient complains of urine loss initiated by an increase in intra-abdominal pressure (e.g. coughing or sneezing). Stress incontinence is also a sign: noted if urine loss is perceived by the physician when the patient coughs. The term *genuine stress incontinence* (GSI) implies urethral sphincter incompetence and is defined as 'involuntary loss of urine when the intravesical pressure exceeds the maximum urethral pressure but in the absence of detrusor activity'. At first glance this might appear to be a cumbersome definition but it describes the condition exactly. Prior to detrusor contraction (normal and sometimes abnormal), there is urethral relaxation, so a sphincter cannot be said to be incompetent if it is relaxed. Therefore it is important to exclude detrusor activity before GSI can be documented and for this reason it can only be diagnosed accurately on the basis of urodynamic studies. Stress incontinence the sign is *not* pathognomonic of GSI as it can often be demonstrated in patients with detrusor instability, or overflow incontinence.

Urge incontinence

Stress incontinence can also be misinterpreted as urge incontinence in that patients may experience urgency and become incontinent only after initiating a sudden movement towards the toilet. For the symptom of urge incontinence, it is important to establish that urgency and then incontinence, occurs in the absence of activities that result in raised intra-abdominal pressure.

Dysuria

There is also confusion over the term dysuria. This is interpreted by some as difficulty in voiding while others understand it to mean painful micturition. The term is best avoided and clinicians should be encouraged to state the patient's actual complaint.

History-taking

History-taking relies on patient recall and unfortunately this is not always reliable. Therefore an assessment of the degree of frequency, nocturia, urgency and incontinence can be made more objective by asking patients to keep a diary or frequency/volume chart (Abrams et al 1983). The extent of the problem may be related to fluid intake and simple advice based on this information can be surprisingly effective. For example, if nocturia is most troublesome then advising the patient to drink less during the evening can often provide a cure.

Clinical judgement is frequently misleading when dealing with lower urinary tract pathology. Symptoms do not faithfully represent the underlying condition and it has been shown by several authors (Cardozo and Stanton 1980, Jarvis et al 1980, Shepherd et al 1982, Versi et al 1990a) that the predictive value of clinical diagnosis is poor. It is for this reason that urodynamic tests are needed, as treatment has to be tailored to suit the pathology if it is to be successful.

URODYNAMIC TESTS

Prior to urodynamic assessment, it is important to ascertain that no urinary tract infection is present. This is important because invasive investigations in the presence of an infection, can result in greater morbidity and also because the urodynamic diagnosis may be unreliable in such a situation (Bergman & Bhatia 1985). Further, the symptoms are sometimes due simply to the presence of an infection and can be eradicated with the appropriate antibiotics.

The different urodynamic tests available range from the very simple and cheap to the enormously complicated and expensive. Many of the tests are really research tools and therefore clinically they range from the essential to the academic. As the urinary tract has a storage and expulsive function urodynamic tests are aimed at assessing continence or voiding. For the purpose of this chapter, the more common tests will be mentioned along with a critique of their usefulness.

Flow studies

The bladder and the urethra function as a unit and during normal micturition the urethra relaxes prior to bladder contraction so allowing efficient voiding; this can be tested by uroflowmetry.

There are many different ways of measuring urine flow and three of the most commonly used are shown in Figure 13.1. The first (Fig. 13.1a)

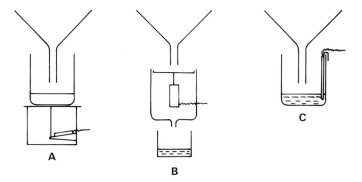

Fig. 13.1 Different methods of measuring flow rate.

records the changes in weight of urine passed and the speed with which it occurs to obtain a flow rate. The second technique (Fig. 13.1b) involves the use of a rotating disk. A servomotor maintains a constant rate and as urine falls on the disk, extra power is required to maintain the spin. This change in wattage is used to determine, electronically, the flow rate. Finally, the capacitance of dipstick type of flowmeter (Fig. 13.1c) is the simplest of all the techniques. It consists of a plastic dipstick coated with metal inserted vertically into the collecting vessel. As the urine collects, so the capacitance decreases. The rate of change in the capacitance is used to measure the urine flow rate.

To obtain a flow measurement, a patient, with a comfortably full

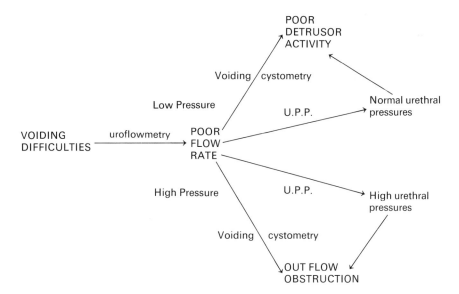

Fig. 13.2 Investigation of voiding difficulties. UPP = Urethral pressure profilometry.

bladder, is asked to void in private on to a modified toilet which has a flowmeter underneath. A peak flow rate greater than 15 ml/s is considered to be normal and indicates that the bladder and urethra are functioning properly and in coordination. However, a poor flow rate may suggest pathology but only if this is reproducible on at least two separate occasions and if prior to voiding, there was more than 200 ml in the bladder (Abrams et al 1983). The latter rider is important because a partially filled bladder does not always allow the detrusor muscle to work efficiently.

A low flow rate may be due to outflow obstruction or poor detrusor contractility (Fig. 13.2). The former can be relative (detrusor-sphincter dyssynergia) or absolute (urethral stricture). A stricture can be detected by urethral pressure profilometry or videocystourethrography (see p. 207 below). Poor detrusor contractility can sometimes be diagnosed by voiding cystometry (see below) in that outflow obstruction should result in high detrusor voiding pressures. However, the detrusor may become decompensated and so there may be a low flow rate and a low voiding detrusor pressure in the presence of outflow obstruction.

Cystometry

This is essentially the measurement of intravesical pressure during dynamic urinary states. Simultaneous intrarectal pressure measurement allows for three channel subtraction cystometry. For a further discussion, see Cardozo (1981). The intrarectal pressure is read as the intra-abdominal pressure and this, subtracted from the intravesical pressure, yields the pressure exerted by the detrusor muscle.

Filling

Fast fill (>100 ml/min) provocative cystometry is designed to elicit aberrant detrusor activity, either detrusor instability or low compliance. The bladder is filled to capacity at a rate of 60–100 ml/min and during this time the patient is asked to cough several times. At cystometric capacity, she undergoes a postural change from the supine to erect position. During this test any inappropriate detrusor contraction or a detrusor pressure rise greater than 15 cm of water, is considered abnormal. A steady detrusor pressure rise towards the end of filling is interpreted as low-compliance of the bladder. However, this may be indistinguishable from a slow detrusor contraction which represents true detrusor instability. It may be that poor compliance is a form of detrusor instability as it often presents with the same symptom complex and responds to the same therapy.

Voiding

Voiding cystometry enables detrusor contractility to be assessed. Normal

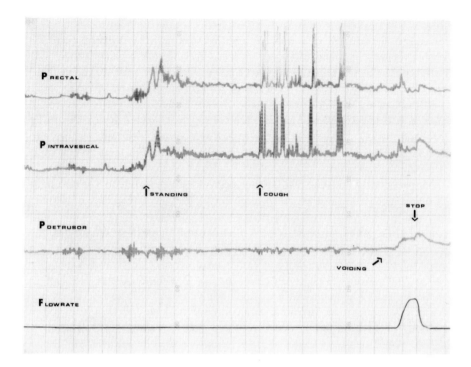

Fig. 13.3 Detrusor pressure rise following the stop test. The urethral sphincter contracts before the detrusor is able to relax resulting in an isometric contraction of the bladder.

women void with a low detrusor pressure because of their short, relatively weak urethrae which produce little outflow resistance; however, measurement of these voiding pressures are difficult to interpret.

During voiding there is a flow of urine and so intravesical pressure measurement may be more a reflection of outflow resistance than detrusor function. This problem can be overcome by asking the patient to stop voiding suddenly. This leads to a rapid closure of the urethral sphincter prior to the relaxation of the detrusor muscle. The resulting rise in intravesical pressure due to isometric contraction of the detrusor muscle is a more realistic measure of the contractile capability of the detrusor (Fig. 13.3). This pressure rise is known as the 'piso' or p. det. maxism.

Quantification of urine loss

The complaint of incontinence should be substantiated by an objective test. Stress incontinence, the sign, is not always easy to elicit. Ideally the patient should be examined in the erect position with a full bladder but in practice this is difficult as women with urinary complaints rarely allow their bladders to become full for fear of incontinence. Objective tests can take the form of a Urilos nappy test (James et al 1971) where the quantity of urine is measured electrically, or a pad test (Sutherst et al 1981, Versi & Cardozo 1986a) where it is measured as an increase in weight of a perineal pad. For both types of tests the patients receive an oral fluid load prior to the test and are asked to carry out a pre-set series of activities and to void after the test.

Both tests are easy to carry out and the simplified pad test is very cheap indeed (Versi & Cardozo 1986a). However, these tests do not yield any information as to the cause of the incontinence and although simple, are not as accurate as the more sophisticated videographic tests (Versi et al 1988) described below.

More recently another test has been developed that detects the presence of urine in the distal urethra (Holmes et al 1985a). It consists of a small catheter probe with two gold-plated brass ring electrodes placed 1 mm apart. This probe is sited in the distal urethra and on coughing, the presence of any urine is detected by increased conductance between the electrodes. The comparability of the distal urethral electrical conductance and pad tests needs to be investigated further (Mayne & Hilton 1988).

All the tests for detection of urine loss have been criticized because they are stress tests in an artificial environment and so for this reason the 24-hour or 48-hour home pad tests have been developed (Jakobsen et al 1987). These tests appear to be more sensitive (Jorgensen et al 1987) and when this information is taken in conjunction with the data from fluid volume charts, the degree of the disability can be more thoroughly assessed (Klevmark et al 1988).

In centres where imaging facilities are not available, the complaint of stress incontinence in the absence of detrusor instability (negative cystometry) is regarded as being due to urethral sphincter weakness or genuine stress incontinence (GSI). Unfortunately, there are many different causes for incontinence (Table 13.1) but only GSI will respond to bladder neck surgery. As misdiagnosis can lead to disastrous consequences, clearly it is important to maximize one's diagnostic acumen. To this end quantification tests should form an essential part of the urodynamicist's armamentarium and because of their simplicity can be employed widely.

Table 13.1   Causes of urinary incontinence in the female

Genuine stress incontinence
Detrusor instability
Urethral instability
Overflow incontinence
Fistula (malignant or iatrogenic)
Congenital malformation
Functional
Miscellaneous, e.g. urethral diverticulum

Videocystourethrography

Videocystourethrography (VCU) is radiological screening of the bladder and urethra during cystometry (Bates et al 1970) and is effectively the 'Rolls Royce' of urodynamic tests. The bladder can be screened during the filling phase of cystometry and also when the bladder is full in the erect oblique position. Morphological abnormalities such as bladder or urethral diverticula can be seen, as can trabeculation, sacculation and congenital abnormalities which occur below the level of the ureters. Fistulae and ureteric reflux (Fig. 13.4) can also be visualized at rest or during the voiding sequence.

During radiological screening urethral sphincter weakness (anatomical incontinence) is diagnosed when contrast medium is seen to streak down the length of the urethra during a cough. However, simultaneous cystometry is essential to prove that there was no detrusor contraction which could be responsible for the incontinence. During micturition there is relaxation of the urethra followed by contraction of the bladder and this urethral relaxation can occur prior to an aberrant detrusor contraction. Therefore, as mentioned before, it is important to exclude detrusor instability for the diagnosis of GSI to be made as a relaxed sphincter cannot be said to be incompetent.

Traditionally, continence has been thought to be maintained by external and internal (bladder neck) sphincters. However, recent work has shown that about 50% of continent post-menopausal women have an incompetent

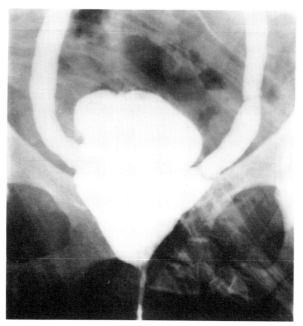

Fig. 13.4 X-ray showing gross bilateral ureteric reflux.

Table 13.2 Information obtained by X-ray screening with an image intensifier

---

X-ray screening at rest
  Diverticula
  —bladder
  —urethra
  Sacculation
  Trabeculation
  Ureteric reflux
  Bladder neck
  —open
  —closed

X-ray screening—on coughing
  Post-surgical tethering
  Bladder base descent
  Incompetent bladder neck
  Genuine stress incontinence

X-ray screening—on voiding
  Ureteric reflux
  Detrusor sphincter dyssynergia
  Bladder base descent
  Urethral stricture
  Voluntary inhibition of stream
  Milkback
  Bladder emptying

---

bladder neck (Versi et al 1986a). There is other evidence in the literature (Hilton & Stanton 1983a) to suggest that bladder neck incompetence is a normal variant. Therefore during VCU testing it is important to see contrast medium traversing past the mid-urethral point for the diagnosis of GSI as in many normal continent women, there will be bladder neck beaking (or Grade I stress).

The advantages of VCU screening are numerous and the information that can be gleaned from such a study is shown in Table 16.2. The major disadvantage is that of expense if radiological screening facilities have to be established specifically for urodynamic tests. However, if the urodynamic tests can be carried out in the X-ray department then the increase in expense is negligible. Radiation is also a potential risk but most women being investigated are not of child-bearing age and 1–2 minutes of image intensifier screening approximates in exposure to a single A-P chest film. Sensitivity to the iodine-containing contrast medium has also been suggested as a disadvantage. This theoretical risk is not evident in practice as the medium is only· instilled into the bladder, is not systemically administered and is voided after a few minutes.

Urethral pressure profilometry

Technique

Incontinence occurs only when the intravesical pressure exceeds the

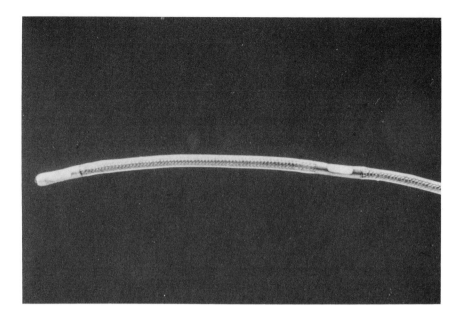

Fig. 13.5   A urethral pressure profile catheter. Note the two solid-state transducers mounted on this flexible silastic 7 French catheter.

intraurethral pressure (Enhorning 1961) so simultaneous measurement of these pressures for the investigation of incontinence is logical on theoretical grounds. Urethral pressure was widely measured using a fluid catheter system (Brown & Wickham 1969) but the response time of this system does not allow for accurate measurements during coughing which is essential if the technique is to be used for detecting urethral sphincter weakness under stress. This problem has been overcome with the advent of solid-state microtransducers (Asmussen & Ulmsten 1975). Two of these transducers are mounted on a silicone catheter at a separation of about 6 cm (Fig. 13.5). Initially this is inserted through the urethra so that both sensors are in the bladder and then by pulling the catheter out at a steady rate the proximal sensor passes along the length of the urethra (Fig. 13.6) and so records the urethral pressure profile. This can be done at rest (Fig. 13.7) or while the patient is coughing (Fig. 13.8). The subtraction trace can be used to plot (dotted line) the stress pressure profile (Fig. 13.9) which represents the superiority of the urethral pressure over that of the bladder. If cough impulses are transmitted equally to the bladder and the urethra, then the stress profile is identical to the resting profile. However, even in continent women, only a part of the urethra is intra-abdominal and so cough impulses will not be transmitted to the distal urethra. This results in negative waves in the subtraction trace of the distal urethra (Fig. 13.9). The consequence

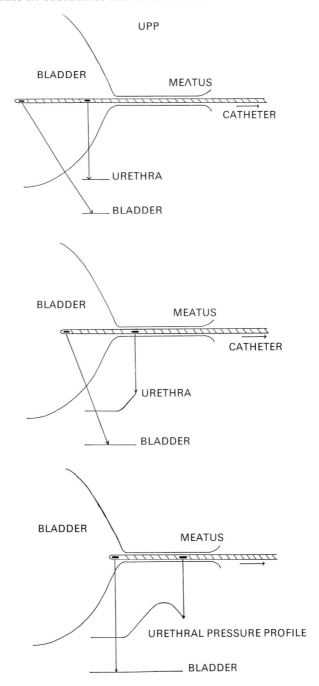

Fig. 13.6   Generation of the urethral pressure profile. The catheter is pulled out at a steady speed (e.g. 2.5 mm/s) while the patient is lying supine and the pressure profile of the urethra is recorded as the transducer traverses its length. Note that the bladder sensor remains intravesical throughout and so registers no change in pressure.

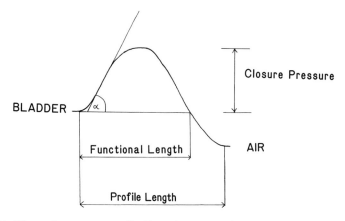

Fig. 13.7   The resting pressure profile. Several measures of urethral pressure can be made from this trace. The closure pressure represents the maximum excess pressure in the urethra over the bladder pressure at rest. The functional urethral length is the length of the urethra over which the pressure is above bladder pressure at rest. The profile length represents the anatomical urethral length. The tangent of alpha is the gradient of the urethral pressure in the proximal urethra and represents the pressure gradient that has to be overcome for incontinence to occur. (From Versi et al 1988b, with permission.)

of this is that the stress profile is shortened (functional length) and that this shortening takes place distally (Fig. 13.9).

Incontinence

The maximum urethral closure pressure prevents incontinence at rest

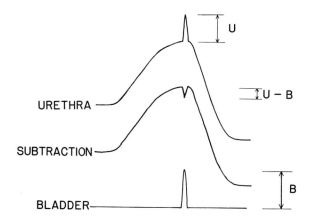

Fig. 13.8   Generation of the stress pressure profile. The catheter is pulled through as far as in Figure 13.7 but this time the patient is asked to cough repeatedly. These cough impulses are registered by both the urethral (U) and bladder (B) transducers. The subtraction trace records the difference between the pressure in the urethra and the bladder (U–B). Only a single cough is depicted for the sake of clarity. The result of repeated coughs are shown in Figure 13.9.

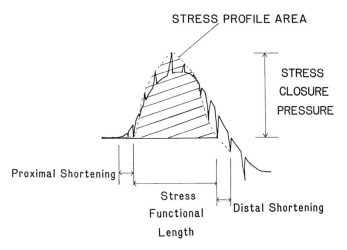

Fig. 13.9 Stress pressure profile. The dotted line on this subtraction trace is the stress pressure profile and as with Figure 13.7, several measurements can be made from this.

(Fig. 13.7) or under stress (Fig. 13.9). Irrespective of the absolute magnitude of the resting maximum closure pressure, if a cough causes transmission of the intra-abdominal pressure equally to the urethra and to the bladder then continence will be preserved as the differential will still be maintained. That is, even during the cough, the intraurethral pressure will exceed the intravesical pressure. Hilton and Stanton (1983a) have suggested that GSI is due to a failure of the transmission of pressure to the proximal urethra and that corrective surgery is aimed at effectively restoring this (Hilton & Stanton 1983b).

Given the above, it would seem that this technique could be used to diagnose GSI. Indeed in a study of 102 normal and 70 women with GSI (VCU diagnosis) 23 out of 30 urethral pressure profile parameters were found to have averages that were significantly different between the normal and incontinent groups (Versi 1990). Unfortunately, this has been interpreted by some to mean that this is a valid method for diagnosing patients with GSI. In our study (Versi et al 1986b) we found that even the most discriminating parameter (area under the stress profile) was not diagnostically accurate. There was a very large overlap in the data (Fig. 13.10) yielding either poor sensitivity or specificity depending upon the positioning of the cut-off point. These results clearly demonstrate that microtransducer urethral pressure profilometry cannot be used for the diagnosis of GSI on the basis of any single parameter (Versi et al 1986b, 1990b). The reason for this is probably artefactual due to catheter movement during the cough. It is possible that in the future, catheters employing circumferential pressure transduction may be more useful.

The accuracy of urethral pressure profilometry can be enhanced by

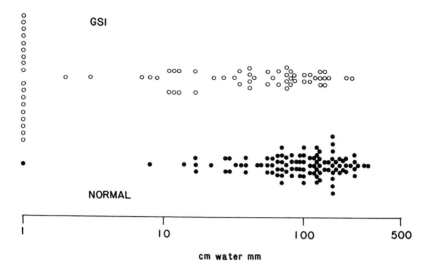

Fig. 13.10 A distribution of the values of total area under the stress profile in normal and GSI patients. Note the semi-log scale. (After Versi 1990, with permission.)

examining several parameters together. Discriminant analysis can be employed to this end (Versi 1990) and reveals a better separation of normal and GSI patients. Unfortunately, some overlap still exists (Fig. 13.11) and those patients with ambiguous results should be referred for VCU studies.

Strictures and diverticula

Microtransducer catheters do have another place in urodynamic studies. They can be used to detect urethral diverticula and strictures and we believe that the presence of the latter should be demonstrated before urethral dilatation is contemplated. In our experience non-iatrogenic strictures in females are rare.

Urethral instability

More recently urethral instability has been recognized as a cause of incontinence (Kulseng-Hansen 1983). This is characterized by the loss of urethral pressure in the absence of detrusor contractions either at rest or after a cough. In some cases of detrusor instability, the abnormal detrusor contraction is preceded by urethral relaxation. Thus it is possible that urethral instability has a similar aetiology to detrusor instability but this remains to be elucidated further. The diagnosis of urethral instability can be made by positioning a microtransducer at the point of maximum urethral pressure. With the patient lying still, if the fluctuation in the maximum urethral pressure exceeds one-third of the resting maximal

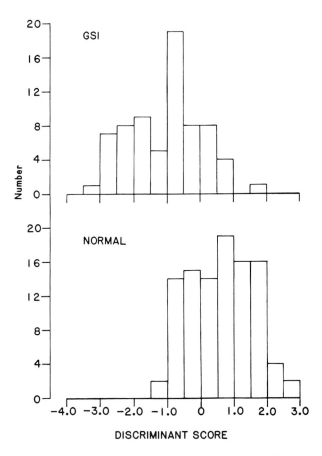

Fig. 13.11   Histograms of the distributions of the discriminant scores for the normal and GSI patients. Note the still considerable overlap. (From Versi 1990, with permission.)

urethral pressure then the diagnosis can be made (Versi & Cardozo 1986b). These fluctuations are seen in the absence of detrusor activity and in cases where there is a total loss of urethral closure pressure, incontinence may occur. However, statistically abnormal fluctuations in urethral pressure have not been correlated with increased symptomatology and so for this reason doubt is cast on the clinical relevance of these abnormal fluctuations (Tapp et al 1986).

Other tests

Ultrasound

As a non-invasive technique, this method may be accepted rapidly for routine investigations. Its primary use is for the detection of post-micturition residual urine and this can be accurately estimated (Griffiths et al 1986). The development of the vaginal probe has allowed clear imaging of the bladder neck even during coughing (Quinn et al 1987). However, as an incompetent bladder neck is not synonymous with urethral sphincter incompetence (Versi et al 1986a), the value of ultrasound for the diagnosis of GSI is limited at present. However the technique has potential.

Electromyography (EMG)

This is a study of bio-electrical potentials generated by smooth and striated muscle. These can be detected by surface or needle electrodes. Use of the former is painless but cannot measure individual motor unit potentials. Needle electrodes are accurate but the technique is invasive and relatively unpleasant for the patient.

Attempts at studying detrusor electromyography have to date been clinically disappointing. Urethral sphincter activity has been studied by examining various muscle groups involved in micturition control. Anal plug surface electrodes are most commonly used as the anal sphincter has a similar supply to the urethral sphincter (S2–4) and the technique is simple. Unfortunately this is not a reliable indicator of urethral sphincter activity as the two sphincters frequently function independently. Recently, the use of single-fibre electromyography has gained prominence as it enables a computation of the motor neurone fibre density (Anderson 1984). This is increased in neuropathies and myopathies and so the technique is promising for investigating such conditions.

Although urethral sphincter EMG is a useful research technique, its clinical application is limited. It can be used for investigating neurological disorders (Kirby et al 1983) and for the diagnosis of detrusor sphincter dyssynergia (Fowler & Kirby 1986) when VCU facilities are not available or in conjunction with them. In general the technique is dogged with artefact and simplified systems using integrated EMG are easier to use but information is lost by the integrating process.

Fluid bridge and electrical conductance tests

The fluid bridge tests pioneered by John Sutherst in 1980, (Sutherst & Brown 1980, Shawer et al 1981) are designed to detect bladder neck incompetence. This may be of little use clinically as normal continent women may have an incompetent bladder neck on coughing (Versi et al 1986a).

A variation of the fluid bridge test has been used to measure the electrical conductivity of the proximal urethra and so determine when the bladder neck opens (Holmes et al 1985b). This new development is promising because it may provide an objective means of assessing the symptoms of urgency and its response to treatment.

Intravenous urogram and cystoscopy

This time-honoured partnership is useful for the investigation of haematuria and for frequency and urgency, especially in the elderly. However, in the younger patient complaining of incontinence, the dangers of iodine allergy, anaesthetic risk and the costs outweigh the benefits of these investigations.

Gold standards

Of all the tests we have discussed, urine culture, uroflowmetry and videocystourethrography alone can be used to diagnose all the common female lower urinary tract conditions. For this reason we refer to these as the Gold Standard and suggest that any new test should be evaluated against the results from these tests as we have done for the simplified pad test (Versi & Cardozo 1986a, Versi et al 1988a) and urethral pressure profilometry (Versi et al 1986b, 1990b).

CLINICAL MANAGEMENT

Presentation

Gynaecologists are confronted with urinary problems which usually fall into one or more of the following categories:

1. Incontinence,
2. Urgency and frequency ± painful micturition,
3. Voiding difficulties.

Assessment

This should consist of history and examination including not only gynaecological but also neurological aspects. Prolapse often co-exists with incontinence but it is important to ascertain which is the more troublesome because curing one will not necessarily help the other. Before proceeding further it is important to ensure that the urine is sterile.

Investigation

If upper urinary tract pathology or bladder neoplasia are suspected then IVU and cystoscopy are indicated. If incontinence is the main complaint then it is due to one of the causes depicted in Table 16.1. Clinical examination may have excluded overflow incontinence and possibly congenital malformation. The next step is to verify objectively that incontinence is present (Fig. 13.12) and in difficult cases one may have to resort to the use of pyridium which stains urine and so makes it identifiable

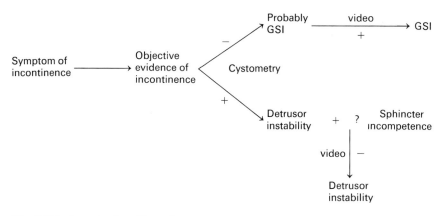

Fig. 13.12   Investigation of incontinence.

on a pad. Cystometry will exclude or confirm detrusor instability. Video-cystourethrography can be used to identify GSI and anatomical malformations. Urethral pressure profilometry will diagnose urethral instability, diverticula and may help towards a diagnosis of GSI. A 'functional' diagnosis should only be made when there is an associated psychiatric history. If the patient has GSI then pre-operative uroflowmetry will help to pick up those patients likely to have post-operative voiding difficulty (Fig. 13.13) as a poor flow rate pre-operatively may predict retention of urine post-operatively (Stanton et al 1978).

If the complaint is of frequency and urgency (Fig. 13.14) then cystometry will show whether this is of motor (detrusor instability) or sensory origin.

Voiding difficulties are either due to outflow obstruction or more likely due to poor detrusor contractility. Non-neuropathic female outflow obstruction is usually iatrogenic following previous surgery or urethral dilatation. Poor detrusor contractility can follow difficult childbirth when epidural analgesia has been used (Tapp et al 1987). Voiding difficulties are

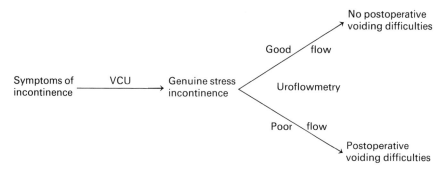

Fig. 13.13   Pre-operative assessment of voiding function.

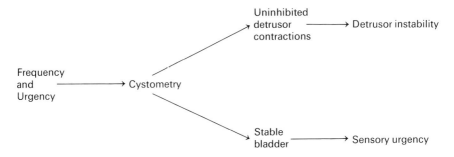

Fig. 13.14 Investigation of abacteruric urinary frequency and urgency.

Table 13.3 Urodynamic assessments: which test? which patients?

	Symptoms		
Tests	Incontinence	Urgency/frequency	Voiding difficulties
History, examination and MSU	●	●	●
Pad test	●		
Uroflowmetry	●		●
Videocystourethrography	●	●	●
Urethral pressure profilometry		●	●

usually investigated with uroflowmetry (Fig. 13.1). If a poor flow rate is confirmed, this is followed by voiding cystometry (Fig. 13.2). High pressures suggest outflow obstruction and a stricture may be detected by the use of urethral pressure profilometry. Low or normal voiding pressures would suggest detrusor hypotonia.

The recommended tests for any given presenting complaint are summarized in Table 13.3. All patients should have a history taken, examinations performed and urinary tract infection excluded. Pad testing is only appropriate in cases of incontinence but uroflowmetry is also useful for predicting post-operative voiding difficulties and possibly can aid in the diagnosis of detrusor sphincter dyssynergia. Videocystourethrography is useful for investigating any complaint. Urethral pressure profilometry may reveal urethral instability as a cause of frequency and urgency and can be used to diagnose a urethral stricture.

Treatment

For the conditions mentioned, the most common methods of treatment are outlined in Table 13.4.

Table 13.4   Treatment of urodynamically diagnosed conditions

Condition	Treatment
Genuine stress incontinence	Bladder neck surgery
	Physiotherapy
	Drugs: Oestrogens $\pm$ adrenergic agents
Detrusor instability	Anticholinergic agents
	Bladder re-training/biofeedback
Urethral instability	Not known
Voiding difficulties	
—poor detrusor contractility	Cholinomimetic agent, e.g. bethanecol
—detrusor sphincter dyssynergia	Phenoxybenzamine
—urethral stricture/bladder	
neck obstruction	Urethral dilatation and/or urethrotomy
Fistula	Corrective surgery
Congenital malformation	Plastic surgery
Functional	Psychiatric referral
Sensory urgency	Oestrogens if atrophic
	Probanthine

Genuine stress incontinence

Retropubic operations are preferable to vaginal procedures in the management of GSI and recently colposuspension has been shown to be more effective than anterior colporrhaphy in a prospective randomized trial (Stanton et al 1985). A Stamey or Pereyra procedure is quicker to perform than a colposuspension but is not as effective in controlling incontinence (Weil et al 1984, Bhatia & Bergman 1985). The sling operation has also gained popularity because of the ease of the technique using either organic (Jarvis & Fowlie 1985) or inorganic (Iosif 1985) material. However, in comparison with the Stamey procedure, there is greater post-operative morbidity and voiding difficulty (Hilton 1986).

Although not as effective as surgery, physiotherapy has been shown to be useful on its own or in combination with electrical stimulation (Wilson et al 1987). Treatment with perineometers (Shepherd et al 1983) confers some benefit and the new vaginal cones (Plevnic 1985) show promise. In post-menopausal women oestrogens alone (Hilton & Stanton 1983c) or combined with adrenergic agents have been advocated (Beisland et al 1984) as medical treatment.

Detrusor instability

Detrusor instability can be treated with anticholinergic agents or bladder retraining or both. However, drug therapy usually has side-effects and has to be continued indefinitely to be effective in its treatment. Fortunately, the condition undergoes spontaneous remission so medical therapy can be intermittent. Bladder retraining and various different forms of biofeedback have also been shown to be promising but they are time consuming (Cardozo et al 1978).

Urethral instability

Urethral instability is a recently recognized condition and its significance is still not understood. As yet no treatment has been evaluated for this condition.

Voiding difficulties

The most common cause of voiding difficulties in women is poor detrusor activity. In such a case the treatment of choice is a cholinomimetic agent such as bethanecol (Downie 1984, Finkbeiner 1985). More recently the use of intermittent self-catheterization is becoming more widely used (Stanton 1984) but requires reasonable dexterity on the part of the patient. The infection rate is fortunately quite low in patients who do it satisfactorily. To diminish urethral resistance adrenergic blocking agents may be used. Phenoxybenzamine is prescribed for detrusor sphincter dyssynergia and the only indication for surgery is urethral stricture or bladder neck obstruction. Inopportune use of urethral dilatation can result in subsequent formation of strictures and possibly an incompetent sphincter. Bladder neck obstruction is rare but when present can be treated by incision with the use of an Otis urethrotome. This procedure has a modest success rate and so some authors would prefer to advocate intermittent self-catheterization (Delaere et al 1983).

Fistula

Fistulae caused by surgery can be repaired immediately if diagnosis is made at operation but otherwise surgery should be delayed for at least 12 weeks.

Congenital

Congenital malformations usually present during childhood but are sometimes only diagnosed during adult life. Here again corrective surgery is indicated.

Functional

When a functional element is thought to underlie the problem of incontinence, treatment of the psychiatric condition results in remission in about one-third of cases (Hafner et al 1977).

Atrophy

Sensory urgency when accompanied by post-menopausal atrophic urethritis will respond to oestrogen replacement therapy. Vaginal oestriol preparations are not thought to significantly affect the endometrium and so are safe. However, other oestrogen preparations should be accompanied by progestogen therapy when there is a uterus in situ. In younger women, sensory urgency can be treated with propantheline.

COST

One of the major drawbacks to setting up a urodynamic unit is the cost of the apparatus, the salaries of trained technical staff and the availability of urodynamicists. As the field is expanding, the increase in the number of manufacturing companies has resulted in a relative decrease in the price of equipment.

The total cost has to be offset against the cost of inappropriate therapy. Inappropriate surgery may result in the worsening of the condition and this in turn leads to recurrent visits by the patient to the outpatients' clinic. The financial cost to the Health Service over a life-time is considerable, while the cost to the patient in terms of morbidity and wasted time is also sizeable. Finally, it should be remembered that the physician will also suffer because 'one's failures always come back'.

CONCLUSIONS

Urodynamic studies have dramatically improved our understanding of lower urinary tract dysfunction and have, in many instances, completely altered our approach to management. Despite the fact that accurate diagnosis prior to treatment must be the logical approach to management, many clinicians still ask 'Do I need to send every patient for tests for which she may have to wait a long time before I treat her?'. Our reply would be an emphatic 'Yes'. Very occasionally, a patient presents whose only complaint is of stress incontinence and in whom stress incontinence is demonstrated on clinical examination. In such a patient it would be safe to operate on the assumption that she has genuine stress incontinence but as such patients constitute only 2.5% of the incontinent population (Haylen & Fraser 1987), this modus operandi has little practical value.

The only group of patients for whom urodynamics may not be necessary as first line management are the elderly in whom an accurate diagnosis might not drastically affect treatment. For them, an algorithmic approach is useful (Hilton & Stanton 1981) and after exclusion of a urinary tract infection, faecal impaction and a large urinary residual, anticholinergic drugs can be prescribed as a therapeutic trial. Should the patient fail to respond then urodynamic studies should be employed to aid diagnosis.

The facilities for sophisticated tests may not be available everywhere but uroflowmetry and subtracted cystometry can be performed in most district general hospitals and referral to a tertiary centre is worthwhile for anyone with complicated problems, or in whom previous incontinence surgery has failed.

ACKNOWLEDGEMENTS

We should like to thank Beverley Poel for typing this manuscript.

REFERENCES

Abrams P, Fenley R, Torrens M 1983 Clinical practice in urology. In: Chisholm G D (ed) Urodynamics, Springer Verlag, Berlin, pp 34

Abrams P, Blavias J G, Stanton S L, Anderson J T 1988 The standardisation of terminology of lower urinary tract function. Scandinavian Journal of Urology and Nephrology. Supplementum 114: 5–19

Anderson R S 1984 A neurogenic element to urinary genuine stress incontinence. British Journal of Obstetrics and Gynaecology 91: 41–45

Asmussen M, Ulmsten V 1975 Simultaneous urethrocystometry and urethral pressure profile measurement with a new technique. Acta Obstetrica et Gynecologica Scandinavica 54: 385–388

Bates C P, Whiteside C G, Turner-Warwick R T 1970 Synchronous cine pressure flow cystourethrography with special reference to stress and urge incontinence. British Journal of Urology 42: 714–723

Beisland H O, Fossberg E, Moer A, Sander S 1984 Urethral sphincter insufficiency in postmenopausal females: treatment with phenylpropanolamine and estriol separately and in combination. Urology International 39: 211–216

Bergman A, Bhatia N N 1985 Urodynamics: effect of urinary tract infection on urethral and bladder function. Obstetrics and Gynecology 66: 366–371

Bhatia N N, Bergman A 1985 Modified Burch versus Pereyra retropubic urethropexy for stress incontinence. Obstetrics and Gynecology 66: 255–260

Bonney V 1923 Diurnal incontinence of urine in women. Journal of Obstetrics and Gynaecology of the British Empire 30: 358–365

Brown, M, Wickham W E A 1969 The urethral pressure profile. British Journal of Urology 51: 211–214

Cardozo L D 1981 The use of cystometry in the understanding of urinary incontinence. In: Studd J W W (ed.) Progress in Obstetrics and Gynaecology vol. 1. Churchill Livingstone, Edinburgh, pp 151–166

Cardozo L D, Abrams P H, Stanton S L 1978 Idiopathic bladder instability treated by biofeedback. British Journal of Urology 50: 521–523

Cardozo L D, Stanton S L 1980 Genuine stress incontinence and detrusor instability: a review of 200 patients. British Journal of Obstetrics and Gynaecology 87: 184–190

Delaere K P J, Debruyne F M J, Moonen W A 1983 Bladder neck incision in the female: a hazardous procedure. British Journal of Urology 55: 283–286

Downie J W 1984 Bethanechol chloride in urology—a discussion of issues. Neurourology and Urodynamics 3: 211–222

Enhorning G 1961 Simultaneous recordings of intravesical and intra-urethral pressure. Acta Chirurgica Scandinavica (suppl) 276: 1–68

Enhorning G, Miller E, Hinman F 1964 Urethral closure studies with cine roentography and simultaneous bladder-urethral pressure recording. Surgical Gynecological Obstetric 118: 507–516

Finkbeiner A E 1985 Is bethanechol chloride clinically effective in promoting bladder emptying? A literature review. Journal of Urology 134: 443–449

Fowler C J, Kirby R S 1986 Electromyography of urethral sphincter in women with urinary retention. Lancet i: 1455–1456

Green T 1962 Development of a plan for diagnosis and treatment of urinary stress incontinence. American Journal of Obstetrics and Gynecology 63: 632–648

Griffiths C J, Murray A, Ramsden P D 1986 Accuracy and repeatability of bladder volume measurement using ultrasonic imaging. Journal of Urology 136: 808–812

Hafner R J, Stanton S L, Guy J 1977 A psychiatric study of women with urgency incontinence. British Journal of Urology 49: 211–214

Haylen B T, Fraser M I 1987 Is the investigation of most stress incontinence really necessary? Neurourology and Urodynamics 6: 3 188–189

Hilton P 1986 A clinical and urodynamic comparison of the sub-urethral sling and Stamey procedures in the treatment of genuine stress incontinence. British Journal of Obstetrics and Gynaecology 93: 291–293

Hilton P, Stanton S L 1981 Algorithmic method for assessing urinary incontinence in elderly women. British Medical Journal 282: 940–942

Hilton P, Stanton S L 1983a Urethral pressure measurement by microtransducer: the results in symptom-free women and in those with genuine stress incontinence. British Journal of Obstetrics and Gynaecology 90: 919–933.

Hilton P, Stanton S L 1983b A clinical and urodynamic assessment of the Burch colposuspension for genuine stress incontinence. British Journal of Obstetrics and Gynaecology 90: 934–939

Hilton P, Stanton S L 1983c The use of intravaginal oestrogen cream in genuine stress incontinence. British Journal of Obstetrics and Gynaecology 90: 940–944

Holmes D M, Plevnic S, Stanton S S L 1985a Distal urethral electric conductance (DUEC) test for the detection of urinary leakage. Proceedings of the 15th International Continence Society Meeting, London, pp 94–96

Holmes D M, Plevnic S, Stanton S L 1985b Bladder neck electrical conductance (BNEC) test in the investigation and treatment of sensory urgency and detrusor instability. Proceedings of 15th International Continence Society Meeting, London, pp 96–97

Iosif C S 1985 Sling operations for urinary incontinence. Obstetrics Scandinavia 64: 187–190

Jakobsen H, Vedel P, Andersen J T 1987 Which pad-weighing test to choose: ICS one-hour test, the 48-hour home test or a 40-minute test with known bladder volume. Proceedings of the 17th International Continence Society Meeting, Bristol. Neurourology and Urodynamics 6: 166–167 (abst 22)

James E, Flack F, Caldwell K, Martin M 1971 Continuous measurement of urine loss and frequency in incontinent patients. British Journal of Urology 43: 233–237

Jarvis G J, Fowlie A 1985 Clinical and urodynamic assessment of the porcine dermis bladder skin in the treatment of genuine stress incontinence. British Journal of Obstetrics and Gynaecology 92: 1189–1191

Jarvis G J, Hall S, Stamp S, Miller D R, Johnson A 1980 An assessment of urodynamic examination in incontinent women. British Journal of Obstetrics and Gynaecology 87: 893–896

Jeffcoate T W A, Roberts H 1952 Stress incontinence. British Journal of Obstetrics and Gynaecology 59: 685–720

Jorgensen L, Lose G, Thunedborg P 1987 Diagnosis of mild stress incontinence in females: 24-hour home pad-weighing test versus the 1-hour ward test. Proceedings of the 17th International Continence Society Meeting. Neurourology and Urodynamics 6: 165–166 (abst 21)

Kirby R S, Fowler C, Gilpin S-A et al 1983 Non-obstructive detrusor failure. A urodynamic electromyographic neurohistochemical and autonomic study. British Journal of Urology 55: 652–659

Klevmark B, Telseth T, Eri L M 1988 Objective assessment of urinary incontinence. The advantages of relating 24-hour pad-weighing test to frequency-volume charts ('combined test'). Proceedings of the 18th International Continence Society Meeting. Neurourology and Urodynamics 7: 170–171 (abst 7)

Kulseng-Hansen S 1983 Prevalence and pattern of unstable urethral pressure in 174 gynecologic patients referred for urodynamic investigations. American Journal of Obstetrics and Gynecology 146: 895–900

Lewis L G 1939 New clinical recording cystometer. Journal of Urology 41: 638–645

Mayne C J, Hilton P 1988 The distal urethral electrical conductance test: standardization of method and clinical reliability. Neurourology and Urodynamics 7: 55–60

Plevnic S 1985 New method for testing and strengthening of pelvic floor muscles. Proceedings of the 15th International Continence Society Meeting. London, pp 267–268

Quinn M J, Beynon J, Mortensen N M, Smith P J B 1987 Transvaginal endosonography in the assessment of urinary stress incontinence. Neurourology and Urodynamics 6: 180–181

Shawer M, Brown M, Sutherst J 1981 Diagnosis of bladder-neck incompetence without use of capital equipment. British Medical Journal 283: 760–761

Shepherd A M, Montgomery E, Anderson R S 1983 Treatment of genuine stress incontinence with a new perineometer. Physiotherapy 69: 113

Shepherd A M, Powell P H, Ball A J 1982 The place of urodynamic studies in the investigation and treatment of female urinary tract symptoms. Journal of Obstetrics and Gynaecology 3: 123–125

Stanton S L 1984 Voiding difficulties and retention. In: Stanton S L (ed) Clinical gynecologic urology. C. V. Mosby, Toronto, p 256

Stanton S L 1985 Surgery for urethral sphincter incompetence. Urogynaecologia 1: 19–23

Stanton S L, Cardozo L D 1979 Results of colposuspension operation for incontinence and prolapse. British Journal of Obstetrics and Gynaecology 86: 693–697

Stanton S L, Cardozo L D, Chaudhury N 1978 Spontaneous voiding after surgery for urinary incontinence. British Journal of Obstetrics and Gynaecology 85: 149–152

Stanton S L, Chamberlain G V P, Holmes D M 1985 Randomized study of the anterior repair and colposuspension operation in the control of genuine stress incontinence. Proceedings of the 15th International Continence Society Meeting, London, pp 236–237

Sutherst J R, Brown M C 1980 Detection of urethral incompetence in women using the fluid bridge test. British Journal of Urology 52: 138–142

Sutherst J R, Brown M, Shawer M 1981 Assessing the severity of urine incontinence in women by weighing perineal pads. Lancet i 1128–1130

Tapp A, Meire H, Cardozo L D 1987 The effect of epidural analgesia on post-partum voiding. Neurourology and Urodynamics 6: 235–236

Tapp A, Versi E, Cardozo L, Studd J W 1986 Urethral instability real or imaginary? Proceedings of 16th International Continence Society Meeting, Boston, pp 40–41

Versi E 1990 The use of discriminate analysis to increase the diagnostic accuracy of urethral pressure profilometry. British Journal of Obstetrics and Gynaecology (In press)

Versi E, Cardozo L D 1986a Perineal pad weighing versus videographic analysis in genuine stress incontinence. British Journal of Obstetrics and Gynaecology 93: 364–366

Versi E, Cardozo L D 1986b Urethral instability: diagnosis based on variation in the maximum urethral pressure in normal climacteric women. Neurourology and Urodynamics 5: 535–542

Versi E, Cardozo L D, Studd J W W, Brincat M, O'Dowd T M, Cooper D J 1986a Internal urinary sphincter in maintenance of female continence. British Medical Journal 292: 166–167

Versi E, Cardozo L D, Studd J W W, Cooper D 1986b Evaluation of urethral pressure profilometry for the diagnosis of genuine stress incontinence. World Journal of Urology 4: 6–9

Versi E, Cardozo L D, Anand G K 1988a The use of pad tests in the investigation of female urinary incontinence. Journal of Obstetrics and Gynaecology 8: 270–273

Versi E, Cardozo L, Brincat M, Cooper D, Montgomery J, Studd J 1988b Correlation of urethral physiology and skin collagen in postmenopausal women. British Journal of Obstetrics and Gynaecology 95: 147–152

Versi E, Cardozo L D, Anand G K, Cooper D 1990a The accuracy of a diagnosis of genuine stress incontinence based on symptoms alone. American Journal of Obstetrics and Gynecology (submitted for publication)

Versi E, Cardozo L D, Studd J W W, Cooper D J 1990b The use of transmission pressure ratios for the diagnosis of genuine stress incontinence. British Journal of Urology (submitted for publication)

von Garrelts B 1956 Analysis of micturition: a new method of recording the voiding of the bladder. Acta Chirurgica Scandinavica 112: 326–340

Weil A, Reyes H, Bischoff P, Rothenberg R D, Krauer F 1984 Modifications of the urethral rest and stress profile under different types of surgery for urinary stress incontinence. British Journal of Obstetrics and Gynaecology 91: 46–55

Wilson P D, Al Samarrai T, Deakin M, Kolbe E, Brown A D G 1987 An objective assessment of physiotherapy for female genuine stress incontinence. British Journal of Obstetrics and Gynaecology 94: 575–582

14. Injury to the bowel during gynaecological surgery

R. H. J. Kerr-Wilson

INTRODUCTION

'The gynaecologist entering the abdomen must be prepared to do surgery involving the gastrointestinal tract' (Schaefer & Graber 1981). Although this maxim is one to be recommended, there are few occasions today when the general gynaecologist is required to carry out major bowel surgery single-handed. An increase in medical methods of treatment for many gynaecological complaints, with early referral and diagnosis in many Western countries, together with fear of litigation, has resulted in a decline in the gynaecologist's general surgical skills. He or she is therefore better advised to appreciate which patients are at risk of bowel injury, to be able to recognize it when it has occurred, and to learn some simple techniques of bowel repair which can easily be remembered, rather than try to keep up to date with the latest advances in gastrointestinal surgery. Perhaps a more appropriate quotation for this chapter would be: 'When in doubt, the gynaecologist should seek the advice of a well-trained general surgeon' (Marchant 1981).

INCIDENCE

Fortunately, the incidence of bowel injury during gynaecological surgery is low. Reported figures range from 0.3–0.8%, depending on the operation. Two-thirds are minor lacerations, and three-quarters involve the small bowel. Perhaps surprisingly, laparoscopy and vaginal surgery appear to carry less risk of injury to the bowel than does abdominal surgery.

Copenhaver (1962) reported a series of 1000 vaginal hysterectomies, with and without repairs, at the Johns Hopkins Hospital between 1948 and 1952 without any record of damage to the bowel. From the same institution, Thompson and Wheeless (1973) described 3600 patients undergoing laparoscopic sterilization between 1968 and 1972. Eleven (0.3%) had gastrointestinal injuries, although 10 of these were attributed to electrical burns.

A more detailed account over the decade following has been given by Krebs (1986). He examined the records of 128 cases of bowel injury which

Table 14.1 Bowel injury according to operation (128 cases). (After Krebs 1986)

Operation	% of total
Entrance into peritoneal cavity	37
Lysis of adhesions or dissection	35
Laparoscopy	10
Vaginal operations	9
D & C or evacuation	9

occurred from 1973–1982 in 17 650 patients having gynaecological surgery at the Medical College of Virginia. The results are given in Table 14.1. The small intestine was involved in 75% of cases, the large bowel in 25%; 69% had minor lacerations, and major injury was only recorded in 31%. However, the majority of bowel injuries (72%) occurred during 'uncomplicated' gynaecological operations.

Gastrointestinal injuries following laparoscopy alone have been estimated to occur in from 0.5–3.0 per 1000 procedures (Borten 1986). The Centre for Disease Control in Atlanta found an even lower figure when they reviewed 5027 women who underwent laparoscopic sterilization from 1978–1982. Twelve (0.24%) had unintended laparotomies for complications, of whom three required bowel resections (Franks et al 1987).

Following Caesarean section, only one case of intestinal injury was recorded in a review of 1319 patients during the years 1978–1980 at Boras in Sweden. About 20 cm of small intestine was inadvertently sewn to the posterior part of the uterus, but was discovered before closing the abdomen. The sutures were removed and the post-operative course was uncomplicated (Nielsen et al 1984).

These figures indicate that in a general gynaecological practice with an average of 15 operations per week (750 per annum), injury to the gastrointestinal tract should only occur once in every 3–4 years. Even with 60 operations per week (3000 per annum), bowel injury should only occur once a year—hardly enough to maintain adequate experience in appropriate techniques.

RISK FACTORS

The major risk factors predisposing to bowel damage are:

1. Obesity,
2. Previous laparotomy,
3. Adhesions from malignancy, endometriosis or infection,
4. Intrinsic bowel problems,
5. Irradiation.

It has been estimated that the incidence of bowel injury during entry into the abdominal cavity is two-and-a-half times higher in obese patients (Schaefer & Graber 1981, Krebs 1986). Likewise, previous laparotomy carries a threefold risk of intestinal injury on entering the abdominal cavity (Hurt & Dunn 1984, Krebs 1986). This seems to apply even if the previous abdominal surgery was a Caesarean section (Franks et al 1987).

Gynaecological conditions which should alert the surgeon to the risk of injury to the bowel are those which may result in adhesions, such as malignancy, endometriosis or pelvic inflammatory disease (Krebs 1986, Mitchell & Massey 1988). Intrinsic bowel problems which result in acute or chronic inflammation, such as Crohn's disease, ulcerative colitis and diverticular disease can also make the bowel more susceptible to injury (Mitchell & Massey 1988). Previous radiation therapy to the pelvis or abdomen can make surgery particularly hazardous. Loops of bowel may become adherent to the anterior abdominal wall, or become matted together, with a loss of distinct tissue planes.

A particular problem that may occur during laparoscopy is perforation of the dilated gastrointestinal tract in cases of obstruction, or of the distended stomach if there has been faulty insertion of the endotracheal tube at general anaesthesia (Thompson & Wheeless 1973, Endler & Moghissi 1976). However, it is important to note that more than half the cases of gastrointestinal injury following laparoscopy do not have any predisposing factors.

TYPES AND SITES OF INJURY

Injury to the bowel may be a perforation, laceration or a crush injury. It may be inflicted by a scalpel, needle, scissors, forceps, diathermy, or even, at least theoretically, by laser. Type and site of injury may vary according to the initial gynaecological operation, so it is important to consider these before discussing management.

Abdominal surgery

Small or large bowel may be injured during the course of open abdominal surgery. The commonest site is the small intestine at the time of opening the abdominal cavity. The rectum and pelvic colon are also vulnerable at the time of hysterectomy, particularly if there is pelvic inflammation, malignancy or diverticulitis. The caecum, ascending and transverse colon are less likely to be damaged.

Laparoscopy

More has been written about injury to the gastrointestinal tract at the time of laparoscopy than after any other gynaecological operation (Thompson & Wheeless 1973, Endler & Moghissi 1976, Hurt & Dunn 1984, Levy et al

1985, Borten 1986, De Cherney 1988). This is not because it carries a greater risk than other gynaecological procedures (see Table 17.1), but probably more because of the traumatic appearance of the procedure, and the fact that it is often performed on otherwise healthy young women.

Bowel injury at laparoscopy may occur as a result of direct trauma or thermal damage (Hurt & Dunn 1984), although the latter is less common with decreasing use of diathermy for sterilization. However, some of the injuries attributed to electrical injury may in fact be traumatic in origin (Levy et al 1985). Traumatic damage may be caused either by the Verres needle, or at insertion of the trocar and cannula. The commonest site for penetrating bowel injury at laparoscopy is the small intestine. Sometimes partial transfixion of the bowel wall with the Verres needle may occur, causing bullous distention on insufflation with gas. This resolves spontaneously without treatment, providing there is no bleeding or spillage of bowel contents. The large bowel is rarely at risk of perforation at laparoscopy because of its lateral position, although gastric perforation has been recorded (see Risk Factors, p. 220).

Laser surgery

Intra-abdominal CO_2 laser surgery for fertility or endometriosis, either by open surgery or laparoscopy, has been used since 1974 (Tadir & Ovadia 1986). More recently, the Nd:YAG laser has been used for endometrial ablation. 'In general, the potential for major gastrointestinal complications with the CO_2 laser laparoscope is the same as with cautery' (Martin 1985). However, Bellina and Bandieramonte (1984) reported over 1000 intra-abdominal microsurgical procedures using the CO_2 laser without complications. Bellina (1986) reports having seen bowel perforations, although few if any of these have yet been documented officially.

Vaginal surgery

The small intestine may be damaged at the time of vaginal hysterectomy, either by laceration or from a crush injury following misapplication of forceps (Isaacs 1988). Injury to the rectum may occur during posterior colporrhaphy (Hurt & Dunn 1984), or in the course of an operation such as the McIndoe procedure for construction of a neovagina (Thompson 1988). Perforation of the lower rectum may also occur when a pelvic abscess is drained from below (Schaefer & Graber 1981).

DIAGNOSIS

Injury to the bowel may be of sufficient size to be recognized immediately by seeing bowel mucosa, bowel contents or bleeding. This will be most obvious after a large perforating injury or laceration. At laparoscopy, direct

Table 14.2   Clinical presentation of unrecognized bowel injuries. (Adapted from Thompson & Wheeless 1973)

Post-operative day	3–7
Physical examination	Mild distention
	Lower quadrant pain
	Decreased bowel sounds
Temperature	37.2–38.3°C
WBC	4000–10 000
X-rays	Not helpful, except ileus

injury to the bowel on insertion of the Verres needle can theoretically be recognized by aspiration if this is carried out prior to insufflation. Thermal injury to the bowel shows as a blanched area.

However, damage may easily go unrecognized, particularly after thermal, crush, or fine penetrating injuries by instruments or laser beam. Thompson and Wheeless (1973) found that only half the electrical injuries to bowel that occurred at the time of laparoscopic sterilization were noticed at the time. If the injury is unrecognized at surgery, it may become apparent after 72 hours with nausea, anorexia, lower abdominal pain and fever, progressing to vomiting, peritonitis and ileus (Table 14.2). Clinical assessment is essential as investigations, such as white cell count and abdominal X-rays, are often unhelpful. If left untreated, a fistula may develop (see Complications, p. 228).

MANAGEMENT

Management of bowel injury in gynaecological surgery will depend on the size and site of the trauma.

Perforating injury

Small perforating injuries with a suture or Verres needle can usually be managed conservatively with observation. If perforation of the stomach is suspected at laparoscopy on insertion of the Verres needle, decompression of the stomach with a nasogastric tube and re-insertion of the Verres needle is recommended. Providing the site of injury is visualized and there is no bleeding nor spillage of bowel contents, further surgical intervention is unnecessary (Endler & Moghissi 1976). If the injury is greater than 5 mm, as when the laparoscopic trocar is inserted into a viscus, then surgical closure is advisable (Borten 1986). If the laparoscope itself is inserted into the bowel, it is probably best to leave the laparoscope in place, perform a laparotomy, identify the defect and then close it appropriately after removing the laparoscope. Leaving the laparoscope in situ will seal the puncture wound and allow easy identification of the site of trauma (De Cherney 1988).

Small intestine

If a laceration of the small intestine involves less than half the circumference of the bowel, and there is no non-viable gut, a simple closure should be adequate (Masterson 1986). Horizontal tears are best closed in the same plane, but vertical and diagonal tears should be closed horizontally to avoid constriction of the lumen. Although a single layer closure, inverting the edges of the mucosa and the adjacent seromuscular layer, is adequate (Mitchell & Massey 1988), a two-layer closure of interrupted sutures, the inner being absorbable, is probably safer for the gynaecologist who operates on bowel only occasionally (Masterson 1986).

If the small intestine is lacerated during vaginal surgery, it may not always be technically feasible to carry out the repair vaginally. In such cases, the visible damage should be tagged with sutures, leaving long ends, and then the repair can be undertaken via a laparotomy (Hurt & Dunn 1984).

If the damage to small bowel is more severe, causing devitalization of tissue, as after extensive tearing, crushing with clamps, or thermal injury greater than 5 mm, then resection of the affected area with end-to-end anastomosis will be necessary. The principles to be remembered in this procedure are:

1. Avoid tension,
2. Ensure adequate blood supply,
3. Ensure that the lumen of the intestine is adequate.

Probably the simplest method for this procedure is that described by Monaghan (1986). The small bowel is elevated and the limits of resection identified so that an adequate blood supply will reach the anastomosis before soft bowel clamps are applied (Fig. 14.1). The damaged bowel is

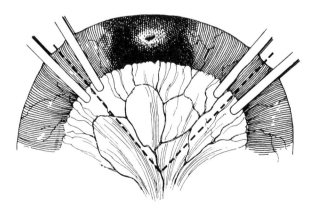

Fig. 14.1   Resecting a damaged segment of small bowel. (Reproduced with permission from Monaghan 1986).

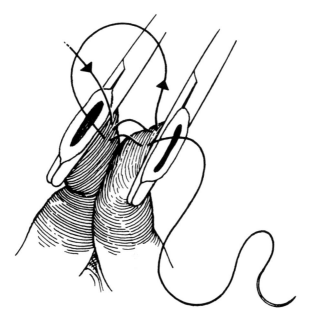

Fig. 14.2   Suturing the serosa of the bowel segments. (Reproduced with permission from Monaghan 1986).

then resected and mesenteric vessels ligated. The bowel clamps are then approximated and rotated laterally before suturing in two layers. The posterior outer serosal layer is sutured first, using either a continuous absorbable suture, such as 2/0 catgut (Fig. 14.2, Monaghan 1986) or, more traditionally, interrupted 3/0 or 4/0 silk (Marchant 1981). The inner mucosal, or all-coats layer should be an absorbable suture, and is continued onto the anterior wall simply by reversing the needle (Fig. 14.3). The anastomosis is completed by suturing the anterior seromuscular layer and closing the mesentery. Intra-operatively, it is advisable to give intravenous prophylactic antibiotics, such as gentamicin and metronidazole, and after the anastomosis is complete, to irrigate the operation site with saline. If the patient's condition is poor, the resection is anticipated to be particularly difficult, or the injuries are multiple, then a side-to-side anastomosis should be considered instead (Mitchell & Massey 1988).

Intestinal staplers are being used with increasing frequency for bowel resection and anastomosis by general gastrointestinal surgeons. They are certainly an acceptable alternative to sutures, since they cause less tissue trauma, take less time, and leave a greater blood flow to the anastomosis (Masterson 1986). However, for the gynaecologist who only performs bowel surgery rarely, it is probably safer to rely on a simple suture technique such as that described above.

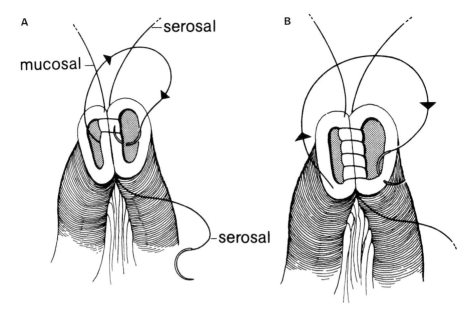

Fig. 14.3A   Suturing the mucosa of the bowel; **B** completing the mucosal suture. (Reproduced with permission from Monaghan 1986).

Large intestine

The ascending colon is similar to the small bowel as regards bacterial flora, so providing there is no non-viable bowel, a simple laceration involving less than half the circumference may be closed in two layers as for the small intestine. Injury to the descending colon may be closed in a similar fashion providing the bowel has been adequately prepared. However, trauma to the descending colon in gynaecological surgery is more likely to occur in patients whose bowel is unprepared, and in these cases a proximal colostomy is also required. A proximal colostomy will also be necessary if the laceration is large, the blood supply to the damaged bowel is in doubt, or the closure is under tension (Hurt & Dunn 1984). Any devitalized tissue will need to be excised and a two-layer anastomosis performed before fashioning a colostomy. The method already described for anastomosing small bowel is also suitable for large intestine (Monaghan 1986).

A simple technique for creating a temporary colostomy is the transverse loop colostomy described by Monaghan (1986, 1987). This avoids siting the stoma in the lower abdomen where further surgery may be required. The steps are as follows:

1. Make a transverse midline incision above the umbilicus (Fig. 14.4),
2. Deliver transverse colon and dissect off greater omentum from the lower border over 10 cm,

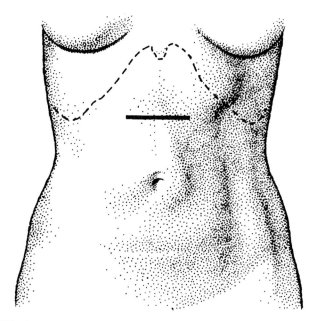

Fig. 14.4   The site of the incision for a temporary transverse colostomy. (Reproduced with permission from Monaghan 1986).

3. Insert bridge or rod through small hole in the mesentery (Fig. 14.5),
4. Close the anterior rectus sheath and skin,
5. Open in theatre along the taenia and apply a bag,
6. Remove the bridge in 4–5 days.

If the bowel has not been adequately prepared, the patient will also require intravenous antibiotics both during and after surgery.

When the anastomosis is considered to have healed, the colostomy is easily reversed by dissecting the bowel free from the abdominal wall, closing the stoma transversely in two layers, re-inserting the colon within the abdominal cavity and closing the abdominal wall. A temporary sigmoid colostomy may be fashioned similarly, using an incision in the left lower quadrant (Marchant 1981). If the colon has been previously irradiated, it is probably wise to wait 6–8 weeks before considering colostomy closure, and then only after preliminary X-ray studies of the distal colon (Masterson 1986).

Rectum

If the rectum is entered below the peritoneal reflection during vaginal surgery, a single- or double-layer closure will usually be sufficient. In the majority of cases this will heal without fistula formation. Only if there is a significant opening above the peritoneal reflection, extensive local damage,

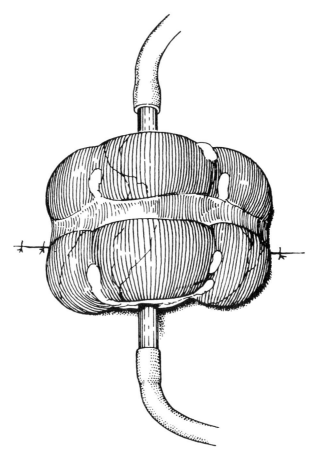

Fig. 14.5   Anchoring the loop of large bowel to the surface. (Reproduced with permission from Monaghan 1986).

or irradiated bowel will it be necessary to consider a temporary diverting colostomy (Mitchell & Massey 1988). Post-operative care should include a stool softener and low-residue diet. Some authors recommend that post-operative tension on the suture line after repair of rectal injury can be avoided by dilating the anal sphincter with two or three fingers at the time of surgery, and for several days post-operatively, to prevent gas collection (Hurt & Dunn 1984).

COMPLICATIONS

Short-term complications following intestinal injury in gynaecological procedures include ileus, peritonitis and leakage from the anastomosis. Fortunately, long term complications are rare. Krebs (1986) reported seven

Table 14.3 Complications following intestinal injury in gynaecological surgery. (Reproduced with permission from Krebs 1986)

Complication	Number
Wound infection	7
Atelectasis, pneumonia	6
Febrile morbidity (not specified)	6
Urinary tract infection	3
Ileus	4
Peritonitis	2
Anastomotic leak	1
Other	2

cases of ileus, peritonitis or anastomotic leak in his series of 128 cases of bowel injury (Table 14.3) but none had long-term problems.

Fistulae involving bowel are usually associated with radical surgery or radiation. However, they may still occur in surgery for benign conditions if the primary repair is unsuccessful, or the original injury was unrecognized. Small intestinal fistulae will usually require early operation because of loss of electrolytes and the irritating nature of the bowel contents. Large bowel fistulae may close spontaneously with conservative management unless complicated by distal obstruction, infection or malignancy. Small rectovaginal fistulae should be excised and closed in two layers, although more complicated ones may require temporary colostomy and delayed closure of the defect. Low rectovaginal fistulae near the external sphincter may be treated by incision of the perineal body to the level of the fistula, followed by closure similar to that of an episiotomy (Hurt & Dunn 1984).

PREVENTION

Avoidance of injury to the bowel will save not only time, anxiety and possible embarrassment for the surgeon at the time of operation, but also prevent post-operative worry, prolonged hospital stay for the patient, and possibly costly litigation. If trauma to the gastrointestinal tract does occur at the time of surgery, a full explanation must be given to the patient by the consultant or most senior doctor present as soon as the patient is able to understand (Mitchell & Massey 1988). For reasons of anaesthesia and analgesia, this may best be left until the day following the operation itself.

Certain operations such as culdoscopy, or transvaginal tubal sterilization are particularly hazardous to the bowel, and are no longer recommended (Krebs 1986). Particular care should be taken with obese patients, those who have had previous abdominal or pelvic surgery, or who have other factors which put them at risk of bowel injury (see above). If direct involvement of the bowel is diagnosed pre-operatively, or there is a strong chance of bowel injury during surgery, pre-operative bowel preparation with enemas and an appropriate antibiotic, such as neomycin, is recommended (Masterson 1986, Mitchell & Massey 1988).

Certain technical procedures may also help to avoid bowel injury:

1. When entering the abdomen through an old incision, it may be advisable to extend the new incision above the old, or else to ensure entry is in the superior part of the incision (Hurt & Dunn 1984);

2. In obese patients, dissect the pre-peritoneal fat down to the level of the peritoneum first, before picking up the peritoneum with non-toothed forceps and rolling it between thumb and index finger to make sure no bowel is included (Schaefer & Graber 1981);

3. When inserting a self-retaining retractor, make sure that the lateral blades are not in a position to compress the bowel (Hurt & Dunn 1984);

4. When packing bowel, do not exert undue pressure, do not handle it directly with forceps, and do not release bowel by blunt dissection (Mitchell & Massey 1988);

5. Use sharp dissection when adhesions are dense or tissue planes are destroyed (Krebs 1986, Mitchell & Massey 1988), as in endometriosis. Adhesions from pelvic inflammatory disease may often be divided by blunt dissection, since the serosa maintains its integrity. In endometriosis, however, the structures become welded together and sharp dissection is indicated (Hurt & Dunn 1984). After radiation therapy, avoid dissecting loops of bowel unless it is absolutely necessary, and then only with extreme caution;

6. Intrafascial enucleation of the cervix or subtotal hysterectomy can always be considered in very obese patients or in cases of particularly dense adhesions. Discretion may be the better part of valour;

7. For laparoscopic sterilization, the existence of clips and rings for tubal occlusion eliminates the need for intra-abdominal coagulation (Thompson & Wheeless 1973).

8. At laparoscopy, if there is a suspicion of gastric distention from inspection, palpation or percussion, insert a nasogastric tube first (Endler & Moghissi 1976).

CONCLUSION

Injury to the bowel during gynaecological surgery is uncommon. The majority of cases occur at laparotomy in the form of lacerations involving the small bowel and can be managed by primary closure. Significant predisposing factors are obesity and previous lower abdominal surgery.

REFERENCES

Bellina J H 1986 Tubal surgery. In: Sharp F, Jordan J A (eds) Gynecological laser surgery. Perinatology Press, Ithaca, New York, pp 217–239
Bellina J H, Bandieramonte G 1984 Principles and practice of gynecologic laser surgery.

Plenum Publishing Corporation, New York, pp 187–212

Borten M 1986 Laparoscopic complications: prevention and management. B C Decker, Toronto

Copenhaver E H 1962 Vaginal hysterectomy: an analysis of indications and complications among 1000 operations. American Journal of Obstetrics and Gynecology 84: 123–128

De Cherney A H 1988 Laparoscopy with unexpected viscus penetration. In: Nichols D H (ed) Clinical problems, injuries and complications of gynecologic surgery 2nd edn. Williams and Wilkins, Baltimore, pp 62–63

Endler G C, Moghissi K S 1976 Gastric perforation during pelvic laparoscopy. Obstetrics and Gynecology 47: 40s–42s

Franks A L, Kendrick J S, Peterson H B 1987 Unintended laparotomy associated with laparoscopic tubal sterilization. American Journal of Obstetrics and Gynecology 157: 1102–1105

Hurt W G, Dunn L J 1984 Complications of gynecologic surgery and trauma. In: Greenfield L J (ed) Complications in surgery and trauma. J B Lippincott, Philadelphia, pp 790–799

Isaacs J H 1988 Unexpected clamping of small bowel during hysterectomy. In: Nichols D H (ed) Clinical problems, injuries and complications of gynecologic surgery 2nd edn. Williams and Wilkins, Baltimore, pp 212–214

Krebs H-B 1986 Intestinal injury in gynecologic surgery: a ten-year experience. American Journal of Obstetrics and Gynecology 155: 509–514

Levy B S, Soderstrom R S, Dail D H 1985 Bowel injuries during laparoscopy. The Journal of Reproductive Medicine 30: 168–172

Marchant D J 1981 Special problems of the intestinal tract. In: Schaefer G, Graber E A (eds) Complications in obstetric and gynecologic surgery. Harper and Row, Hagerstown, New York, ch 35

Martin D C 1985 Laser safety. In: Keye W R Jr (ed) Laser surgery in gynaecology and obstetrics. Castle House Publications, Tunbridge Wells, p 49

Masterson B J 1986 Management of bowel injuries in gynecologic surgery. In: Manual of gynecologic surgery 2nd edn. Springer Verlag, New York, ch 22

Mitchell G W, Massey F M 1988 Injury to the bowel during pelvic surgery. In: Nichols D H (ed) Clinical problems, injuries and complications of gynecologic surgery 2nd edn. Williams and Wilkins, Baltimore, pp 207–211

Monaghan J M 1986 Operations on the intestinal tract for the gynaecologist In: Bonney's gynaecological surgery 9th edn. Baillière Tindall, London, pp 241–250

Monaghan J M 1987 Formation of a colostomy and construction of a urinary conduit. In: Rob and Smith's Operative Surgery: Gynaecology and Obstetrics 4th edn. J M Butterworth, London, pp 213–222

Nielsen T F, Hokegård K-H 1984 Caesarean section and intra-operative surgical complications. Acta Obstetrica et Gynecologica Scandinavica 63: 103–108

Schaefer G, Graber E A 1981 Complications in obstetric and gynecologic surgery. Harper and Row, Hagerstown, New York, pp 445–466

Tadir Y, Ovadia J 1986 Laser endoscopy in gynaecology In: Sharp F, Jordan J A (eds) Gynaecological laser surgery. Perinatology Press, Ithaca, New York, pp 241–249

Thompson B H, Wheeless C R 1973 Gastrointestinal complications of laparoscopy sterilization. Obstetrics and Gynecology 41: 669–676

Thompson J D 1988 McIndoe procedure with rectal penetration. In: Nichols D H (ed) Clinical problems, injuries and complications of gynecologic surgery 2nd edn. Williams and Wilkins, Baltimore, pp 87–91

15. A second look at second-look surgery

C. W. E. Redman   K. K. Chan

INTRODUCTION

In the first volume of this series, the role of second-look operations in the management of epithelial ovarian cancer (EOC) was reviewed (Singer 1981). It was concluded that the place of these procedures was controversial but on balance, of value. The passage of time has allowed further appraisal of the role of second-look procedures in conjunction with the developments that have occurred in the management and monitoring of EOC. In general there has been increasing scepticism about this once fashionable approach (Luesley et al 1988, Chambers et al 1988) but considerable debate continues, evidenced by the sustained, if not increasing, amount of related literature (Fig. 15.1). In the light of these changes, this chapter re-addresses the question of whether second-look procedures, and in particular second-look laparotomy (SLL), have any value in the management of EOC.

Second-look surgery should be differentiated from other forms of

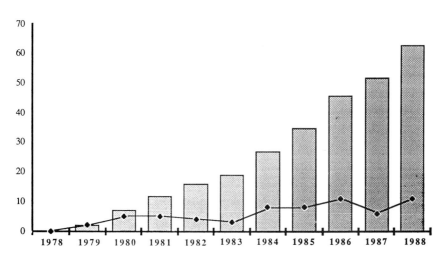

Fig. 15.1 Number of publications on second-look surgery since 1978. Diagram shows the number of publications each year and the cumulative total of publications since 1978.

secondary surgery. For the purposes of this review, second-look surgery is considered to be an operation performed electively at the end of primary induction therapy, whether or not the presence of disease was suspected pre-operatively. The surgical objectives are to assess disease status and to resect residual tumour. In recent years these procedures have largely been performed in patients without clinically and radiologically detectable disease (Schwartz et al 1983).

PRIMARY THERAPY IN EOC

Although the concept of second-look surgery was first described in 1951 (Wangensteen et al 1951), it was only during the 1970s that second-look surgery, usually laparotomy, became a widely incorporated part of primary radical therapy for EOC (Copeland 1985). It was also during this time that active chemotherapy (Bagley et al 1972, Smith & Rutledge 1970) and the surgical principles of primary cytoreductive surgery were introduced (Griffiths 1975). More recently the advent of cis-platinum has had a major impact in primary treatment schedules and response rates (Vogl et al 1982, Edmondson et al 1979). Thus any overall improvement in the outcome for patients with ovarian cancer during this time could be due to any one of these treatment factors. However, no such improvement has been noted and the overall prognosis for EOC remains poor, particularly for the majority of ovarian cancer patients who present with extensive disease that is not amenable to surgical extirpation (Smith & Day 1979, Kottmeier 1982).

MORBIDITY

Any discussion about the value of second-look surgery has to take account of both the potential benefits and the undoubted morbidity of such surgical intervention, which is particularly relevant to laparotomy. The majority of published studies of second-look procedures are primarily survival studies without any meaningful assessment of associated morbidity. However, when listed, the most common complications are blood loss requiring transfusions, wound and urinary tract infections, ileus, bowel injury and pulmonary complications (Schwartz & Smith, 1980, Phibbs et al 1983). The active search for alternatives to second-look surgery, particularly laparotomy, emphasizes the reservations many have.

In the performance of SLL, many have stressed the importance of extensive biopsies and detailed exploration of the peritoneal cavity (Barber 1984, Smith et al 1976, Wharton 1978, Phillips et al 1979, Smith 1980). Such prolonged procedures are necessarily associated with morbidity. In a recent series of 97 patients, 63% of patients undergoing laparotomy experienced some complication (Chambers et al 1988). The median post-operative hospital stay was 12 days which is very similar to the results of the

West Midlands Ovarian Cancer Group (WMOCG), reported by Luesley et al (1984). In this series 70% of patients had a prolonged ileus, and 70% required blood transfusion. In view of these dangers and because of the obvious difficulty of repeating such operations at regular intervals, some attention has been paid to laparoscopy, although there remains a significant complication rate, and there is a high false-negative rate varying from 20–77% (Rosenoff et al 1975, Smith et al 1977, Piver et al 1980, Quinn et al 1980, Berek et al 1981, Ozols et al 1981, Lele & Piver 1986).

MONITORING OF DISEASE

The majority of patients with EOC will have residual disease after primary surgery. In our own experience, approximately 80% of patients will have macroscopic residual disease and half this number will have disease residuum that exceeds 2 cm in maximum diameter. [These figures are perhaps higher than those reported from some specialist gynaecological oncology centres and reflect the fact that in the West Midlands the vast majority of primary laparotomies are performed by surgeons who do not have a particular expertise in this field]. When there is residual disease, further therapy is conventionally given, and currently available evidence would suggest that chemotherapy is the most appropriate. Despite the advent of active chemotherapeutic agents, the increased response rates have not yet been translated into significant gains in long-term survival. Such therapy is, however, associated with significant short- and long-term toxicity. Thus the ability to monitor response accurately and conveniently is potentially important. For example, by the early selection of poor or non-responders to first-line therapy, it would enable a more timely change in therapy and thereby minimize toxicity. The monitoring of response has also been considered to be important for assessing the duration of therapy and influencing the selection of further treatment in responding patients. Surgery, particularly laparotomy, suffers from the disadvantage that it is not easily repeated, although Copeland et al (1983) have reported third- and fourth-look laparotomies.

Clinical examination

One reason why second-look surgery was widely adopted was because of the recognized shortcomings of the currently available alternatives. Clinical examination is inaccurate and insensitive, particularly with small-volume disease. A compilation of second-look laparotomy results shows that macroscopic residual disease was detected in 33% (range 0–59%) of patients in complete clinical remission (Table 15.1). When documented, microscopic residual disease was present in a further 17%. The timing of the second-look procedure will influence disease-detection rates. Thus in our own series where laparotomy was performed approximately 6 months

Table 15.1   Findings at second-look laparotomy in patients with no clinical disease

Study	Total	Macroscopic (%)	Microscopic (%)	Negative (%)
Berek et al 1984	56	53	14	32
Bertelsen et al 1988	157	45	15	40
Cohen et al 1983	63	35	17	48
Curry et al 1981	27	26	11	63
Free & Webb 1987	34	59	18	23
Ho et al 1988	39	41	15	44
Luesley et al 1984	68	37	31	32
Miller et al 1986	88	36	18	43
Phibbs et al 1983	36	44	8	47
Raju et al 1982	16	—	25	75

after the primary surgery, 68% of patients had evidence of disease (macroscopic 37%, microscopic 31%), a higher figure than other reported series. However, in those series when the interval was greater, a smaller proportion of clinically negative cases had residual disease, as some of those patients who harboured occult residual disease at 6 months would have relapsed.

Imaging

Recent years have seen the development and improvement of imaging techniques of ultrasonography, computed axial tomography, magnetic resonance, and radioimmunolocalization. These techniques have replaced traditional radiography in the evaluation of pelvic cancers but remain less sensitive than surgery for the detection of small-volume macroscopic residual disease (Pussell et al 1980, Saunders et al 1983, Goldhirsch et al 1983, Brenner et al 1985, Epenetos et al 1985, Shepherd et al 1987, Chatel et al 1987). In addition surgery can detect microscopic disease. Thus these non-invasive and repeatable procedures have significant false-negative rates but they do provide some useful information if positive.

Tumour markers

In the absence of accurate non-invasive techniques for the detection and monitoring of small-volume disease in ovarian cancer, attention has been focused on the use of serum markers. Although there are no tumour-specific antigens in ovarian cancer, monoclonal antibodies have been developed to recognize a number of tumour-associated antigens (TAA) that are expressed by certain types of cancer cells but few non-malignant cells.

A number of markers have been evaluated but currently serum CA125 has shown the greatest promise in this context. CA125 is a high molecular weight glycoprotein that is detected by the monoclonal antibody OC125. This antibody was developed by Bast et al (1981) using somatic hybridization of spleen cells from mice, immunized with an epithelial ovarian carcinoma cell line (OVCA 433). It can be detected in serum using a radioimmunoassay (Klug et al 1984) and is present in the serum of normal women. If an arbitrary cut-off point of 35 U/l is adopted, only 1% of normal subjects have elevated levels, whereas elevated levels are found in 82% of ovarian cancer patients, and in 6% of patients with non-malignant conditions (Bast et al 1983). Elevated serum levels are also found in a number of non-malignant conditions, especially when the peritoneum is inflamed, as in pelvic inflammatory disease or when there are serous effusions (Niloff et al 1984, Bergmann et al 1987, Halila et al 1986, Barbieri et al 1986, Cruickshank et al 1987). Serum CA125 levels rise post-operatively, possibly as a result of peritoneal trauma (Krebs et al 1986), supported by the observation that peritoneal CA125 levels are significantly higher when performed at laparotomy than if done at laparoscopy (Redman et al 1988). In addition, elevated CA125 levels are found with a number of other malignancies including non-epithelial ovarian tumours, cancer of the endometrium, endocervix, stomach, and pancreas (Altaras et al 1986, Duk et al 1986, Kivinen et al 1986, Peters et al 1986, Quentmeier et al 1987).

In EOC serum CA125 levels are influenced by stage and the bulk of disease (Krebs et al 1986). There is considerable variation in serum levels for a given tumour burden, perhaps reflecting the wide cellular heterogeneity observed in ovarian cancers and the effect of peritoneal involvement which is not necessarily related to tumour burden. Nevertheless, rising or falling levels of CA125 correspond with progression or regression of disease (Bast et al 1983, Canney et al 1984). Despite this excellent correlation, up to 50% of patients who have negative values will be found to have residual disease up to 2 cm in diameter at second-look procedures (Niloff et al 1985, Berek et al 1986, Krebs et al 1986, Atack et al 1986, Schilthuis et al 1987). Serum CA125 therefore lacks sensitivity for small-volume disease and is inferior to SLL for the detection of sub-clinical disease.

The ability to predict prognosis and response to therapy would theoretically enhance management and serum CA125 has been evaluated in this respect. Overall, it would appear that pre-treatment CA125 values are not sufficiently prognostic so as to influence management (Kivinen et al 1986, Parker et al 1988, Lavin et al 1985, Cruickshank et al 1987). In a multivariate analysis, controlling for stage and residual disease, Canney (1985) did not find that pre-treatment serum CA125 influenced survival.

Another approach relates to the rate at which antigen levels decline during treatment. When a tumour is completely removed, CA125 levels decline with an apparent half-life of 4.5 days (Canney et al 1984). In patients with residual disease and who respond to chemotherapy, the apparent half-life is 9.2 days (± 4.9 days), whereas it is 22.2 days (± 2.2 days) when the response is static. In a study of 27 EOC patients with residual disease, it was noted that the failure of serum CA125 levels to return to normal within 3 months of first-line treatment was associated with a poor prognosis (Lavin et al 1987). In a further study it was seen that failure of CA125 to normalize (< 35 U/ml) by 3 months after initiation of treatment was associated with the presence of disease at second-look operation. Even when CA125 had returned to normal prior to the operation, only those patients who had normal CA125 levels at 3 months were free of disease at second-look (Bast et al 1987). Vergote et al (1987) confirmed these findings in a similar study of 227 patients and in addition reported that only patients who had a fall of greater than 30% after the first course of chemotherapy would respond to therapy.

In the absence of completely effective but toxic therapy, the main role of monitoring is to limit toxicity. In poor prognostic patients these data suggest that serum CA125 can provide early prognostic information which is of potential value in sparing patients, unlikely to derive benefit from further aggressive therapy, unwarranted toxicity. In this respect serum CA125 has undoubted advantages over surgery. An important aspect of damage limitation in good prognostic patients (for example patients with no macroscopic residual disease) may be to treat only selected patients rather than give global adjuvant therapy. Sensitivity is highly important in this context and serum CA125 is certainly less sensitive than surgery. However, surgery cannot be performed repeatedly and, in any event, the therapeutic efficacy of early disease detection is limited by the effectiveness of available treatment.

The negative second-look laparotomy

The standard by which any monitoring method is judged is therefore that of laparotomy. The only way of evaluating laparotomy is to examine relapse rates after negative procedures. Survival of patients with no documented residual is significantly better than those with macroscopic residual disease (Berek et al 1983). However, a review of the literature shows that 4–53% of patients who had histologically negative second-look procedures, subsequently relapsed (Table 15.2). Small patient numbers, short follow-up intervals and non-standardized therapy render comparisons and interpretation difficult. It is semantic to try and differentiate true recurrences from inadequate sampling since from a practical point of view all these relapses represent false negatives. In any event there seems to be little difference in survival in pathologically negative cases compared with patients with microscopic residual disease (Copeland et al 1983).

The chances of relapse after a negative SLL appear to be influenced by a number of tumour characteristics, such as initial tumour residuum, histological type and degree of differentiation (Gerhenson et al 1985, Free & Webb 1987). The timing of the SLL can also influence the proportion of

Table 18.2   Recurrence after histologically negative second-look laparotomy

Reference	No. of histologically negative cases	Recurrence rate (%)
Berek et al 1984	18	22
Chambers et al 1988	38	18
Copeland & Gershensen 1986	86	44
Curry et al 1981	17	17
Free & Webb 1987	55	11
Greco et al 1981	17	5
Ho et al 1988	17	53
Jones et al 1981	23	4
Luesley et al 1984	23	30
Miller et al 1986	38	21
Roberts et al 1982	36	16
Rubin et al 1988	83	25
Schwartz & Smith 1980	58	12
Webb et al 1982	32	12

relapses subsequently observed. Thus relapse rates fall the further SLL is performed from the commencement of treatment (Berek et al 1981) but this reduces its usefulness in influencing management. However, it is clear that recurrence after a negative SLL is high in studies with adequate follow-up. The implication of this is that more recurrences will occur the longer one waits. This is reinforced by the observation of Neijt et al (1986) who observed that the relapse rate for patients in pathological complete remission had not flattened out after 72 months' follow-up. Thus SLL provides limited prognostic information.

The value of second-look surgery in monitoring

In terms of disease detection, second-look surgery would appear to be the most sensitive method available. One must question, however, whether this ability to detect disease is of value. Certainly this information can direct and select further treatment. Thus patients who have > 5 mm residual disease are not suitable for total abdominal irradiation (Rizel et al 1985). Similarly, intraperitoneal chemotherapy or immunotherapy only has therapeutic potential in patients with minimal residual disease (Ozols 1985). However, the potential advantage of this presupposes that further treatment in this group of patients is of benefit. Following primary *cis*-platinum therapy, continuing high dose treatment (Neijt et al 1984) or changing to alternative consolidation treatments has not been shown to confer any survival benefit (Blackledge et al 1987, Luesley et al 1988). Randomized studies evaluating the therapeutic role of further therapy compared with observation alone have not been performed. Therefore as there is no proven therapeutic benefit in the further treatment of patients with advanced ovarian cancer, the value of second-look surgery in this context is dubious.

On the basis of these observations it has been concluded that, as a means of monitoring, secondary surgery should be reserved for use in only experimental protocols in which exact measurement of tumour size may be important (Ho et al 1988, Chambers et al 1988).

SECONDARY CYTOREDUCTION

The majority of patients with EOC will have advanced disease at presentation that is not amenable to complete surgical extirpation at primary surgery. The presence and amount of post-operative residual disease is a major adverse prognostic factor. Many factors may contribute to the inability to excise all the tumour at the primary operation. These include the nature and extent of disease, and the general condition of the patient.

Chemotherapy regimens, especially those containing *cis*-platinum, are active in EOC and responses can be achieved in approximately 80% (Williams et al 1982, Vogl et al 1983, Neijt et al 1984). There is a theoretical possibility that primary surgical resection, active first-line chemotherapy and then secondary surgical cytoreduction might improve overall patient survival. A short-term survival advantage has been demonstrated in patients totally debulked at a second operation (Luesley et al 1984, Berek et al 1983) although this has not been the experience of others (Raju et al 1982, Free & Webb 1987, Podratz et al 1985, Ho et al 1988, Chambers et al 1988). The interpretation of these data is made difficult in that many of the patients undergoing second-look operations were a selected group and post-operative management was heterogeneous. The therapeutic benefit of such secondary cytoreduction is limited by the efficacy of post-surgical therapy.

West Midlands Ovarian Cancer Group (WMOCG) prospective randomized study

The necessity for a prospective, randomized assessment of the survival benefit of second-look surgery in ovarian cancer patients with post-operative residual disease, was addressed by the West Midlands Ovarian Cancer Group (Luesley et al 1988). This study also compared total abdominal and pelvic irradiation with a single agent alkylating agent as post-second-look management. From October 1981 to June 1985, 166 previously untreated patients with advanced EOC (FIGO stages IIb–IV) were entered into this study. The study design is shown in Figure 15.2 and patients, stratified by stage and residual disease, were entered into one of three arms. Primary chemotherapy in all treatment groups was single agent high-dose *cis*-platinum (100 mg/m² × 5 at three-weekly intervals).

Groups A and B underwent secondary surgery. This was performed 6

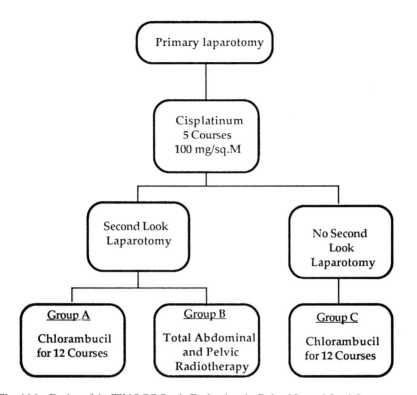

Fig. 15.2   Design of the WMOCG Study Evaluating the Role of Second-Look Laparotomy.

weeks after completion of primary chemotherapy (20–24 weeks after primary surgery) if there was no clinical evidence of progression of disease. If disease was found, an attempt was made to excise as much as possible.

Patients in Groups A ($n = 53$) and C ($n = 57$) received cyclical oral chlorambucil (0.2 mg/kg orally for 14 days every 28 days × 12). Patients in Group B ($n = 56$) received moving strip abdominopelvic irradiation if found to have < 2 cm disease at SLL (Dembo et al 1979). Thirty-nine (36%) patients did not undergo SLL as planned. The reasons for exclusion were disease progression (19), patient or clinician's refusal (16) or toxicity from chemotherapy. Treatment toxicity and disease progression rates in both the SLL and no SLL arms were similar.

The design of this study allowed a comparison between two randomized groups (A and C) treated identically except for the inclusion of second-look laparotomy in one treatment arm. With a median follow-up of 46 months no difference in survival was demonstrated (Fig. 15.3). This was still the case when complete and partial clinical responders were evaluated.

It is conceivable that there may be a subgroup of patients who do actually

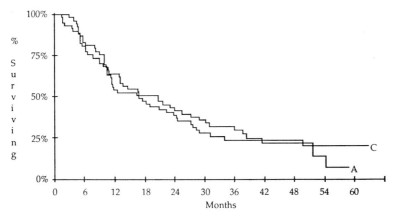

Fig. 15.3   The influence of second-look laparotomy on EOC patients receiving sequential *cis*-platinum/chlorambucil (A = second-look laparotomy, C = no second-look laparotomy) (from Luesley et al 1988, with permission).

benefit from SLL. For example, some have advocated that patients with small volume residual disease and negative cytology had a favourable prognosis (Schwartz & Smith 1980, Free & Webb 1987, Ho et al 1988). It is not possible to conclude from these retrospective analyses whether this better outcome is in any way related to surgery. In the WMOCG study there was no significant difference between patients who had no macroscopic disease at operation compared with those who had < 2 cm (Fig. 15.4). It would therefore appear that cytoreduction of < 2 cm group is not likely to be contributory to the outcome. These findings do not support the routine inclusion of second-look surgery in the management of ovarian cancer, either for debulking or diagnostic purposes.

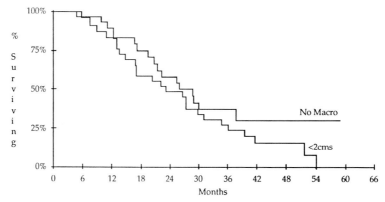

Fig. 15.4   Residual disease status at second-look laparotomy and survival (from Luesley et al 1988, with permission).

In view of these important but negative findings, it is important to consider why secondary cytoreduction, performed at the end of a planned course of chemotherapy, does not confer any survival benefit in patients with chemosensitive tumours. One explanation concerns the timing of secondary surgery. The Goldie-Coldman model of the development of acquired chemoresistance from spontaneous mutation suggests that the likelihood of the development of a clone of chemoresistant cells within a tumour is a function of the number of cell divisions that have occurred. Thus, the larger the tumour or the longer it has been in situ, the greater is the chance that a chemoresistant clone of cells will develop. This may account for the poor results associated with secondary resection carried out after a completed course of chemotherapy, perhaps 6–12 months after the onset of treatment. Potentially earlier secondary surgery, combined with active debulking chemotherapy, may improve patient outcome because the greater and more rapidly achieved cytoreductive treatment may preclude the development of chemoresistance.

EARLY SECONDARY CYTOREDUCTIVE SURGERY

Early secondary cytoreductive surgery should be differentiated from second-look surgery as it is performed during, rather than at the end of, primary induction therapy. Nevertheless, this surgical approach warrants discussion in this review as it has evolved from second-look surgery and its results will throw further light on the value of secondary surgery as a whole.

Neijt et al (1984) indicated that the outcome for patients with suboptimal primary surgery can be improved if early secondary surgery (termed intervention-debulking surgery) is performed during primary induction chemotherapy. These observations prompted the WMOCG to incorporate early secondary cytoreductive surgery during primary, intensive chemotherapy. As almost all responses to chemotherapy will occur within three cycles (Lawton et al 1987) it was attempted to perform the secondary surgery after only two or three cycles of treatment.

In an initial pilot study (Lawton et al 1989), 36 patients with EOC, incompletely resected at primary laparotomy, were recruited. The intention was to perform early secondary cytoreductive surgery after two or three cycles of platinum combination therapy in patients responding to treatment. Patients were treated with one of two chemotherapy regimes. Twenty-two patients received a combination of cis-platinum 75 mg/m² doxorubicin 50 mg/m² and bleomycin mg/m², while 14 were treated with cis-platinum 75–100 mg/m², and mitoxantrone 12–14 mg/m². All patients had gross residual disease, 23 (64%) patients having residual disease with greater than 5 cm.

Secondary surgery was performed in 28 (78%) patients, who had had sufficient response to chemotherapy. The median interval from the primary surgery to the second operation was 12.7 weeks (range 5.7–24.8) weeks. The surgical objectives were to complete a total abdominal hysterectomy, bilateral salpingo-oophorectomy, and infra-colic omentectomy if not already done, and to excise all macroscopic tumour. As a result of this surgery 16 out of the 28 patients (57%) were left with no macroscopic residual disease, and 9 (32%) were debulked to less than 2 cm residuum. These surgical results were achieved with few surgical complications, with a median post-operative stay of 10 days. The median survival for patients optimally debulked (20.8 months) at the second operation was significantly longer when this was not possible (7.1 months). This, of course, is a predictable finding. However, it was encouraging to note that those patients optimally debulked at secondary surgery had a similar survival as in 93 patients optimally debulked at primary surgery (27.4 months). Nevertheless, when survival was compared with that of 132 patients with advanced EOC who had bulky residual disease but who did not undergo early secondary surgery (15.6 months), no significant survival was noted. At present the impact of the incorporation of early secondary surgery remains unknown. The WMOCG have activated a randomized study which is evaluating this approach. Patients with more than 2 cm of residual disease after primary surgery are randomized to undergo early secondary surgery after three cycles of platinum combination chemotherapy or receive chemotherapy alone.

CONCLUSIONS

Since the last review in this series, there has been a critical reappraisal of the value of second-look operations. There have been a number of analyses, including a prospective randomized study, that have failed to demonstrate any therapeutic benefit for these procedures when performed at the end of primary therapy. In addition, the advent of new modes of monitoring disease status, in particular tumour markers such as serum CA125, may enable valuable prognostic information to be obtained non-invasively and at an earlier stage in treatment.

The question of whether early secondary cytoreductive surgery may confer survival benefit is at present unanswered but is currently being addressed by a number of collaborative groups, including the WMOCG. It is quite possible that such early surgery may, in fact, not confer any survival benefit as chemoresistant clones of cells may already exist prior to even the first operation.

It is salutary to recall that secondary cytoreductive surgery was considered to be potentially beneficial as a logical extension of the perceived value of primary cytoreduction. Whilst the value of secondary surgery has been submitted to evaluation in properly designed clinical studies, as yet, this is not the case for primary surgery.

REFERENCES

Altaras M M, Goldberg G L, Levin W, Darge L, Bloch B, Smith J A 1986 The value of cancer antigen CA125 as tumor marker in malignant germ cell tumours of the ovary. Gynecologic Oncology 25: 150–159

Atack D B, Nisker J A, Allen H H, Tustanoff E R, Levin L 1986 CA125 surveillance and second-look laparotomy in ovarian carcinoma. American Journal of Obstetrics and Gynecology 154: 287–289

Bagley C M, Young R C, Canellos G P, De Vita V T 1972 Treatment of ovarian carcinoma; possibilities for progress. New England Journal of Medicine 287: 856–862

Barber H R K 1984 Ovarian cancer: diagnosis and management. American Journal of Obstetrics and Gynecology 150: 910–916

Barbieri R L, Niloff J M, Bast R C Jr, Schaetzl E, Kistner R W, Knapp R C 1986 Elevated serum concentrations of CA125 in patients with advanced endometriosis. Fertility and Sterility 45: 630–634

Bast R C Jr, Feeney M, Lazarus H, Nadler L M, Colvin R B, Knapp R C 1981 Reactivity of a monoclonal antibody with human ovarian carcinoma. Journal of Clinical Investigation 68: 1331–1337

Bast R C Jr, Klug T L, St John E et al 1983 A radioimmunoassay using a monoclonal antibody to monitor the course of epithelial ovarian cancer. New England Journal of Medicine 309: 883–887

Bast R C Jr, Hunter V, Knapp R C 1987 Pros and cons of gynecologic tumor markers. Cancer 60: 1984–1992

Berek J S, Griffiths C T, Leventhal J M 1981 Laparoscopy for second-look evaluation in ovarian cancer. Obstetrics and Gynecology 58: 192–198

Berek J S, Hacker N F, Lagasse L D, Nieberg R K, Elashoff R M 1983 Survival of patients following secondary cytoreductive surgery in ovarian cancer. Obstetrics and Gynecology 61: 189–193

Berek J S, Hacker N F, Lagasse L D, Poth T, Resnick B, Nieberg R K 1984 Second-look laparotomy in stage III epithelial ovarian cancer; clinical variables associated with disease status. Obstetrics and Gynecology 64: 207–212

Berek J S, Knapp R C, Malkasian G D et al 1986 CA125 serum levels correlated with second-look operations among ovarian cancer patients. Obstetrics and Gynecology 67: 685–689

Bergmann J-F, Bidart J-M, George M, Beaugrand M, Levy V G, Bohoun C 1987 Elevation of CA125 in patients with benign and malignant ascites. Cancer 59: 213–217

Bertelsen K, Hansen M K, Pedersen P H et al 1988 The prognostic and therapeutic value of second-look laparotomy in advanced ovarian cancer. British Journal of Obstetrics and Gynaecology 95: 1231–1236

Blackledge G, Lawton F, Luesley D et al 1987 The relative merits of chemotherapy and radiotherapy following debulking chemotherapy. In: Sharp F, Soutter P (eds) Ovarian cancer—the way ahead. Royal College of Obstetricians and Gynaecologists, London, pp 427–440

Brenner D E, Shaff M I, Jones H W, Grosh W W, Greco F A, Burnett L S 1985 Abdominopelvic computed tomography in the management of ovarian cancer. Obstetrics and Gynecology 65: 715–719

Canney P A 1985 Tumour-associated antigens CA125 and CA19-9. An assessment of their value as tumour markers in ovarian adenocarcinoma. MD Thesis, University of Manchester

Canney P A, Moore M, Wilkinson P M, James R D 1984 Ovarian cancer antigen CA125: A prospective clinical assessment of its role as a tumour marker. British Journal of Cancer 50: 765–769

Chambers S, Chambers J T, Kohorn E I, Lawrence R, Schwartz P E 1988 Evaluation of the role of second-look surgery in ovarian cancer. Obstetrics and Gynecology 72: 404–408

Chatel J-F, Fumoleau P, Saccavini J-F et al 1987 Immunoscintigraphy of recurrences of gynecologic carcinomas. Journal of Nuclear Medicine 28: 1807–1819

Cohen C J, Goldberg J D, Holland J F et al 1983 Improve therapy with cisplatin regimens for patients with ovarian carcinoma (FIGO Stages III and IV) as measured by surgical and staging (second-look operations). American Journal of Obstetrics and Gynecology 145: 955–965

Copeland L J, Wharton J T, Rutledge F N, Gershenson D M, Seski J C, Herson J 1983 The role of third-look laparotomy in the guidance of ovarian cancer treatment. Gynecologic Oncology 15: 145–149

Copeland L J 1985 Second-look laparotomy for ovarian carcinoma. Clinical Obstetrics and Gynecology 28: 816–823

Copeland L J, Gershenson D M 1986 Ovarian cancer recurrences in patients with no macroscopic tumor at second-look laparotomy. Obstetrics and Gynecology 68: 873–874

Cruickshank D J, Fullerton W T, Klopper A 1987 The clinical significance of pre-operative serum CA125 in ovarian cancer. British Journal of Obstetrics and Gynaecology 94: 692–695

Curry S L, Zembo M M, Nahas W A et al 1981 Second-look laparotomy for ovarian cancer. Gynecologic Oncology 11: 114–118

Dembo A J, Bush R S, Beale F A et al 1979 The Princess Margaret Study of ovarian cancer stages I, II, and asymptomatic stage presentations. Cancer Treatment Reports 63: 249–254

Duk J M, Aalders J G, Fleuren G J, de Bruijn H W A 1986 CA125: a useful marker in endometrial cancer. American Journal of Obstetrics and Gynecology 155: 1097–1102

Edmondson J H, Fleming T R, Decker D G et al 1979 Different chemotherapeutic sensitivities and host factors affecting prognosis in advanced ovarian carcinoma versus minimal residual disease. Cancer Treatment Reports 63, 241–247

Epenetos A, Shepherd J, Britton K E et al 1985 ^{123}I radioiodinated antibody imaging of occult ovarian cancer. Cancer 55: 984–987

Fleuren G J, Nap M, Aalders J G, Trimbos J B, de Bruijn H W A 1987 Explanation of the limited correlation between tumour CA125 content and serum CA125 antigen levels in patients with ovarian tumours. Cancer 60: 2437–2442

Free K E, Webb M J 1987 Second-look laparotomy—clinical correlations. Gynecologic Oncology 23: 290–297

Gerhenson D M, Copeland L J, Wharton J T et al 1985 Prognosis of surgically determined complete responders in advanced ovarian cancer. Cancer 55: 1129–1133

Goldhirsch A, Triller J K, Greiner R, Dreher E, Davis B W 1983 Computed tomography prior to second-look laparotomy for ovarian cancer. Obstetrics and Gynecology 62: 630–634

Greco F, Julian C G, Richardson R et al 1981 Advanced ovarian cancer: brief intensive combination chemotherapy and second-look operations. Obstetrics and Gynecology 58: 199–205

Griffiths C T 1975 Surgical resection of tumour bulk in the primary treatment of ovarian carcinoma. National Cancer Institute Monograph 42: 101–104

Halila H, Stenman U-H, Seppala M 1986 Ovarian cancer antigen CA125 levels in pelvic inflammatory disease and pregnancy. Cancer 57: 1327–1329

Heinonen P K, Tontti K, Koivula T, Pystynen P 1985 Tumour-associated antigen CA125 in patients with ovarian cancer. British Journal of Obstetrics and Gynaecology 92: 528–531

Ho G, Beller U, Speyer J L, Columbo N, Wernz J, Beckman E M 1988 A reassessment of the role of second-look laparotomy in advanced ovarian cancer. Journal of Clinical Oncology 5: 1316–1321

Jones S, Khoo I S, Whitaker S 1981 Evaluation of ovarian cancer by second look laparotomy after treatment. Australian and New Zealand Journal of Surgery 51: 30–33

Kivinen S, Kuoppala T, Leppilampi M, Vuori J, Kaupilla A 1986 Tumor-associated antigen CA125 before and during the treatment of ovarian carcinoma. Obstetrics and Gynecology 67: 468–472

Kottmeier H (ed) 1982 Annual report on the results of treatment in gynecological cancer, vol 18. FIGO, Stockholm.

Klug T L, Bast R C Jr, Niloff J M, Knapp R C, Zurawski V R 1984 Monoclonal antibody immunoradiometric assay for an antigenic determinant (CA125) associated with human epithelial ovarian carcinomas. Cancer Research 44: 1048–1053

Krebs H B, Goplerud D R, Kilpatrick S J, Myers M B, Hunt A 1986 Role of CA125 as a
  marker in ovarian cancer. Obstetrics and Gynecology 67: 473–477
Lavin P T, Knapp R C, Malkasian G, Whitney C W, Berek J C, Bast R C Jr 1987 CA 125 for
  the monitoring of ovarian carcinoma during primary treatment. Obstetrics and Gynecology
  69: 223–227
Lawton F G, Kelly K, Sant-Cassia L, Blackledge G 1987 Speed of response to platinum-
  based chemotherapy: implications for the management of ovarian cancer. European
  Journal of Cancer and Clinical Oncology 23: 1071–1075
Lawton F G, Redman C W E, Luesley D M, Chan K K, Blackledge G 1989 Neoadjuvant
  (cytoreductive) chemotherapy combined with intervention debulking surgery in advanced,
  unresected epithelial ovarian cancer. Obstetrics and Gynecology 73: 61–65
Lele S B, Piver M S 1986 Interval laparoscopy as predictor of response to chemotherapy in
  ovarian carcinoma. Obstetrics and Gynecology 68: 345–347
Luesley D M, Chan K K, Fielding J W L, Hurlow R, Blackledge G R, Jordan J A 1984
  Second-look laparotomy in the management of epithelial ovarian carcinoma: an evaluation
  of fifty cases. Obstetrics and Gynecology 64: 421–426
Luesley D, Lawton F, Blackledge G et al 1988 Failure of second-look laparotomy to influence
  survival in epithelial ovarian cancer. Lancet ii: 599–603
Miller D S, Ballon S C, Teng N N H et al 1986 A critical reassessment of second-look
  laparotomy in epithelial ovarian carcinoma. Cancer 57: 530–535
Neijt J P, Van Der Burg M E L, Vriendorp R et al 1984 Randomised trial comparing two
  combination chemotherapy regimens (HEXA-CAF versus CHAP-5) in advanced ovarian
  cancer. Lancet ii: 594–600
Neijt J P, Ten Bokkel-Huinink W W, Van Der Burg M E L, Van Oosterom A T 1986
  Complete remission at laparotomy: still a gold standard in ovarian cancer? Lancet i: 1028
Niloff J M, Knapp R C, Schaetzl E, Reynolds C, Bast R C Jr 1984 CA125 levels in obstetric
  and gynecologic patients. Obstetrics and Gynecology 64: 703–707
Niloff J M, Bast R C Jr, Schaetzl E M, Knapp R C 1985 Predictive value of CA125 antigen
  levels in second-look procedures for ovarian cancer. American Journal of Obstetrics and
  Gynecology 151: 981–986
Niloff J M, Klug T L, Schaetzl E, Zurawski V R Jr, Knapp R C, Bast R C Jr 1984 Elevation
  of serum CA125 in carcinomas of the fallopian tube, endometrium and endocervix.
  American Journal of Obstetrics and Gynecology 148: 1057–1058
Ozols R F, Fisher R I, Anderson T, Makuch R, Young R C 1981 Peritoneoscopy in the
  management of ovarian cancer. American Journal of Obstetrics and Gynecology 140:
  611–619
Ozols R F 1985 Intraperitoneal chemotherapy in the management of ovarian cancer.
  Seminars in Oncology 12: 75–80
Parker D, Patel K, Alred E J, Harnden-Mayor P, Naylor B 1988 CA125 and survival in
  ovarian cancer: preliminary communication. Journal of the Royal Society of Medicine 81:
  22
Peters W A, Bagley C M, Smith M R 1986 CA125: use as a marker with mixed mesodermal
  tumors of the female genital tract. Cancer 58: 2625–2627
Phibbs G D, Smith J P, Stanhope C R 1983 Analysis of sites of persistent cancer at 'second-
  look' laparotomy on patients with ovarian cancer. American Journal of Obstetrics and
  Gynecology 147: 611–617
Phillips B P, Buchsbaum H J, Lifshitz S 1979 Re-exploration after treatment for ovarian
  cancer. Gynecologic Oncology 8: 339–345
Piver M S, Lele S B, Barlow J J, Gamarra M 1980 Second-look laparoscopy prior to
  proposed second-look laparotomy. Obstetrics and Gynecology 55: 571–573
Podratz K C, Malkasian G D, Hilton J F et al 1985 Second look laparotomy in ovarian
  cancer: Evaluation of prognostic variables. American Journal of Obstetrics and Gynecology
  152: 230–238
Pussell S J, Cosgrove D O, Hinton J, Wiltshaw E, Barker G H 1980 Carcinoma of the
  ovary—correlation of ultrasound with second-look laparotomy. British Journal of
  Obstetrics and Gynaecology 87: 1140–1144
Quentmeier A, Schlag P, Geisen H P, Schmidt-Gayk H 1987 Elevation of CA125 as a tumour
  marker for gastric and colo-rectal cancer in comparison to CEA and CA19-9. European
  Journal of Surgical Oncology 13: 197–201

Quinn M A, Bishop G J, Cambell J J, Rodgerson J, Pepperel R J 1980 Laparoscopic follow-up of patients with ovarian cancer. British Journal of Obstetrics and Gynaecology 87: 1132–1139

Raju K F, McKinna J A, Barker G H, Wiltshaw E, Jones J M 1982 Second-look operations in the planned management of advanced ovarian cancer. American Journal of Obstetrics and Gynecology 144: 650–654

Redman C W E, Jones S, Luesley D M et al 1988 Peritoneal trauma releases CA125? British Journal of Cancer 58: 502–504

Rizel S, Biran S, Anteby S et al 1985 Combined modality treatment for stage III ovarian cancer. Radiotherapy and Oncology 3: 237–241

Roberts W S, Hodel K, Rich W M et al 1982 Second-look laparotomy in the management of gynecological malignancy. Gynecologic Oncology 13: 345–355

Rosenoff S H, Devita V T, Hubbard S, Young R C 1975 Peritoeoscopy in the staging and follow-up of ovarian cancer. Seminars in Oncology 3: 223–228

Rubin S C, Hoskins W J, Hakes T B, Markman M, Cain J M, Lewis J L Jr 1988 Recurrence after negative second-look laparotomy for ovarian cancer: analysis of risk factors. American Journal of Obstetrics and Gynecology 159: 1094–1098

Saunders R C, McNeil B J, Finberg H J et al 1983 A prospective study of computed tomography and ultrasound in the detection and staging of pelvic masses. Radiology 162: 278–281

Schilthuis M S, Aalders J G, Bouma J et al 1987 Serum CA125 levels in epithelial ovarian cancer: Relation with findings at second look operation and their role in the detection of tumour recurrence. British Journal of Obstetrics and Gynaecology 94: 202–207

Schwartz P E, Smith J P 1980 Second-look operations in ovarian cancer. American Journal of Obstetrics and Gynecology 138: 1124–1130

Schwartz P E 1983 Current status of the second-look operation in ovarian cancer. Clinical Obstetrics and Gynecology 10: 245–259

Shepherd J H, Granowska M, Britton K E et al 1987 Tumour-associated monoclonal antibodies for the diagnosis and assessment of ovarian cancer. British Journal of Obstetrics and Gynaecology 94: 160–167

Singer A 1981 Second-look operations in the management of ovarian cancer. In: Studd J (ed) Progress in Obstetrics and Gynaecology vol. 1. Churchill Livingstone, Edinburgh, pp 240–252

Smith J P, Rutledge F 1970 Chemotherapy in the treatment of cancer of the ovary. American Journal of Obstetrics and Gynecology 107: 691–703

Smith J P, Delgrado G, Rutledge F 1976 Second-look operation in ovarian carcinoma. Cancer 38: 1438–1442

Smith J P, Day T G 1979 Review of ovarian cancer at the University of Texas Systems Cancer Center, MD Anderson Hospital and Tumor Institute. American Journal of Obstetrics and Gynecology 135: 984–993

Smith J P 1980 Surgery for ovarian cancer. In: Newman C E, Ford D H J, Jordan J (eds) Advances in the biosciences—ovarian cancer. Pergamon Press, Oxford, p 317

Smith W G, Day T G, Smith J P 1977 The use of laparoscopy to determine the results of chemotherapy for ovarian cancer. Journal of Reproductive Medicine 18: 257–260

Van Der Berg M E L, Lammes F B, Van Putten W L J, Stoter G 1988 Ovarian cancer: the prognostic value of the serum half-life of CA125 during induction chemotherapy. Gynecologic Oncology 30: 307–312

Vergote I B, Bormen O P, Abeler V M 1987 Evaluation of serum CA125 levels in the monitoring of ovarian cancer. American Journal of Obstetrics and Gynecology 157: 88–92

Vogl S E, Pagano M, Kaplan B 1982 Cyclophosphamide, hexamethylmelamine, adriamycin and diamminodichloroplatin, 'CHAD' versus melphalan in advanced ovarian carcinoma. Proceedings of the American Association of Clinical Oncology 22: 473

Vogl S E, Pagano M, Kaplan B, Greenwald E, Arseneau J, Bennett B 1983 Cisplatin-based combination chemotherapy in advanced ovarian cancer. High overall response rate with curative potential only in women with small tumor burdens. Cancer 51: 2024–2030

Wangensteen O H, Lewis F J, Tongen L A 1951 Second-look in cancer surgery. Lancet ii: 303–307

Webb M J, Snyder J A, Williams T J et al 1982 Second-look laparotomy in ovarian cancer. Gynecologic Oncology 14: 285–293

Wharton T 1978 Managing ovarian cancer: the second-look operation. Contemporary
    Obstetrics and Gynaecology 12: 137
Williams C J, Mead B, Arnold A, Green J, Buchanan R, Whitehouse M 1982 Chemotherapy
    of advanced ovarian cancer; initial experience using a platinum-based combination. Cancer
    49: 1778–1783

16. The treatment of endometriosis

Chris Sutton

INTRODUCTION

Between 10% and 25% of women undergoing laparotomy in the UK and the USA are found to have endometriosis, making it the second-most common gynaecological disorder after uterine fibroids (Shaw 1988). Nevertheless, it remains a condition that is shrouded in mystery. In spite of the vast amounts of energy, ingenuity and research devoted to the study of endometriosis, our understanding of its aetiology or pathogenesis has progressed little during the past 70 years (Meyer 1919, Sampson 1927a, 1927b). The clinical presentation bears little relationship to the severity of the disease, the natural history is unpredictable and attempts to provide rational treatment are often based on anecdote and intuition rather than on scientific logic. It is therefore not surprising that there are many different approaches to treatment, often straying beyond the confines of orthodox medicine, and to add to the confusion, most of the treatments are based on studies that have been largely uncontrolled and retrospective. Against this background it is not surprising that both patients and doctors often find themselves confused. Before embarking on any plan of patient management it is essential that the diagnosis is made correctly.

DIAGNOSIS

Although about a quarter of patients with endometriosis are completely asymptomatic (O'Connor 1987), most present with one or other of the classic quartet of symptoms—congestive dysmenorrhoea, deep dyspareunia, pelvic pain, and infertility. Clinical examination may reveal a fixed uterus with tenderness in the adnexae and sometimes the presence of painful nodules in the cul-de-sac or at the insertion of the uterosacral ligaments. Sometimes rocking the cervix forwards with the examining finger can result in severe pain and often mimics the discomfort felt at intercourse during deep penetration. A normal pelvic examination does not exclude the diagnosis and the only way to be certain that endometriosis is present is to perform a diagnostic laparoscopy.

Laparoscopy

The diagnosis of endometriosis carries significant implications for any woman and it is therefore important that the procedure should be performed by an experienced gynaecologist rather than delegated to a junior member of the team. A systematic and thorough inspection of the entire pelvis and abdomen should be made employing a double portal technique with an aspiration cannula inserted suprapubically in the mid-line. A single-puncture technique is to be deprecated, although it is still used by a depressingly large number of gynaecologists according to the findings of the RCOG Confidential Enquiry into Laparoscopy (Chamberlain & Carron-Brown 1978). The aspiration cannula is used to suck out the yellow serous fluid, so often associated with endometriosis, from the pouch of Douglas so that the peritoneal surface can be visualized and also to elevate the ovary so that the ovarian fossa can be inspected for the presence of endometrial implants or adhesions. If an ovarian endometrioma is suspected needle aspiration should be performed to test for the presence of the characteristic thick chocolate fluid sequestered in the ovarian stroma.

It is important to inspect closely the peritoneal surface using the laparoscope as a magnifying instrument and to be aware of the appearances associated with acute endometriosis, rather than merely looking for haemosiderin which often represents 'burnt out' or inactive disease. There appears to be a relationship between the colour and the age of the endometrial implants and, indeed, even with the age of the patient as seen in the non-haemorrhagic lesions more usually found in young women and the black deposits laden with haemosiderin more common in the older patients (Redwine 1987). Jansen and Russell (1986) drew attention to a number of characteristic appearances which are associated with endo-metriosis and have been confirmed by histological inspection of the peritoneal biopsy. These non-pigmented lesions are:

1. White opacified peritoneum (endometriosis in 81% of biopsies)
2. Red flamelike lesions (endometriosis in 81% of biopsies)
3. Glandular lesions resembling endometrium at hysteroscopy (67% of biopsies).

Other lesions such as sub-ovarian adhesions, yellow-brown peritoneal patches and circular peritoneal defects had endometriosis in half of the biopsies. Any gynaecologist who is seriously involved in the treatment of endometriosis should read this article.

Documentation

All these lesions and vascular appearances should be carefully marked on a rubber stamp diagram of the pelvis and supplemented, if the equipment is available, by a Polaroid® photograph from a still camera or a video printer. Ideally the laparoscopy and any operative procedures performed at laparoscopy should be recorded on videotape since this is the only reliable way to monitor the response to treatment at subsequent second-look laparoscopy.

An attempt should be made to grade the severity of the disease using the revised American Fertility Society (AFS) scale (1985) which, although by no means perfect, is probably the best available classification at the present time. The clinician must be aware that the attainment of a high numerical grade on a scoring system does not necessarily correlate with the degree of pain experienced by the patient. Recent studies has shown that the pain in endometriosis is linked to prostaglandin metabolism, particularly prostaglandin F (Vernon et al 1986). Even small lesions are capable of producing large amounts of prostaglandin F which accounts for the finding that patients with mild or moderate disease on the AFS scale can often have more pain than those with extensive disease (sometimes found incidentally at laparotomy for a pelvic mass in an otherwise asymptomatic patient).

TREATMENT

Principles

It is important to individualize the approach to treatment because circumstances and situations vary enormously and will depend on the severity of symptoms, previous treatment, the age of the patient, and her fertility expectations. If endometriosis is discovered incidentally as, for example, at the time of laparoscopic sterilization it might be entirely appropriate to advise no treatment at all, especially if the patient is asymptomatic. In the present medico-legal climate, however, it would be prudent to discuss this with the patient because untreated endometriosis may become more severe and give rise to future problems (Thomas & Cooke 1987b).

There is also a definite place for expectant management particularly in the infertile patient with minimal or mild disease. Increased volumes of peritoneal fluid and higher concentrations of macrophages have been implicated in endometriosis-associated infertility (Haney et al 1983) and removal of this fluid at diagnostic laparoscopy as well as chromopertubation of the fallopian tubes have resulted in higher conception rates than those achieved with hormonal suppression (Olive et al 1985).

The rationale behind medical therapy for endometriosis is based on two aspects of the natural history of the disease and a third pharmacological observation:

1. Endometriosis usually goes into remission during pregnancy;
2. Endometriosis invariably disappears after the menopause;
3. Androgens appear to cause regression of endometriosis.

Drug treatment therefore aims to mimic the hormonal state of pregnancy, an androgenic state or the menopause with the inevitable side-effects associated with all these conditions.

Surgical treatment aims to remove the endometriotic implants and can be conservative if further pregnancies are desired, or radical, with removal of the ovaries, to create a menopausal state. Such treatment is usually performed as a last resort when medical therapy has failed.

The most exciting development in endometriosis therapy in recent years has been the use of different lasers to destroy ectopic endometrial implants and this approach has the overwhelming advantage that treatment can be performed laparoscopically at the same time as the diagnosis is made.

Laparoscopic treatment

Before the advent of lasers the only method of removing endometrial implants endoscopically was by relatively crude cutting techniques, heating the endometrial implants by endocoagulation (Semm & Mettler 1980) or destroying them by the passage of an electric current. Although this is an increasingly popular treatment, it is important to realize that it has no proven efficacy and it is potentially dangerous. The confidential enquiry of the Royal College of Obstetricians and Gynaecologists drew attention to the hazards of electrodiathermy burns to the bowel (Chamberlain & Carron-Brown 1978) and this is particularly important in endometriosis since the implants are often adjacent to viscera and other easily damaged structures, including the ureter (Cheng 1976, Sutton 1974).

These techniques inevitably result in bleeding or are so imprecise that there is considerable destruction of surrounding tissue with subsequent fibrosis and scarring. In contrast, the carbon dioxide laser has the advantage of being able precisely to vaporize abnormal tissue so that, although there is some cellular damage up to 500 microns from the impact point, the zone of thermal necrosis is usually less than 100 microns (Bellina et al 1984). Since all the tissue debris is evacuated as smoke in the laser plume there is minimal fibrosis or scar tissue formation, and laser wounds heal with virtually no contracture or anatomical distortion (Allen et al 1983). These characteristics make the carbon dioxide laser particularly suitable for the vaporization of endometriosis and its associated adhesions, especially in patients who are infertile or who may wish to have children in future. Endometrial implants in hazardous situations such as the bowel, bladder or ureter, can also be vaporized providing the surgeon is careful and is aware of the depth of penetration of the laser on different tissues, adjusting the power density accordingly. With good eye-hand coordination and careful irrigation of charred material it is possible to limit the depth of vaporization to as little as 0.1 mm (Wilson 1988).

Carbon dioxide laser laparoscopy

The first reports of laser laparoscopy came from Clermont-Ferrand in

France (Bruhat et al 1979) but prototype instruments and techniques were developed independently in Israel (Tadir et al 1981), the USA (Daniell & Brown 1982), the UK (Sutton 1986) and Belgium (Donnez 1987).

We started using this technique at St Luke's Hospital, Guildford in October 1982 and have treated over 500 patients for a variety of conditions ranging from endometriosis and adhesions to neosalpingostomies, ovarian cysts, polycystic ovarian syndrome and unruptured ectopic pregnancies. The time in hospital is relatively short (day case or overnight stay) and complications are few and usually minor. So far we have had no injury or morbidity due to the effects of intraperitoneal laser energy.

We have recently reviewed 228 consecutive patients with endometriosis who were treated by laser laparoscopy between 1982 and 1987 and have been followed up for between 1 and 6 years (Sutton & Hill 1989). Patients were classified according to the presenting symptoms of pain, infertility or both and all had consented to laser treatment if endometriosis was found at the time of diagnostic laparoscopy. The results are summarized in Figure 16.1.

Symptomatic improvement was seen in 126 of 181 (70%) of patients complaining of pelvic pain and the benefit was sustained in all but 17 patients who relapsed, usually after about 6 months. It is tempting to

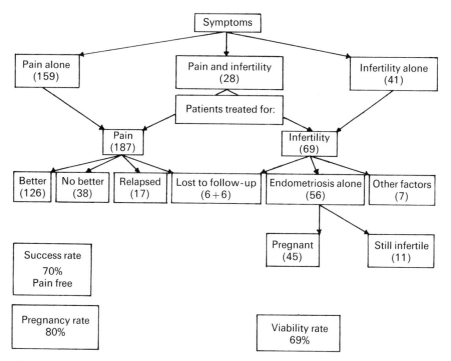

Fig. 16.1   Results of laser laparoscopy in 228 patients with endometriosis. (Sutton & Hill 1989).

ascribe this success to the placebo effect of the laparoscopy but almost one-third of these patients had undergone previous laparoscopies or medical therapy without relief of their pain. We managed to persuade 33 patients in this group to have a second-look procedure to evaluate the result of the original laser laparoscopy. In 15 patients there was no evidence of recurrent endometriosis although the charcoal deposits remaining from the laser vaporization could be clearly seen underneath the peritoneum. Careful inspection with the laparoscope lens held close to the peritoneal surface revealed a characteristic appearance with no inflammatory reaction and biopsy showed inactive carbon particles with no evidence of endometrial glands or stroma. Eighteen patients had formed endometriosis at different sites but there was no evidence of endometriosis at the sites previously lasered. Obviously this small sub-group of patients with recurrent disease needs long term drug treatment or bilateral oophorectomy to halt further progression of endometriosis.

Although there is little doubt that the anatomical distortion caused by severe endometriosis is responsible for infertility, some authors have suggested that the relationship with early stage disease is incidental rather than causal (Lilford & Dalton 1987). In the Guildford series there were 56 patients with endometriosis as the only abnormal factor implicated in their infertility which ranged from 6 months to 10 years. Forty-five (80%) of these patients have become pregnant following laser laparoscopy without adjuvant drug treatment, the majority (73%) within 8 months of the procedure. The pregnancy-procedure interval and the relationship of the outcome to the severity of endometriosis is shown in Tables 16.1 and 16.2.

The Guildford data compares favourably with results from the United States (Daniell 1984; Feste 1985; Davis 1986; Nezhat et al 1986) and Europe (Donnez 1987). Nezhat obtained 62 pregnancies in 102 patients which included one elective termination and nine spontaneous abortions. This high abortion rate is reflected in our series although unfortunately our abortion rate is even higher (24%). This probably reflects the high abortion rate noted among endometriosis sufferers which has been reported to be as high as 49% (Malinak & Wheeler 1985). If the results are presented as

Table 16.1 Guildford Laser Laparoscopy Project. October 1982—October 1987. Pregnancy procedure interval (Sutton & Hill 1989)

Number of months	Pregnancies (number)	Percentage
0– 6	33	73
8–12	7	16
12–18	4	9
> 18	1	2
	Total = 45	

Table 16.2   Guildford Laser Laparoscopy Project. October 1982—
October 1987. Severity of endometriosis related to pregnancies

Stage (AFS scale)	No. of patients	Other factors*	Pregnancies	%
Minimal I	19	3	15	94
Mild II	25	1	17	71
Moderate III	16	3	11	85
Severe IV	2	0	2	100
TOTAL	62	−7 = 55	45	

* Other factors: Oligospermia 6, cervical fibroid 1. (Sutton & Hill 1989.)

pregnancies resulting in full-term infants our viability rate of 69% is similar to that of Donnez in Belgium (Donnez 1987). The results of several recent studies are published in Table 16.3. They can all be criticized on the basis that they are retrospective studies and there is a great need for a double-blind prospective study comparing laser treatment with placebo in one arm and medical therapy in another.

The only prospective study in the literature followed one group of 64 patients treated by carbon dioxide laser laparoscopy and another control group of 44 patients who received a variety of medical treatments or laparoscopic electrocoagulation. The laser group achieved pregnancy at a higher overall rate and also had shorter post-treatment intervals. Using life-table analysis the monthly fecundity rate for the laser group was 6.7% and the control group was 4.5% (Adamson et al 1988).

Laser laparoscopy for advanced disease

One of the most interesting developments in laser laparoscopy in recent

Table 16.3   Results of laser laparoscopy for endometriosis

	Patients (No.)	Pregnancies		Viability (%)
		(No.)	(%)	
Daniell (1984)	75	48	62	—
Feste (1985)	29	21	72	—
Davis (1986)	65	37	—	57
Nezhat et al (1986)	102	62	61	51
Martin & Olive (1986)	80	33	41	—
Donnez (1987)	70	40	—	57
Sutton* (1989)	56	45	80	69
Feste (1989)	178	93	73	—
Feste* (1989)	64	52	81	—
Nezhat (1989)	243	168	69	—

* Endometriosis only, no other infertility factors.

Table 16.4 Endometriosis patients by stage of disease and pregnancy rates (Nezhat et al, 1989)

	All patients	Stage I	Stage II	Stage III	Stage IV[a]
No.	243	39	86	67	51
Age* Years*	29.4 ± 4.1	26.8 ± 2.2	27.6 ± 2.4	30.5 ± 1.9	31.5 ± 4.1
infertile	3.6 ± 1.9	3.3 ± 1.9	3.6 ± 2.1	3.8 ± 1.2	3.6 ± 2.0
Pregnant	168 (69.1%)	28 (71.8%)	60 (69.8%)	45 (67.2%)	35 (68.6%)

[a] American Fertility Society 1979 Classification of Endometriosis. Fertility and Sterility 32: 633
* 95% Confidence limit.

years has been the growing tendency to push the technique 'to the limits'. At first there was a tendency to limit treatment to early-stage disease and schedule patients with advanced disease for conservative surgery with a pre- or post-operative course of medical therapy. With increasing experience and the realization that high pregnancy rates can be achieved with laparoscopic surgery, even with the gross anatomical distortion of Stage IV disease, there is now an increasing tendency to use laser laparoscopy as first-line therapy even although these procedures are very lengthy and require direct video operating to avoid undue strain on the surgeon's back. Nezhat has produced some very impressive results with this technique and life-table analysis gives comparable results for all stages of endometriosis (see Table 16.4) (Nezhat et al 1989). Martin and Olive, using laser laparoscopy without adjunctive drug therapy, had fecundity rates for mild and moderate disease of 3.33% and 2.51% respectively but for severe disease the rate was an amazing 5.79% (Olive & Haney 1986). These impressive results for Stage IV endometriosis now being reported from many different centres convince me that laser laparoscopy is the most significant recent advance in the treatment of this disease.

Argon and KTP/532 laser laparoscopy

The main advantage of the carbon dioxide laser is its precision but, at the present time, commercially available laser beams of this type can only be passed down rigid delivery systems using multiple mirrors. This tends to be rather cumbersome, can cause loss of beam alignment and can be awkward to use in places where access is difficult, such as the posterior surface of an ovary that is adherent to the broad ligament. The neodymium-YAG (Nd:YAG), the argon and the KTP/532 laser beams can all be passed down flexible fibres and have the added advantage that they will work in haemorrhagic fields, whereas carbon dioxide laser energy is absorbed by blood which renders it ineffective.

As can be seen, the argon and the potassium-titanyl-phosphate laser

(KTP/532, a frequency-doubled YAG laser) are of virtually the same wave length and are in the blue-green portion of the spectrum; as such, there is selective absorption of energy by haemoglobin and haemosiderin, both of which are present in abundant amounts within the endometrial implants. It is a myth, however, to think that this laser-tissue interaction prevents damage to surrounding structures because the primary tissue reaction is coagulation with lateral thermal damage of 0.5–2 mm, less than with the Nd:YAG but more than that produced by the carbon dioxide laser. In addition, at higher energy levels when tissue vaporizes and carbon builds up, further attempts at lasing through this will result in incandescence as tissue heats with an orange glow to over 1500°C. This could cause extensive thermal damage resulting in a branding-iron type of burn and ultimate scarring of tissue (Absten 1990). In view of these problems and the eye hazards inherent in their use these lasers should only be used by laparoscopists already adept at carbon dioxide laser laparoscopy.

The first animal and human studies with the argon laser used laparoscopically were performed by William Keye at the University of Utah and with the KTP/532 laser by Jim Daniell in Nashville, Tennessee. Keye reported a prospective study involving 92 consecutive patients who were evaluated for ability to conceive and reduction of pain. Many of the patients had additional sub-fertility factors and 34% became pregnant (a monthly fecundity rate of 2.5%), 64% of which within 6 months of treatment. More dramatic was the relief of pain in 92% of 50 women who were complaining of dyspareunia, dysmenorrhoea and pelvic pain due to endometriosis (Keye et al 1987).

Using the KTP/532 laser combined with LUNA (laser uterine nerve ablation) Daniell achieved a 75% relief of dysmenorrhoea in endometriosis patients (Daniell 1989). Nezhat compared the carbon dioxide, argon and KTP/532 lasers in three groups of 40 patients and found the best outcome in terms of pain relief and pregnancy rate was with the carbon dioxide laser (Nezhat 1988).

Neodymium-YAG (Nd:YAG) laser laparoscopy

This is a solid-state laser in which the crystal of yttrium aluminium garnet is deliberately contaminated with neodymium ions which then become the actual lasing medium. It can be passed down flexible fibres, works in a liquid medium and generates less smoke than the carbon dioxide laser. It is absorbed by all tissues to a depth of 3–5 mm and therefore is excellent for haemostasis; unfortunately, there is up to 40% of back-scatter which at this wavelength can permanently damage the macula portion of the retina and lead to blindness so special goggles have to be worn by all theatre personnel.

Lomano first reported its use on 60 cases of early endometriosis with acceptable results (Lomano 1987) and Corson has recently reported 100 patients, 60 of whom had Stage III and IV disease, and many of whom had failed to respond to medical or surgical treatment. 41% conceived within 9 months and 63% had complete pain relief with partial relief in a further 29% (Corson 1990).

We have used the Neodymium-YAG laser laparoscopically in Guildford for the past 2 years. It has the slight disadvantage that the equipment takes more time to set up and requires more stringent safety precautions than the carbon dioxide laser, which can be a problem during a busy surgical schedule. The problem of beam scatter and the laser-tissue interaction means that it is less precise but this can be partially overcome by the use of artificial sapphire laser scalpels. These are particularly useful in situations where bleeding can be expected but they have a limited life span, are expensive and tend to stick to tissue if not used correctly. All fibre lasers generate less smoke and are particularly useful in laparoscopic ovarian surgery.

Laser laparoscopy for ovarian endometriomas

Ovarian endometriomas (chocolate-cysts) are notorious for their poor response to danazol and progestogens. They can be removed laparo-scopically by scissors and blunt dissection but the procedure is time-consuming, difficult, and at the same time relatively crude. A more sophisticated approach is to make a linear incision over the thinnest part of the endometrioma capsule with an argon, KTP or Nd:YAG laser at a power setting of 10–15 watts. The old blood and haemosiderin (chocolate fluid) inside the cyst is sucked out and the cavity repeatedly irrigated with heparinized Hartmann's solution. The laser fibre is then introduced inside the cyst to photocoagulate the cyst wall at 5–10 watts. There is no need for the insertion of endosutures and the cyst can be left open to heal over.

An interesting new technique for dealing with ovarian endometriomas has recently been described by Brosens and Puttemans (1990). For ovarian cystoscopy (ovarioscopy) a double optic laparoscope is used which is a combination of an operating laparoscope and a 2.6 mm rigid endoscope inside a 5 mm sheath which is introduced down the operating channel of the laparoscope. The sheath is necessary to provide a 1 mm channel for the passage of biopsy forceps, laser fibres and irrigating solutions.

The cyst is punctured and the contents aspirated and sent for cytological examination. The ovarioscope is then introduced through the puncture hole and the cyst distended with a continuous flow of saline until the solution becomes clear so that the inner wall can be inspected and biopsied. Once the operator is satisfied that this is a benign ovarian cyst, an argon laser fibre is introduced to photocoagulate the superficial vessels and haemorrhagic areas lining the cyst wall to a depth of 1–2 mm. In a 6-month follow up of 11 patients treated by this technique there have been no recurrences of ovarian endometriomas (Brosens & Puttemans 1989).

Medical treatment of endometriosis

Pseudopregnancy treatment

In 1938 Joe Meigs, expounding on the various aetiological factors in endometriosis, advocated early marriage and childbearing as a way of avoiding the disease. Realizing that such measures were a little drastic and could lead to profound sociological consequences, Kistner mimicked the pregnant state pharmacologically by giving his patients ethinyloestradiol in combination with a progestin on a continuous basis (Kistner 1959). Between 30% and 50% of patients showed objective improvement in the disease and the symptomatic improvement was slightly higher, although subsequent pregnancy rates were poor and side-effects such as nausea and breast tenderness were common (Barbieri & Kistner 1984). Although this type of therapy has been superseded by modern anti-endometriosis drugs there are still many patients who are unable to tolerate the side-effects of these agents and continuous therapy with a medium-dose combined oral contraceptive pill is often used to prevent the disease from progressing. It must, however, be given continuously in order to suppress menstruation. To prescribe the oral contraceptive on a cyclical basis makes no rational sense since the ectopic endometrial implants will still be stimulated as in the normal ovarian cycle.

Progestogen treatment

To avoid the side-effects of oestrogen and still partially mimic the hormonal milieu of pregnancy, progestogens such as norethisterone, dydrogesterone and medroxyprogesterone acetate can be given continuously. These drugs act by causing initial decidualization and growth of endometrial tissue which is followed after several months by atrophy. Side-effects include weight gain, acne and irregular menstrual bleeding although 50–70% have symptomatic improvement and 40–60% objective improvement (Barbieri & Kistner 1984). Pregnancy rates vary from 46–53% (Moghissi & Boyce 1976, Johnston 1976). These agents are relatively cheap but their general acceptance is limited because many patients feel generally unwell with a continuous 'pre-menstrual syndrome' feeling. Oddly enough, a progestogen such as provera used in very high doses (400 mg daily) to prevent metastases in endometrial carcinoma rarely seems to produce any side effects and although most patients so treated belong to an older age group they often admit to a distinct feeling of well-being whilst taking this preparation.

If patients tolerate oral medroxyprogesterone acetate without side-effects they can be given Depo-Provera injections every 3 months (Moghissi & Boyce 1976) but irregular bleeding can be a problem and fertility can be impaired as it can take up to 2 years for one injection to be cleared completely from the body. This type of therapy is usually reserved for patients who get recurrent disease after discontinuing drug therapy and is appropriate for long-term maintenance, unlike danazol and LHRH analogues which can cause potentially serious metabolic disturbances if used for more than 6 months.

Androgen treatment

Before the days of diagnostic laparoscopy an injection of testosterone propionate was administered by some clinicians as a therapeutic test for endometriosis. If the symptoms were alleviated then a diagnosis could be made and a laparotomy often avoided. Early investigators concluded that although it could relieve pain associated with endometriosis, it was ineffective in enhancing fertility (Hamblen 1957). Testosterone implants can be used in a few patients who have persistent endometriosis following hysterectomy but who steadfastly refuse to have their ovaries removed—not uncommon with some patients nowadays. The pain is alleviated within days of insertion (usually in association with an oestradiol implant to prevent cyclical activity of the ovary) and the pain usually returns about 6 months later when the implant has been completely absorbed, Oestradiol and testosterone implants are an effective way of relieving climacteric symptoms after hysterectomy and bilateral salpingo-oophorectomy for endometriosis. They can be inserted at the time of wound closure and this combined approach prevents the problems associated with oestrogen deficiency, avoids repeated surgery and, as long as all the ovarian tissue has been removed, is not associated with recurrent disease (Studd & Montgomery 1987).

Danazol

Danazol, probably the most widely prescribed drug in the treatment of endometriosis, is itself an androgen, an isoxazole derivative of 17-alpha-ethinyl testosterone. It also causes a rise in free testosterone by reducing the synthesis of sex-hormone binding globulin per se and also by displacing testosterone from the carrier protein (Dowsett et al 1986). It thus produces androgenic side-effects and, in addition, binds to progesterone receptors to produce progestational side effects. It also interferes with pulsatile gonadotrophin secretion, inhibits several enzymatic processes involved in ovarian steroidogenesis and competitively blocks androgen, oestrogen and progesterone receptors in the ovaries and endometrium (Barbieri & Ryan 1985).

Its efficacy is due largely to the marked anti-oestrogenic milieu thus created (Barbieri et al 1979) and treatment should be continued for 6–9 months, usually in a dose of 200 mg twice daily. Subsequent menstrual suppression is more likely to occur if treatment is started on the first day of the period but it is not necessary to achieve complete amenorrhoea for the treatment to be effective (Doberl et al 1984). Low-dose therapy tends to be associated with less side-effects but sometimes it is necessary to increase the dose to 800 mg daily in divided doses to obtain symptomatic relief.

Danazol has been shown to be effective in reducing most peritoneal implants but a significant recurrence or persistence rate of 29–39% has been noted (Dmowski & Cohen 1978, Greenblatt & Tzingounis 1979). The value of this drug in enhancing fertility is questionable and collected series give an average pregnancy rate of only 36.9% (range = 0–60%) with a monthly fecundity rate never higher than 0.068 (Olive & Haney 1986). Although this drug is in widespread use it is questionable whether the fecundity rate in mild disease is greater than that anticipated with expectant management (Seibel et al 1982) and the delay incurred while taking the drug may actually prove detrimental to fertility.

Side-effects are common (Table 16.5) and patients should be warned and advised to persist with therapy in order to eradicate the disease. Weight-gain is often one of the most distressing side-effects and since this is largely due to sodium retention it can be ameliorated by the avoidance of salty foods and increasing the intake of water. It has recently been observed that patients who partake of 2–3 hours of vigorous exercise each day report a

Table 16.5 Adverse events reported during therapy with danazol and Buserilin (from Jelley 1986)

	Buserilin group n = 40, (%)		Danazol group n = 39, (%)
Androgenic			
Acne	1	(p < 0.01 D2)	9 (23)
Maculo-papular rash	6 (15) (month 1 only)	(n/s)	11 (28)
Seborrhoea	0		7 (18)
Myalgia (cramps)	3	(p < 0.005 D2)	16 (41)
Appetite increase	0	(p < 0.05 D2)	10 (26)
Weight gain	1	(p < 0.007 D2)	15 (38)
Weight loss	1		1
Altered follicular activity			
Hot flushes	37 (93)	(p < 0.001 Bs)	13 (33)
Vaginal dryness/vaginitis	26 (65)	(p < 0.005 Bs)	11 (28)
Superficial dyspareunia	6 (15)		2 (5)
Vulvovaginitis	3 (7.5)		2 (5)
Libido decreased	8 (20)	(n/s)	10 (26)
Pre-menstrual-like symptoms	12 (30)	(n/s)	6 (15)
Breast pain	7 (20)		3 (8)
Breast atrophy	0		3 (8)
Miscellaneous			
Nausea	12 (30)	(n/s)	20 (51)
Abdominal swelling	3 (7.5)		5 (13)
Depression	4 (10)	(n/s)	11 (28)
Malaise	4 (10)	(p < 0.02 D2)	14 (36)
Insomnia	8 (20)	(n/s)	4 (10)
Headaches	24 (60)	(p < 0.002 Bs)	9 (23)

significant reduction in side-effects, particularly weight-gain and muscle aches, whilst at the same time promoting muscle development. This is possibly due to the anabolic steroid effect associated with the marked rise in free testosterone and is a novel way to get round the problem of side-effects (Rock 1988).

Patients should also be warned that they must not become pregnant during therapy because danazol is potentially teratogenic and could cause masculinization of a female fetus (Shaw & Farquhar 1984). They should use barrier methods of contraception but it is pointless to prescribe the oral contraceptive because that defeats the purpose of therapy which is to create a low-oestrogen state to prevent the development of endometrial tissue.

Danazol therapy should not be prescribed for longer than 6 months because it causes adverse changes in serum lipids (Fahreus et al 1984, Booker et al 1986). These changes are reversible on cessation of therapy but could have serious implications in patients at high risk from cardiovascular disease.

Gestrinone

Gestrinone is a trienic-19-norsteroid which has undergone clinical trials in this country and is expected to be available for general use in the near future. Gestrinone abolishes the mid-cycle surge although basal gonadotrophin secretion is not significantly altered. It is markedly anti-progestogenic and anti-oestrogenic and causes progressive endometrial atrophy. It differs from danazol by progressively reducing sex hormone binding globulin (SHBG) levels by about 85%, whilst the total serum concentration of testosterone and oestradiol is reduced by 30% and 40% respectively, resulting in an increase in the free testosterone index (Kaupilla et al 1985).

Gestrinone appears to be an effective drug with good patient tolerance although the side-effects are similar to danazol. It has a long half-life and is given in a dose of 2.5–5 mg twice weekly; this will induce amenorrhoea and endometrial atrophy in 85–90% of patients. In controlled studies it appears to compare favourably with danazol in terms of symptomatic relief and pregnancy outcome (Coutinho 1982, Thomas & Cooke 1987a).

Pseudo-menopause treatment: LHRH analogues

For many years now it has been realized that the natural menopause or surgical extirpation of ovarian tissue are the most effective ways of halting the progression of endometriosis. In patients still wishing to retain child-bearing potential this is clearly undesirable so the possibility of achieving a reversible menopause state with the LHRH analogues was an exciting breakthrough in endometriosis therapy (Meldrum et al 1982). The continued use of these preparations produces down-regulation of pituitary function with low circulating levels of gonadotrophins with no determinant pusatile patterns, together with suppression of ovarian steroidogenesis with levels of oestradiol-17B in the post-menopausal range (Shaw 1988).

Studies have shown objective improvement of endometriosis with buserilin 200 μg daily as an intranasal spray (Shaw & Matta 1986), naferilin 400 μg twice daily (Schriock et al 1985) and Zoladex as a depot-preparation given in a monthly dose of 3.6 mg (Shaw 1988). Zoladex depot produced a more profound and consistent suppression of FSH and LH than buserilin and there was less breakthrough bleeding. Compared with danazol it appears that buserilin achieves a greater reduction in active endometriotic deposits at second-look laparoscopy but actual symptomatic relief is much the same (Lemay 1988).

In 1986 Jelley reported a multicentre study from Guildford and four other hospitals in the south-east of England comparing danazol and buserilin over a 7-month treatment period. About 60% of patients obtained symptomatic relief and at second-look laparoscopy there was a marked decrease in the AFS score. Some 20% of patients on buserilin had irregular bleeding during treatment but there was adequate resolution of endometriotic deposits in spite of the fact that oestradiol levels had not been reduced to post-menopausal levels. The side-effects in both groups were quite impressive and are listed in Table 16.5.

Since LHRH analogues are so effective at producing a pseudo-menopause it is not surprising that the symptoms are similar—hot flushes, night sweats, headache, dry vagina and superficial dyspareunia. Some advocates of this type of therapy claim that these side-effects are well tolerated by the patients but this is not always the case and the headaches, in particular, can be unpleasant. In addition patients should be warned about an increase in pelvic pain soon after the commencement of treatment otherwise they may discontinue the medication. A further worry is the increased loss of bone calcium and trabecular density similar to that occurring at the time of the menopause (Matta et al 1987). This bone loss is reversible after 6 months of treatment but may be a limiting factor on the length of time LHRH analogues can be used for benign gynaecological conditions such as fibroids and endometriosis.

A large multicentre study comparing nafarelin with danazol and placebo is currently in progress and initial reports show an 80% improvement in AFS scores in both treatment groups and an overall pregnancy rate of 59% (Henzl et al 1988). Although the AFS scores were reduced they did not show eradication of the disease and this study confirms my view that primary treatment should aim for extirpation of the endometriotic implants by laser laparoscopy whilst drug therapy, with its attendant side-effects and expense, should be reserved for those patients who suffer recurrent disease.

Gossypol

In the 1950s Chinese scientists noted that cooking with crude cotton seed oil could lead to male infertility. Gossypol acetate is a phenolic compound extracted from the seed, stem and root of the cotton plant and has been used in China for the treatment of endometriosis, fibroids and menorrhagia in a dose of 20 mg daily for 2 months and 25 mg twice-weekly for maintenance therapy (Cheng Kuo-Fen et al 1980). It is a suppressor of FSH and LH, producing endometrial atrophy in about 50% of patients after 3 months and although the results improve with prolonged therapy so does the time taken to restore normal menstruation. It produces symptomatic improvement in 80% of patients with dysmenorrhoea but side-effects can sometimes be serious and include electrolyte disturbances, especially hypokalaemia, and alterations in hepatic and renal function (Han 1980, Zhou 1981, Zhu et al 1984).

Clomiphene

Although anovulation is not usually a feature of endometriosis, a recent retrospective cohort study used clomiphene in 30 women with infertility and minimal endometriosis as the only abnormal finding. Over 8 months the cumulative pregnancy rate was 31% which was similar to their conception rate in patients with luteal phase defects, anovulation and unexplained infertility (Koninckx et al 1984).

Alternative medicine therapies

The profusion of medical drugs and regimes already discussed suggests, even to the uninitiated, that the search for the ideal anti-endometriosis drug has a long way to go. It is not surprising therefore that many patients resort to the ministrations of practitioners of alternative medicine such as acupuncturists, chiropractors and homeopaths to try to obtain relief from their symptoms. I personally have no objection to this and if the patient improves as a result of these techniques I am delighted. Inevitably in a disease with such diffuse clinical symptoms many patients will derive benefit from an unconventional approach and, unlike the situation with malignant disease, such therapy is unlikely to do any harm. Equally, many patients derive benefit from a self-help group such as The Endometriosis Society where meeting with fellow sufferers can show them that they are not alone with their problems. Unfortunately some of the 'horror stories' that are exchanged can have an adverse effect on patients who have a high psychoneurotic index or a tendency to hypochondria. The book *Overcoming Endometriosis* (Ballweg & Deutsch 1987) provides a well-balanced review of the disease from the patients' point of view.

Some of the alternative treatments have a sound pharmacological basis and can be very helpful in the management of the symptoms or even of the disease itself. Evening Primrose Oil, available from health food stores as Efamol, is a precursor of prostaglandin E1; selenium-ACE probably has an anti-inflammatory action and vitamin B6 acts as a co-enzyme in the production of progesterone which will assist in the suppression of endometriosis. Even exercise, which seems to give relief to some endometriosis sufferers, should be encouraged as some female marathon runners have a similar hypo-oestrogenic state to patients on LHRH analogues (Editorial, Lancet 1986).

Surgical treatment of endometriosis

Radical surgery

In order to eradicate endometriosis completely surgery must be radical and that entails total abdominal hysterectomy, the removal of as much endometriotic tissue as possible and bilateral oophorectomy. This may sound relatively straightforward but in patients with advanced disease the surgeon is confronted with densely scarred and thickened tissues, ovaries distorted by large chocolate cysts glued to the pelvic side wall, adhesions involving bowel and bladder and complete obliteration of both cul-de-sacs. In these cases surgery can be very taxing and arduous and is fraught with as many complications and difficulties as radical cancer surgery. It requires a high level of competence and experience: the ureter is at considerable risk during these operations and it can be extremely difficult to be certain of the removal of all ovarian tissue, without which the disease will continue—the ovarian remnant syndrome. Such treatment is reserved for those patients who have failed to obtain pain relief from other therapies and have no further wish to retain their childbearing potential. Although patients, particularly the younger ones, have an entirely understandable wish to retain at least one ovary such a plea should be resisted by reasoned explanation of the consequences of such a course of action. Leaving the hormonal support for endometriosis means that many patients will present with recurrent disease (Luciano 1982, Schneider 1983, Studd & Montgomery 1987). These patients will need hormone replacement therapy (Luciano 1982, Schneider 1983) but oddly enough the disease does not usually recur if oestrogen alone, or combined with testosterone, is given but it is not necessary or desirable to give additional progesterone. My own approach is to wait for 3 months following surgery to give any residual endometriosis time to regress and then give hormone replacement therapy by implant (ostradiol plus testosterone), transdermally or orally using oestrogen alone.

Conservative surgery

This type of surgery is usually reserved for patients with moderate or severe disease who wish to retain or improve their fertility prospects. The rationale behind this approach must be seriously questioned because the only two studies providing monthly fecundity rates demonstrate a much lower rate of conception than those treated with danazol or even expectant management (Rock et al 1981, Olive & Lee 1986). Microsurgical techniques should be employed wherever possible and this implies gentle tissue handling, meticulous haemostasis, the use of some form of magnification and constant irrigation to prevent dessication of tissues and subsequent adhesion formation. There is possibly still an indication for this type of surgery for removal of ovarian endometriomata or for performing uterine ventrosuspension, but both of these procedures can be performed more simply by laparoscopy with less risk of adhesion formation and less morbidity. Pre-sacral neurectomy can relieve central pelvic pain and dysmenorrhoea in up to 75% of patients (Polan & De Cherney 1980) but this can be achieved much more simply by laser uterine nerve ablation (vaporization of the uterosacral ligaments) performed laparoscopically (Daniell 1990). Lasers have been used at laparotomy via an operating microscope (Chong & Baggish, 1984) but the results are not significantly better than those obtained by laser laparoscopy or even by conventional operative laparoscopy (Reich & McGlynn 1986).

SUMMARY

The study of the treatment of endometriosis has suffered from a plethora of poorly designed and uncontrolled trials which makes it difficult to provide clearly defined guidelines for the management of our patients. Several double-blind randomized prospective studies are now underway but it will be several years before these provide meaningful data.

At this time it appears that it is advantageous to treat the visible endometriotic implants with laser vaporization at the same time as the laparoscopic diagnosis is made. The monthly fecundity rate is high, regardless of the stage of the disease, and the patient avoids having to delay conception and take drugs that are expensive and have numerous physical and biochemical side-effects. If laser equipment is not available then endocoagulators or bipolar diathermy is a possible alternative as long as caution is exercised in the vicinity of bowel, bladder and ureter.

If patients relapse or fail to get pregnant after a year, consideration should be given to drug therapy or assisted conception techniques. If pain is the dominant symptom and laparoscopic or conservative surgery fails then danazol or LHRH analogues are often effective for short-term therapy and progestogens are suitable for long-term suppression. The final eradication of the disease awaits the menopause either naturally or surgically, but if the latter is employed it is essential to remove all ovarian tissue; in the presence of dense endometriotic adhesions and the proximity of the ureter, this is not always easy to achieve.

This fascinating and perplexing disease has suffered from a surfeit of anecdotal data gleaned from retrospective and uncontrolled trials against a background pregnancy rate and the difficulties in sorting out the physical and psychological elements associated with the perception of pelvic pain. There is an urgent need for randomized prospective controlled studies to help us determine the best treatment options available to our patients.

REFERENCES

Absten G 1990 Physics of light and lasers. In: Sutton C (ed) Lasers in gynaecology. Chapman and Hall, London, (in press)

Adamson G D, Lu J, Subak L L 1988 Laparoscopic CO_2 laser vaporization of endometriosis compared with traditional treatments. Fertility and Sterility 50(5): 704–710

American Fertility Society 1985 Classification of endometriosis. Fertility and Sterility 43: 351–352

Allen J M, Stein D S, Shingleton H M 1983 Regeneration of cervical epithelium after laser vaporisation. Obstetrics and Gynecology 62: 700–704

Barbieri R L, Kistner R W 1984 In: Raynaud J-P, Ojasoo T, Martini L (eds) Medical management of endometriosis. Raven, New York, pp 27–40

Barbieri R L, Evans S, Kistner R W 1979 Danazol in the treatment of endometriosis: analysis of 100 cases with a four year follow-up. Fertility and Sterility 37: 737–746

Barbieri R L, Ryan K J 1985 Medical therapy for endometriosis: endocrine pharmacology. Seminars in Reproductive Endocrinology 3: 339–352

Bellina J H, Hemmings R, Voros I J, Ross L F 1984 Carbon dioxide laser and electrosurgical wound study with an animal model. A comparison of tissue damage and healing patterns in peritoneal tissue. American Journal of Obstetrics and Gynecology 148: 327

Bergqvist A, Ljungberg O, Myhre E 1984 Human endometrium and endometriotic tissue obtained simultaneously: a comparative histological study. International Journal of Gynaecological Pathology 3: 135–145

Booker M W, Lewis B, Whitehead M I 1986 A comparison of the changes in plasma lipids and lipoproteins during therapy with danazol and gestrione for endometriosis. Proceedings of the 42nd annual meeting of the American Fertility Society, Birmingham. American Fertility Society, Atlanta. p 66

Brosens I A, Puttemans P J 1989 Double optic laparoscopy. In Sutton C (ed) Laparoscopic surgery. Bailliere's Clinical Obstetrics and Gynaecology Vol. 3(3). Bailliere Tindall, London

Bruhat M A, Mage C, Manhes M 1979 Use of the carbon-dioxide laser via laparoscopy. In: Kaplan I (ed) Laser Surgery III, Proceedings of the Third Congress of the International Society for Laser Surgery. International Society for Laser Surgery, Tel Aviv, p. 275

Buttram V C, Reiter R C, Ward S 1985 Treatment of endometriosis with danazol: report of a six-year prospective study. Fertility and Sterility 43: 353–360

Chamberlain G V P, Carron-Brown J 1978 Gynaecological laparoscopy. The Report of the Working Party of the Confidential Enquiry into Gynaecological Laparoscopy. Royal College of Obstetricians and Gynaecologists, London

Cheng V S 1976 Ureteral injury resulting from laparoscopic fulguration of endometriosis implants. American Journal of Obstetrics and Gynecology 126: 1045–1046

Chen Kuo-Fen W U, Wei Y'u, T'ang Min-Yi, Chu Peng-Ti 1980 Endometrial changes after the administration of gossypol for menorrhagia. American Journal of Obstetrics and Gynecology 138: 1227–1229

Chillik C F, Rosenwaks Z 1985 Endometriosis and in-vitro fertilisation. Seminars in Reproductive Endocrinology 3, 353–359

Chillik C F, Acosta A A, Garcia J E et al 1985 The role of in-vitro fertilisation in infertile patients with endometriosis. Fertility and Sterility 44, 56–61

Chong A P, Baggish M S 1984 Management of endometriosis by means of intra-abdominal carbon dioxide laser. Fertility and Sterility 1: 14–19

Corson S L 1990 Laparoscopic applications of the Nd: YAG laser. In Sutton C (ed) Lasers in gynaecology. Chapman and Hall, London (in press)

Coutinho E M 1982 Treatment of endometriosis with gestrinone (R-2323), a synthetic anti-oestrogen, anti-progesterone. American Journal of Obstetrics and Gynecology 144: 895–898

Daniell J F, Brown D H 1982 Carbon dioxide laser laparoscopy: initial experience in experimental animals and humans. Obstetrics and Gynecology 59: 761

Daniell J F 1984 Laser laparoscopy for endometriosis. Colposcopy and Gynaecological Laser Surgery 3: 185–192

Daniell J F 1990 Advanced operative laser laparoscopy. In: Sutton C (ed) Lasers in gynaecology. Chapman and Hall, London (in press)

Davis G D 1986 Management of endometriosis and its associated adhesions with the carbon dioxide laser laparoscope. Obstetrics and Gynecology 68: 422–425

Dmowski W P, Cohen M R 1978 Antigonadotropin (danazol) in the treatment of endometriosis: evaluation of post-treatment fertility and three-year follow-up data. American Journal of Obstetrics and Gynecology 130: 41–47

Doberl A, Bergqvist A, Jeppson S et al 1984 Regression of endometriosis following shorter treatment with, or lower dose of danazol. Acta Obstetrica et Gynaecologica Scandinavica (suppl) 123: 51–58

Donnez J 1987 Carbon dioxide laser laparoscopy in infertile women with endometriosis and women with adnexal adhesions. Fertility and Sterility 3: 390–394

Dowsett M, Forbes K L, Rose G L, Mudge J E, Jeffcoate S L 1986 A comparison of the effects of danazol and gestrinone on testosterone binding to sex hormone binding globulin in vitro and in vivo. Clinical Endocrinology 24, 555–563

Fahraeus L, Larsson-Cohn U, Ljungberg S, Wallentin L 1984 Profound alterations of the lipo-protein metabolism during danazol treatment in premenopausal women. Fertility and Sterility 42: 52–57

Feste J R 1985 Laser laparoscopy. A new modality. Journal of Reproductive Medicine 5: 413–418

Feste J R 1990 Carbon dioxide laser laparotomy. In: Sutton C (ed) Lasers in Gynaecology. Chapman and Hall, London (in press)

Greenblatt R B, Tzingounis V 1979 Danazol treatment of endometriosis: Long term follow-up. Fertility and Sterility 32: 518–524

Guzick D S, Rock J A (1983) A comparison of danazol and conservative surgery for the treatment of infertility due to mild to moderate endometriosis. Fertility and Sterility 40: 580–584

Hamblen E C 1957 Androgen treatment of women. Southern Medical Journal 50: 743–747

Han M 1980 Preliminary results of gossypol treatment in the menopausal functional uterine bleeding, myoma and endometriosis. Acta Medica Chinese Academy of Medical Science 2: 167

Haney A F, Misukonis M A, Weinberg J B 1983 Macrophages and infertility: Oviductal macrophages as potential mediators of infertility. Fertility and Sterility 39: 310

Henzl M R, Corson S L, Moghissi K, Buttram V C, Bergquist C, Jacobson C 1988 Administration of nasal nafarelin as compared with oral danazol for endometriosis. New England Journal of Medicine 318: 485–489

Jansen R, Russell P 1986 Nonpigmented endometriosis: Clinical, laparoscopic and pathologic definition. American Journal of Obstetrics and Gynaecology 155: 1154–1159

Jelley R, Magill P J 1986 The effect of LHRH agonist therapy in the treatment of endometriosis (English experience). Progress in Clinical Biological Research 225: 227–238

Johnston W I H 1976 Dydrogesterone and endometriosis. British Journal of Obstetrics and Gynaecology 83: 77–79

Kaupilla A, Insomoa V, Ronnberg L, Vierikko P, Vihko R 1985 Effect of Gestrinone in endometriosis tissue and endometrium. Fertility and Sterility 44: 466–470

Keye W R, Hansen L W, Astin M, Marsh Poulson A 1987 Argon laser therapy of endometriosis: a review of 92 consecutive patients. Fertility and Sterility 47(2): 208–212

Kistner R W 1959 The treatment of endometriosis in inducing pseudo-pregnancy with ovarian hormones: a report of 58 cases. Fertility and Sterility 10: 539

Koninckx P R, Muyldermans M, Brosens I A 1984 Unexplained infertility: 'Leuven' considerations. European Journal of Obstetrics, Gynecology and Reproductive Biology 18: 403

Editorial 1986 LHRH analogues in endometriosis. Lancet ii, 1016–1018

Lemay A 1988 Comparison of GnRH analogues to conventional therapy in endometriosis. Abstract 020. International Symposium on GnRH analogues, Geneva, 18–21 February 1988

Lilford R J, Dalton M E 1987 Effectiveness of treatment for infertility. British Medical Journal 295: 6591

Lomano J M 1987 Nd: YAG laser ablation of early pelvic endometriosis: a report of 61 cases. Lasers in Surgery and Medicine 7: 56–60

Luciano A A 1982 A guide to managing endometriosis. Contemporary Obstetrics and Gynaecology 19: 211–234

Malinak L R, Wheeler J M 1985 Association of endometriosis with spontaneous abortion: prognosis for pregnancy and risk of recurrence. Seminars in Reproductive Endocrinology 3: 361–369

Martin D C, Olive D L Unpublished data

Matson P L, Yovich J L 1986 The treatment of infertility associated with endometriosis by in vitro fertilisation. Fertility and Sterility 46: 432–434

Matta W H, Shaw R W, Hesp R, Katz D 1987 Hypogonadism induced by LHRH agonist analogues: effects on bone density in pre-menopausal women. British Medical Journal 294: 1523–1524

Meigs J V 1938 Endometriosis, a possible etiological factor. Surgery, Gynaecology and Obstetrics 67: 253 (editorial)

Meldrum D R, Chang R J, Lu J, Vale W, Rivier J, Judd H L 1982 'Medical Oophorectomy' using a long-acting GNRH agonist—a possible new approach to the treatment of endometriosis. Journal of Clinical and Endocrinological Metabolism 54: 1081–1083

Meyer R 1919 Uber den Staude der Frage der adenomyosites Adenoma in Allgemeinen und Adenomyometitis Sarcomastosa. Zentralblatt fur Gynakologie 36: 745–759

Moghissi K S, Boyce C R 1976 Management of endometriosis with oral medroxyprogesterone acetate. Obstetrics and Gynecology 47: 265–267

Nezhat C, Crowgey S R, Garrison C P 1986 Surgical treatment of endometriosis via laser laparoscopy. Fertility and Sterility 6: 778–783

Nezhat C, Winer W, Nezhat F 1988 A comparison of the carbon dioxide, Argon and KTP/532 lasers in the videolaseroscopic treatment of endometriosis. Colposcopy and Gynaecologic Laser Surgery 1: 41–47

Nezhat C, Crowgey S R, Nehzat F 1989 Videolaseroscopy for the treatment of endometriosis associated with infertility. Fertility and Sterility 51(2): 237–240

O'Connor D T 1987 Endometriosis. Current Reviews in Obstetrics and Gynaecology No. 12. Churchill Livingstone, Edinburgh

Olive D L, Haney A F 1986 Endometriosis-associated infertility: a critical review of therapeutic approaches. Obstetrical and Gynaecological Survey 41: 538–555

Olive D L, Lee K L 1986 Analysis of sequential treatment protocols for endometriosis associated infertility. American Journal of Obstetrics and Gynecology 154: 613–619

Olive D L, Stohs G F, Metzger D A et al 1985 Expectant management and hydrotubations in the treatment of endometriosis associated infertility. Fertility and Sterility 44: 35

Older J 1984 Endometriosis. Charles Scribner, New York

Redwine D B 1987 Age-related evolution in colour appearance of endometriosis. Fertility and Sterility 48: 1062

Reich H, McGlynn F 1986 Treatment of ovarian endometriomas using laparoscopic surgical techniques. Journal of Reproductive Medicine 31: 577–584

Rock J A, Guzick D S, Sengos C 1981 The conservative surgical treatment of endometriosis: evaluation of pregnancy success with respect to the extent of disease as categorized using contemporary classification systems. Fertility and Sterility 35: 131

Rock J A 1988 New concepts in the treatment of endometriosis. In Rock J A, Schweppe K W (eds) Recent advances in the management of endometriosis. Proceedings of the First Congress of the International Society of Gynaecological Endocrinology. Parthenon Publishing, Carnforth, pp 91–101

Sampson J A 1921 Perforating haemorrhagic cysts of ovary. Archives of Surgery 3: 245–323

Sampson J A 1927a Peritoneal endometriosis due to menstrual dissemination of endometrial tissue into peritoneal cavity. American Journal of Obstetrics and Gynecology 14: 422

Sampson J A 1927b Metastatic or embolic endometriosis due to menstrual dissemination of endometrial tissue into the venous circulation. American Journal of Pathology 18: 571–592

Schmidt D L 1985 Endometriosis; a reappraisal of pathogenesis and treatment. Fertility and Sterility 44: 157–173

Schneider G T 1983 In: Studd J (ed) Progress in obstetrics and gynaecology. Churchill Livingstone, Edinburgh, pp 246–256

Schriock E, Monroe S E, Henzl M, Jaffe R B 1985 Treatment of endometriosis with a potent agonist of gonadotropin-releasing hormone (nafarelin). Fertility and Sterility 44: 583–585

Seibel M M, Berber M J, Weinstein F G, Taymor M L 1982 The effectiveness of danazol on subsequent fertility in minimal endometriosis. Fertility and Sterility 38: 534–537

Semm K, Mettler L 1980 Technical progress in pelvic surgery via operative laparoscopy. Amercian Journal of Obstetrics and Gynecology 138: 121–127

Shaw R W, Farquhar J W 1984 Female pseudo-hermaphroditism associated with danazol exposure in utero: Case report. British Journal of Obstetrics and Gynecology 91: 386–389

Shaw R W, Matta W 1986 Reversible pituitary ovarian suppression induced by an LHRH analogue in the treatment of endometriosis—comparison of two dose regimens. Clinical Reproduction and Fertility 4: 329–336

Shaw R W 1988 LHRH analogues in the treatment of endometriosis—comparative results with other treatments. Bailliere's Clinical Obstetrics and Gynaecology Vol. 2, No. 3

Strathy J H, Molgaard C A, Coulam C B, Melton L J 1982 Endometriosis and infertility: a laparoscopic study of endometriosis among fertile and infertile women. Fertility and Sterility 38: 667–672

Studd J W W, Montgomery J C 1987 Oestradiol and testosterone implants after hysterectomy for endometriosis. In: Bruhat M A, Canis M (eds) Contributions to gynaecology and obstetrics: endometriosis. Karger, Basel Vol. 16, pp 241–246

Sutton C J G 1974 Limitations of laparoscopic ovarian biopsy. British Journal of Obstetrics and Gynaecology 81: 317–320

Sutton C J G 1986 Initial experience with carbon dioxide laser laparoscopy. Lasers in Medical Science 1: 25–31

Sutton C J G, Hill D 1989 Laser laparoscopy in the treatment of endometriosis: a five year study. British Journal of Obstetrics and Gynaecology (in press)

Tadir Y, Kaplan I, Zuckerman K 1981 A second puncture probe for laser laparoscopy. In: Atsumi K, Nimsakul N (eds) Laser Surgery IV, Proceedings of the Fourth Congress of the International Society for Laser Surgery, pp 25–26

Thomas E J, Cooke I D 1987 Impact of gestrinone on the course of asymptomatic endometriosis. British Medical Journal 294: 272–274

Thomas E J, Cooke I D 1987 Successful treatment of endometriosis: does it benefit infertile women? British Medical Journal 294: 1117–1119

Vernon M W, Beard J S, Graves K, Wilson E A 1986 Classification of endometriotic implants by morphologic appearance and capacity to synthesise prostaglandin F. Fertility and Sterility 46: 801–806

Wardle P G, Mitchell J D, McLaughlin E A, Ray B D, McDermott A, Hull M G 1985 Endometriosis and ovulatory disorder: reduced fertilisation in vitro, compared with tubal and unexplained infertility. Lancet ii: 236–239

Wilson E A 1988 Surgical therapy for endometriosis. Clinical Obstetrics and Gynecology 4: 857–865

Zhou S 1981 Clinical use of gossypol in gynaecology. Chinese Journal of Obstetrics and Gynecology 16: 137

Zhu P, Sun Y, Cheng J 1984 Electron microscopic observations of the effects of gossypol on the human endometrium. American Journal of Obstetrics and Gynecology 149: 780

17. Active management of infertility

Hossam Abdalla   Rod Baber   John Studd

INTRODUCTION

Infertility is best defined as the inability to conceive after one year of unprotected intercourse (Hammond 1987). Using this definition, the incidence of infertility in Western communities is between 15% and 20% of all couples (Guttmacher 1956), more and more of whom are now seeking professional assistance for their condition.

Several factors contribute to this increased demand for infertility investigation including (i) increased numbers of women in the reproductive age group, (ii) a trend towards later age of child bearing which increases the span of years of exposure to infections or toxins as well as age-specific reductions in fertility (iii) a greater public awareness of the availability and scope of such services (Aral 1983) and (iv) the availability of new technology and drugs for the treatment of previously hopeless causes of infertility.

Unfortunately, the investigation and management of infertility is often slow, time-consuming and although inadequately funded, is paradoxically costly. The infertile couple are seldom seen together. Investigations are performed in a piecemeal fashion rather than as part of an overall strategy whereby diagnosis (or the lack of it) is specified and effective management is initiated. It is also customary in the majority of general hospitals for patients to be seen by junior doctors with little experience of infertility management and who are themselves new to the patient. Consequently, with no answers to give, the unfortunate patient is often told to come back in 6 months time when the doctor has moved on to another consultant and the patient is left to see yet another unfamiliar inexperienced face. Patients may also put their doctors under pressure to do something. Trivial symptoms and abnormalities may indicate repeated laparoscopies or other investigations. Myomectomies may be performed for small fibroids and ovarian cystectomy and wedge resections are performed on simple cysts that could have been treated conservatively. These procedures commonly induce adhesions and damage in a hitherto normal pelvis.

Regardless of the recommendations of the Warnock Committee (Warnock 1984) specialized regional infertility services are seldom available

273

and those that do exist are deprived of resources. This drives more patients into the private sector and investigations are needlessly repeated and resources wasted. Insurance companies, faced with a rising demand for infertility treatment, have recently declared that infertility is not a disease and therefore no cover is available for any definitive treatment.

Both patient and doctor suffer from the inefficient treatment of this problem. The patients are by nature secretive, believing their problems to be personal and are left to cope alone with their anxiety and sadness. Feelings of inadequacy, guilt and depression become long-standing with consequent marital disharmony. Infertility is not only a physical disorder but a social one as well, affecting the productivity of the individual and ultimately of society.

The doctor also feels inadequate and unable to help his patient. Trust between doctor and patient breaks down as the doctor is faced with the difficulties of explaining negative results after exhaustive repeated investigations whilst the couple 'continue trying'. The temptation to try many empirical, possibly useless medical treatments is considerable as time passes and the patient realizes the poverty of the offered advice.

The current investigation and treatment of infertility is mostly inadequate and it will be argued in this chapter that it needs to be streamlined with a division of responsibility between properly-trained primary physicians at the District General Hospital (DGH) level and regional centres where more sophisticated infertility procedures may be employed.

AETIOLOGY OF INFERTILITY

Causes of infertility vary between countries, and even regions, and a knowledge of local disease patterns is essential if appropriate investigations are to be performed and inappropriate ones omitted. Table 17.1 shows the common causes reported in three recent series together with those seen at The Lister Fertility Clinic in 1988. The reduced incidence of anovulation and the increased incidence of unexplained infertility in the latter series may be because The Lister is a secondary referral centre.

Table 17.1 Common causes of infertility

	Rowland 1980	Katayama et al 1979	Pepperell 1983 (Australia)	Lister 1988 (UK)
Anovulation	24%	23%	10–15%	5%
Male factor	13%	18%	15–25%	25%
Tubal disease	34%	12%	20–30%	30%
Endometriosis	—	25%	10–15%	5%
Unexplained	29%	22%	15–25%	35%

Unexplained infertility

Why is unexplained infertility unexplained? The answer lies in two main areas. Firstly, investigations may have been inadequate and the true aetiology missed. For example, in a recent study of 95 couples allegedly suffering from unexplained infertility, Haxton et al (1987) found abnormal sperm parameters in 22 cases and endocrine abnormalities in another 10. Secondly, there remain factors which are either unknown or untestable using any conventional methods; the only sure evidence of ovulation is conception, yet we measure indirect parameters such as a rise in serum progesterone (Hull et al 1982), a rise in basal body temperature (Lenton 1977) or secretory endometrium in a premenstrual biopsy. However, all these parameters will be suggestive of ovulation in both the luteinized unruptured follicle syndrome (Brosens et al 1978, Marik 1978) and in cases of failed oocyte release at ovulation (Stanger & Yovich 1984, Abdalla et al 1987). Even ultrasound, which may be the most reliable indirect test of ovulation (Vermesh et al 1987) cannot detect the latter.

The testing of tubal patency by hysterosalpingogram or laparoscopy will confirm tubal patency but cannot confirm normal ciliary action of the tubal mucosa. Also, tubal patency tests do not test the ability of a fallopian tube to pick up oocytes, yet there is evidence that in only 60% of ovulatory cycles is this pickup mechanism functioning (Croxatto et al 1978). Although a normal semen analysis should include a sperm count, motility and morphology assessment and function tests such as sperm mucus contact tests (Kremer 1965) and hamster egg-penetration tests (Hewitt et al 1987), no test can assess the fertilizing ability of sperm in vivo. Finally, it is often impossible to judge the adequacy of coital exposure and the veracity of information given—to paraphrase a well-known dictum—truth is the first casualty of infertility. Most couples will claim to have coitus 2–3 times per week but it is only later that the wife will admit that intercourse is a most infrequent event. Such is the penalty of the chronic anxiety of the high pressure globe-trotting 20th century life-style. This must be a common cause of 'unexplained infertility'.

Assisted conception

Gamete intrafallopian transfer (GIFT) and in vitro fertilization (IVF) help to answer many of these questions of diagnosis as well as providing therapy. Pregnancy following GIFT was first reported by Asch et al in 1984 and the technique is now recognized as the most successful treatment for patients with unexplained infertility, mild endometriosis and some male-factor infertility (Leeton et al 1987). The success rate of in vitro fertilization, although lower than the GIFT procedure, is improving with rates over 25% per oocyte collection recently being reported (Abdalla et al 1988a, Rutherford et al 1988). In vitro fertilization also allows an assessment of the quality of the oocytes produced, the fertilizing capability of the sperm and the characteristics of the early embryo. The patients who undergo such procedures are often older than the average fertile population. It is for them a last resort as increasing age brings with it reduced fecundity (Dor et al 1980). It is certain that, if patients were treated with such procedures earlier in their reproductive life, better results would be obtained.

Assisted conception (IVF and GIFT) is rarely available on the NHS as the service is considered expensive and does not come within the priorities of the regional health authorities. These procedures are expensive because they are inefficiently used and incorporation of these new developments into the routine investigation and management of infertile couples should make the infertility management more cost-efficient.

IVF is considered to be expensive because (i) it requires a 7-day operating theatre to be available and theatre availability for non-emergency procedures is notoriously difficult to acquire in NHS hospitals; (ii) it needs well-trained clinical personnel for ovulation induction and oocyte retrieval, including a highly trained embryologist; (iii) the capital cost of equipment in setting up and maintaining an IVF laboratory is considerable. The cost of the drugs used for ovulation induction is also considerable but most of all the cost is great if the results are poor. The failure to apply this cost of failure to tubal surgery while assuming successful IVF and GIFT programmes to be expensive is a predictable failure of administrative wisdom.

These expenses are over and above the normal expenses that already cover the conventional investigations of the infertile couple. However, some of these investigations are unnecessary and can be incorporated with or replaced by GIFT or IVF. For more efficient infertility services there will be the need for (i) a speedy diagnosis and management to save clinic and doctor time and saving unnecessary repetitive investigations and/or operations; (ii) centralizing specialized treatment for more efficient training of medical staff and patient management; (iii) combining as much as possible therapeutic and diagnostic procedures to decrease repetition.

ACTIVE MANAGEMENT OF INFERTILITY

We outline below our approach to the management of infertility which is both cost-effective and efficient. For this approach to be adopted radical changes in the management of infertility should occur based on the following principles:

1. Couples should always be seen together and speedy initial investigations performed on both partners;
2. GIFT is the most successful method for treating couples with unexplained infertility, cervical factors and those with minimal male factors;

Table 17.2   Results of operative procedures, Lister Fertility Clinic 1988

Total patients	309
Total cycles of ovarian stimulation with LHRH analogue and HMG	409
Total Diagnostic laparoscopies	10
Total Hysterosalpingograms	98
Total receiving no further investigation of tubal status after initial referral indicated no pelvic pathology	201
Cycles cancelled due to poor response to stimulation	31
Total oocyte collections	378
Collections changed from laparoscopic to vaginal technique during the operative procedure	13
Failed oocyte collections	3

3. GIFT does not require the same technical and laboratory equipment necessary for IVF;
4. Patients with blocked fallopian tubes may be treated by both in vitro fertilization or tubal surgery. Assessment of which procedure is indicated should be performed in a centre that conducts both IVF and tubal surgery. The establishment of these multidiscipline regional centres, as recommended in The Warnock report (1984), is critical to the success of this scheme of management.
5. Assessment laparoscopy and dye insufflation is usually an unnecessary diagnostic procedure and should be replaced by hysterosalpingogram to assess the state of the tubes. Either GIFT or IVF will be performed as a next step depending on whether the tubes are patent or not.

This approach, which we would call an active management of infertility, saves time because of efficient counselling of the couple and avoidance of unnecessary tests and worthless avenues of therapy. For the same reasons it saves money and the avoidance of the initial diagnostic laparoscopy in preference to the treatment laparoscopy is a radical change of policy. If this system is also efficient in producing pregnancy then there is much to commend it. It is!

Table 17.2 outlines the results of patients treated following the application of these principles at The Lister Fertility Clinic during 1988.

The scheme of investigation and treatment

Figure 17.1 outlines the scheme of management.

The first visit

At the first visit the couple should be seen together, preferably in an infertility clinic at the DGH. Complete histories should be taken from both partners with particular reference to the following: length of marriage;

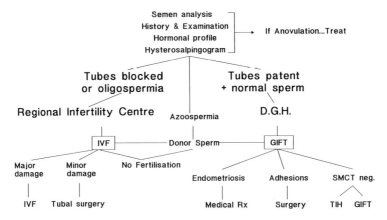

Fig. 17.1   The active management of infertility.

length of infertility; previous contraception; previous pregnancies; coital frequency; developmental and menstrual histories; medical and surgical histories; and exposure to toxins and drugs. Physical examination of the woman should pay particular attention to signs of endocrine disturbances. Her weight should be recorded and compared with her ideal weight for height, as both excessive obesity and weight-loss will adversely affect ovulation (Knuth et al 1977). The pelvic examination should seek uterine abnormalities, ovarian and tubal masses, uterosacral nodularity, pelvic organ mobility and the presence or absence of pain. The cervix should be examined for infection. Blood should be taken for FSH, LH, oestradiol, prolactin, day-21 progesterone and thyroid-function tests. Lastly, a hysterosalpingogram should be arranged for day 6–12 of her next cycle. We do not advocate a laparoscopy for tubal evaluation at this time.

A fresh semen sample, obtained prior to the consultation, should be assessed by the hospital semenologist. This assessment should include quantitative and qualitative tests mentioned previously, a MAR test and sperm wash and swim-up (Kerin et al 1984). Sperm survival should also be assessed over the ensuing 48 hours.

Any abnormality in the semen analysis should lead to a careful physical examination of the male partner with particular attention to secondary sexual characteristics, perineal sensation and anal sphincter tone. The genital examination should include examination of the penis, the meatus and the testes. The epididymis should be palpated throughout its length, a varicocele should be sought and the prostate and seminal vesicles examined. Men with abnormal physical findings or an abnormal semen analysis should have blood taken for FSH, LH and testosterone levels and then be referred to an andrologist for further management. Other tests should be based on clinical suspicion.

The second visit

This should be within 6 weeks of the first so that all results from previous tests are available and definitive treatment can commence.

Where a disorder of ovulation is present the further evaluation should be directed towards abnormal findings; for example a skull X-ray/CT scan of the pituitary fossa are indicated if prolactin levels are elevated and androgen assays if hirsutism is present. Patients with elevated prolactin levels usually ovulate on bromocryptine therapy (Pepperell et al 1977), those with abnormal thyroid function tests usually ovulate when these return to normal and those with low or normal FSH and LH usually ovulate when treated with clomiphene citrate, gonadotrophin-releasing hormone or human menopausal gonadotrophins (HMG) (Pepperell 1983). Patients with significantly elevated FSH levels very rarely respond to any form of ovulation induction (O'Herlihy et al 1980) and for these patients ovum donation is the only practical treatment. Any patients receiving treatment with ovulation-induction agents should preferably have their response monitored with serial pelvic ultrasound scans and/or oestradiol and progesterone levels. Treatment should continue for 6–12 months.

Male factors are best dealt with by an andrologist or urologist. Varicoceles may be found in 10–23% of normal men (Verstoppen & Steeno 1977) and surgery may not improve the semen parameters. Antisperm antibodies occur in 3–13% of infertile men (Hargreaves et al 1980) and although corticosteroid treatment often results in lower antibody titres this is only occasionally associated with increased pregnancy rates (Baker et al 1983) and has a relatively high incidence of serious side-effects (Schulman & Schulman 1982).

Men with endocrinological abnormalities represent no more than 3% of the infertile male population (Aafjes & Van der Vijver 1976). Hypo-gonadotrophic disorders may be chromosomal, infective, metabolic, traumatic and neoplastic, and efficacy of treatment with replacement therapy will depend on the cause. Nevertheless, pregnancies have been reported following this therapy. Male hyperprolactinaemia can result in reduced androgen production. Treatment of affected males with testosterone or bromocryptine may result in increased androgen levels and sexual potency (Franks et al 1978) but subsequent pregnancy rates have been disappointing (Hovatto et al 1979).

Men with idiopathic infertility have been treated with a variety of substances including clomiphene citrate (Ronnberg 1980), tamoxifen (Comhaire 1976), gonadotrophins (Lunenfield et al 1967) and androgens (Lamensdorf et al 1975) but, with the possible exception of tamoxifen, little benefit has derived.

There is an obvious role for therapeutic insemination with husband's sperm (TIH) in cases of coital difficulty, retrograde ejaculation and relative oligospermia (due to a high volume). True oligospermia is also treated with

TIH but pregnancy rates remain low (Wiltbank et al 1985). Severe oligospermia, asthenospermia, teratospermia, combined defects and azoospermia are best treated with therapeutic insemination by donor, IVF or a combination of both techniques. Recent advances in IVF have identified a subset of men whose semen analyses are apparently normal yet whose sperm are unable to penetrate the zona pellucida, oocyte membrane or both (Acosta et al 1986). These findings confirm what has long been suspected and explain why TIH is often unsuccessful.

The next step

Tubes are patent. If all initial investigations are normal and the fallopian tubes were found to be patent on the HSG, a GIFT cycle should be performed and laparoscopic assessment of the pelvis made at the time of oocyte recovery. This procedure may be performed at the DGH. The success and relative simplicity of the GIFT procedure has encouraged more NHS gynaecology departments to try to adopt such a technique as the procedure of oocyte collection and tubal catheterization at laparoscopy is relatively easy to learn. The major difficulty that prevents such a successful procedure from being widely available within the facilities of the NHS is that operative procedure cannot be timed to the convenience of the surgical team, and so the daily availability of an operating theatre is required.

To obviate this problem many authors have attempted to manipulate the menstrual cycle in order to fix the date of oocyte retrieval. Wardle et al (1986) first described the use of progestogens in the pre-treatment cycle in a clinical IVF programme. A withdrawal bleed could be expected between 3 and 5 days after stopping progestogen. The patient is then stimulated with a standard drug regimen normally using clomiphene citrate and human menopausal gonadotrophins (HMG) followed by human chorionic gonadotrophins (HCG) administered 2 days prior to the fixed operation day which is normally day 12 or 13 of the cycle. There are many modifications of this approach which seem to be effective (Templeton et al 1984, Frydman et al 1986).

However, the planning of cycles by progestogens still has problems. The first is that menstruation may not start within the expected time although this was not believed to be any disadvantage in the study by Bates et al (1988). Another disadvantage is that ovulation induction performed by a combination of clomiphene citrate and exogenous gonadotrophins elevates the LH:FSH ratio (Jeffcoate 1984, Abdalla 1988b), and requires monitoring of urinary LH and oestradiol as premature luteinization can occur in 30% of women and premature ovulation occurs in 15% of cycles leading to cancellation of the planned oocyte collection (Steptoe et al 1986). The elevated LH is also associated with the occurrence of post-mature oocytes, poor fertilization rates and poor embryonic development which ultimately is responsible for a reduction in pregnancy rates (Stanger & Yovich 1985, Howles et al 1986, Punnonen et al 1988).

In 1984 Porter et al reported on the successful use of the LHRH analogue Buserelin (Hoechst) plus HMG for induction of ovulation using a so-called 'long protocol of stimulation' in which analogue treatment began on day 23 of the cycle prior to HMG stimulation. Rutherford et al (1988), using a similar protocol, and Abdalla (1988b) using a short protocol both reported an increased number of oocytes collected per procedure and an increased pregnancy rate. Abdalla also showed lower circulating levels of endogenous LH at the time of embryo transfer and a reduced early miscarriage rate.

In the short protocol, LHRH analogue is commenced on day 1 of the treatment cycle and HMG stimulation is begun on day 3 to take advantage of the initial agonistic phase of analogue activity, thus keeping drug usage to a minimum. This regimen will also suppress the mid-cycle LH surge, eliminating the problem of spontaneous ovulation, obviating the need for routine LH and oestradiol assays, and allowing oocyte collection to be timed for routine operating lists at the surgeon's convenience. Abdalla et al (1989) took advantage of this fact and electively delayed oocyte pickup by 1 or 2 days for all patients who would, using normal criteria, have had their oocyte collection performed on a weekend or a non-routine operating day. These procedures were then performed on the next available routine operating list. They found that this technique may be associated with an increased pregnancy rate and will certainly result in improved flexibility and cost-effectiveness of assisted conception programmes. The results of all patients treated at The Lister Fertility Clinic in 1988 are shown in Table 17.3 and results related to time of oocyte collection are shown in Table 17.4.

Follicular development is best monitored using serial pelvic ultrasound (Hackeloer et al 1979, Smith et al 1980, Marrs et al 1983). The first should be performed on day 3 to exclude pelvic pathology and to seek evidence of polycystic ovarian syndrome (Adams et al 1985) followed by two or three others as clinically indicated from about day 8. In our experience over 85% of patients will have a leading follicle of 18 mm on day 11 of the treatment

Table 17.3 Results of IVF or GIFT treatment, Lister Fertility Clinic 1988 following ovarian stimulation with LHRH analogue and HMG

	IVF–ET (n = 116)	GIFT (n = 244)	Total (n = 360)
Age	34.0±4.7	33.3±4.7	33.6±4.7
No. of eggs	7.0±4.7	10.0±6.1	9.0±5.8
Mature	2.7±2.5	4.3±3.4	3.7±3.2
Mature %	38%±2.9	43%±3.4	42%±2.7
Fertilized %	72%±2.7	44%±3.6	54%±3.6
GIFT no.		3.4±1.0	
ET no.	3.1±1.1		
Pregnant	28	78	106
Pregnant %	24.1%	31.9%	29.5%

Table 17.4 Results in all patients (GIFT and IVF), Lister Fertility Clinic 1988 with outcome of treatment in relation to time of oocyte collection

	Total ($n = 360$)	Delayed ($n = 119$)	Not delayed ($n = 241$)
Pregnancy	106 (29.5%)	44 (37.0%)	62 (25.7%)*
Ongoing/delivered	75 (70.7%)	32 (72.7%)	43 (69.3%)
Miscarriage	30 (28.3%)	12 (27.3%)	18 (29.0%)
Ectopic	1 (0.9%)	—	1 (1.6%)

* = $P < 0.02$.

cycle and oocyte collection is planned at about this time according to follicular size, endometrial thickness and endometrial reflectivity (Smith et al 1984, Hull et al 1986). The administration of HCG for final follicular maturation after this stage may then be timed to coincide with the operating list.

At laparoscopy, the pelvis is examined in detail to exclude any associated pathology, as is usual with any assessment laparoscopy and dye (the only difference is that the patency of the tubes is not tested since it has already been tested by HSG). Oocyte collection is performed in the presence of a trained technician who should have received the husband's sperm sample pre-operatively and prepared it in the usual manner (Diamond & De Cherney 1987). Almost all district general hospitals employ a semenologist and training such persons to identify and prepare eggs is not difficult. Following successful egg collection the gametes are transferred to the Fallopian tubes.

At the completion of the procedure a sample of cervical mucus is obtained and a sperm mucus-contact test performed (Kremer 1965). Any sperm mucus penetration problems can be treated by intrauterine artificial insemination following ovulation induction or by a repeat GIFT. If pregnancy does not ensue, further management should be determined by the laparoscopic findings; endometriosis may be treated with the appropriate medical or surgical modality. Mild endometriosis may require no further treatment apart from a repetition of the GIFT procedure (Chillik & Rosenwaks 1985). Periovarian and peritubular adhesions, if not amenable to removal at laparoscopy, should be treated by a separate procedure.

Tubes are blocked. Detection of tubal blockage at HSG should result in the patient being referred to a regional centre with facilities for all forms of assisted conception and tubal microsurgery. Such a centre should have a fully equipped IVF laboratory and embryologist. IVF patients should undergo ovarian stimulation as previously described. Oocyte pickup for IVF may be achieved using the laparoscope or ultrasound guidance (Baber et al 1988), but for the initial attempt we advocate laparoscopic oocyte collection with ultrasound back-up. This allows assessment of the patient's tubal disease and her suitability for tubal microsurgery to be made by the surgeon who may be required to perform such procedures. At the completion of laparoscopy, a sperm mucus contact test should be performed again as its result may influence the decision as to whether the patient should have tubal surgery or continue with IVF

Oocytes and sperm are prepared in the usual way and fertilized embryos are transferred after 48 hours. Should there be no evidence of fertilization after 24 hours it is our policy to recommend the application of donor sperm (of known fertilizing potential) to a proportion of the oocytes to determine whether the apparent problem with fertilization is of male or female origin.

If pregnancy does not ensue, further management will depend on the findings obtained at the first IVF attempt. For example, those suitable for tubal surgery should be so treated; those whose sperm was unable to fertilize their partners' oocytes should be offered treatment with donor sperm and those in whom no reason for failure was apparent and in whom tubal repair is not possible should be offered a second IVF attempt. The subsequent oocyte collections for IVF should be performed using the transvaginal ultrasound-guided approach.

Women who are prematurely menopausal, carriers of inheritable disorders or chromosomal abnormalities, who fail to respond to ovarian stimulation or whose oocytes cannot be fertilized by partner or donor sperm may now be offered a donated oocyte (Lutjen et al 1984). As cryopreservation of embryos has been successfully employed for many years (Whittingham et al 1972) and numerous pregnancies have been reported since 1983 (Trounson & Mohr 1983), regional centres should also be equipped with this facility thus minimizing the need for repeated oocyte collection in patients with extra embryos from GIFT and IVF cycles and also to enable extra oocytes obtained during DGH GIFT procedures to be transferred, fertilized, frozen and stored for future transfer.

CONCLUSION

Properly conducted, such a scheme for the efficient investigation and management of infertility should take no more than 3 months to complete with information having been obtained regarding:

1. Male factor,
2. Menstrual cycle and cervical mucus,
3. Response to ovulation induction,
4. Tubal patency,
5. Pelvic status and suitability for microsurgery,
6. Fertilizing capacity of sperm and oocytes.

Furthermore, each patient will have received definitive treatment in the form of GIFT or IVF/ET.

In this scheme no substantial extra cost has been incurred by the DGH as the GIFT procedure simply replaces the assessment laparoscopy currently performed and the extra equipment required for GIFT is minimal, inexpensive and often already available within the hospital. The other main limiting factor, timing of oocyte collection, is overcome by the use of LHRH analogue.

The centralization of tubal surgery and IVF expertise in regional centres has the advantage of providing centralized training of staff in both disciplines, ensuring the highest quality of care and impartial assessment of treatment options. It should also lead to a reduction in the number of patients requiring tubal microsurgery by that number who become pregnant on their first IVF attempt and avoidance of repetition of surgery inappropriately undertaken elsewhere. These units would also centralize continuing research in tubal surgery, in vitro fertilization and cryopreservation.

REFERENCES

Aafjes J A, Van der Vijver J C M 1976 Men with reduced fertility. Dutch Journal of Medicine 120: 865–867

Abdalla H I, Baber R J, Leonard T et al 1989 Timed oocyte collection in an assisted conception programme using LHRH analogue. Human Reproduction (in press)

Abdalla H I, Ah-Moye M, Brinsden P, Lim Howe D, Craft I 1987 The effect of the dose of human chorionic gonadotrophins and the type of gonadotrophin stimulation on oocyte recovery rate in an IVF programme. Fertility and Sterility 48: 5–8

Abdalla H I, Leonard T, Baber R J et al 1988a IVF. British Medical Journal 296: 1470

Abdalla H I, Ahuja K, Leonard T et al 1988b Reduced fetal loss with the use of LHRH analogue in an assisted conception programme. Proceedings of European Society of Human Reproduction and Embryology, 4th Annual meeting, Barcelona, p 1023

Acosta A A, Chillik C F, Brugo S et al 1986 In vitro fertilisation and the male factor. Urology 28: 1–9

Adams J, Polson D W, Franks S 1985 Prevalence of polycystic ovaries in anovulatory women and those with idiopathic hirsutism. Journal of Endocrinology 104 (suppl): 37–41

Aral S O, Cates W Jr 1983 The increasing concern with infertility; why now? Journal of the American Medical Association 250: 2327

Asch R H, Ellsworth L R, Balmaceda J P et al 1984 Pregnancy following translaparoscopic gamete intrafallopian transfer (GIFT). Lancet ii: 1034

Baber R, Porter R, Picker R, Robertson R, Dawson E, Saunders D 1988 Transvaginal ultrasound directed oocyte collection in an IVF programme; successes and complications. Journal of Ultrasound Medicine 7: 377–379

Baker H W, Clarke G N, Hudson B, McBain J C, McGowan M P, Pepperell R J 1983 Treatment of sperm autoimmunity in men. Clinical Reproduction and Fertility 2: 55–71

Bates R G, Fielding P M, Lindsay K S, White N J, Edmonds D K 1988 Programmed Gamete Intrafallopian Transfer (GIFT). British Journal of Obstetrics and Gynaecology 95: 1220–1225

Brosens I A, Konnickx P R, Corveleyn P A 1978 A study of plasma progesterone, oestradiol, prolactin and LH levels and of the luteal phase appearance of the ovaries in patients with endometriosis and infertility. British Journal of Obstetrics and Gynaecology 85: 246–250

Chillik C, Rosenwaks Z 1985 Endometriosis and in vitro fertilisation. Seminars in Reproductive Endocrinology 3: 377–381

Comhaire F 1976 Treatment of oligospermia with Tamoxifen. International Journal of Fertility 21: 232–238

Croxatto H B, Ortiz M E, Diaz S, Hess R, Balmaceda V, Croxatto H D 1978 Studies on the duration of egg transport by the human oviduct II. Ovum location at various intervals following luteinising hormone peak. American Journal of Obstetrics and Gynecology 132: 629–634

Diamond M P, De Cherney A H 1987 In vitro fertilization and gamete intrafallopian transfer. Obstetric and Gynecology Clinics in North America 14(4): 1087–1098

Dor J, Itzkowic D J, Moshiach S et al 1980 Cumulative conception rates following gonadotrophin therapy. American Journal of Obstetrics and Gynecology 136: 102–105

Franks S, Jacobs H S, Martin N, Nabarro J D N 1978 Hyperprolactinaemia and impotence. Clinical Endocrinology 8: 277–287

Frydman R, Forman R, Rainborn J D, Belaisch-Allart J, Hazout A, Testart J 1986 A new approach to follicular stimulation for in vitro fertilization: programmed oocyte retrieval. Fertility and Sterility 46: 657–662

Guttmacher F 1956 Factors affecting normal expectancy of conception. Journal of the American Medical Association 161: 856–858

Hackeloer B J, Fleming R, Robinson H P, Adams A H, Coutts J R T 1979 Correlation of ultrasonic and endocrinologic assessment of human follicular development. American Journal of Obstetrics and Gynecology 135: 122–128

Hammond M G 1987 Evaluation of the infertile couple. Obstetric and Gynecology Clinics of North America 14(4): 821–830

Hargreaves T B, Haxdon M, Whitelas J, Elton R, Chisholn C O 1980 The significance of sperm agglutinating antibodies in men with infertile marriages. British Journal of Urology 52: 566–567

Haxton M J, Fleming R, Hamilton M P R, Yates R W, Black W P, Coutts J R T 1987 Unexplained infertility: results of secondary investigations in 95 couples. British Journal of Obstetrics and Gynaecology 94: 539–542

Hewitt J, Cohen J, Steptoe P 1987 Male infertility and in vitro fertilization. In: Studd J W W (ed) Progress in Obstetrics and Gynaecology Vol. 6. Churchill Livingstone, Edinburgh, pp 253–276

Hovatto O, Koskimies A I, Ranta T, Stenman U H, Seppala M 1979 Bromocryptine treatment of oligospermia: a double-blind study. Clinical Endocrinology 11: 377–382

Howles C M, MacNamee M C, Edwards R G, Goswamy R, Steptoe P C 1986 Effect of high tonic levels of luteinising hormone on outcome of in vitro fertilization. Lancet ii: 521–522

Hull M G R, Savage P E, Bromham D, Ismail A A, Morris A F 1982 The value of a single serum progesterone measurement in the mid-luteal phase as a criterion of a potentially fertile cycle (ovulation) derived from treated/untreated conception cycles. Fertility and Sterility 37: 355–360

Hull M E, Moghissi K S, Magyar D M, Hayes M F, Zador I, Olson J M 1986 Correlation of serum estradiol levels and ultrasound monitoring to assess follicular maturation. Fertility and Sterility 46(1): 42–45

Jeffcoate S 1984 The endocrine control of ovulation. In: Thompson W, Joyce D N, Newton J R (eds) In vitro fertilization and donor insemination. Proceedings of the Royal College of Obstetricians and Gynaecologists pp 1–12

Katayama K P, Jo K, Manuel M et al 1979 Computer analysis of aetiology and pregnancy rates in 636 cases of 10 infertility. American Journal of Obstetrics and Gynecology 135: 207–214

Kerin J F P, Peck J, Warnes G M et al 1984 Improved conception rate after intra uterine insemination of washed spermatozoa from men with poor quality semen. Lancet i: 533–535

Knuth U A, Hull M G R, Jacobs H S 1977 Amenorrhoea and loss of weight. British Journal of Obstetrics and Gynaecology 84: 801–807

Kremer J 1965 A simple sperm penetration test. International Journal of Fertility 10: 209–210

Lamensdorf H, Compere D, Begley G 1975 Testosterone rebound therapy in the treatment of male infertility. Fertility and Sterility 26: 469–472

Leeton J F, Rogers P, Caro C, Healy D, Yates C 1987 A controlled study between the use of gamete intrafallopian transfer (GIFT) and in vitro fertilization and embryo transfer in the management of idiopathic and male infertility. Fertility and Sterility 48: 605–608

Lenton E, Weston G D, Cooke I D 1977 Problems in using basal body temperature recordings in an infertility clinic. British Medical Journal 1: 803–805

Lunenfield B, Mor A, Mani M 1967 Treatment of male infertility. I: human gonadotrophins. Fertility and Sterility 18: 581–592

Lutjen P, Trounson A, Leeton J, Findley J, Wood C, Renou P 1984 The establishment and maintenance of pregnancy using IVF and embryo donation in a patient with primary ovarian failure. Nature 307: 174–175

Marik J, Hulka J F 1978 Luteinized unruptured follicle syndrome, a subtle cause of infertility. Fertility and Sterility 29: 270–274

Marrs R P, Vargyas J M, March C M 1983 Correlation of ultrasonic and endocrinologic measurements in human menopausal gonadotrophin therapy. American Journal of Obstetrics and Gynecology 145: 417–421

O'Herlihy C, Pepperell R J, Evans J H 1980 The significance of FSH elevation in young women with disorders of ovulation. British Medical Journal 281: 1447–1450

Pepperell R J, McBain J C, Healy D L 1977 Ovulation induction with bromocriptine in patients with hyperprolactinaemia. American Journal of Obstetrics and Gynecology 17: 181–191

Pepperell R J 1983 A rational approach to ovulation induction. Fertility and Sterility 40: 1–14

Punnonen R, Ashorn R, Vilja P, Heinonen P, Kujansuu E, Tuohimaa P 1988 Spontaneous luteinizing hormone surge and cleavage of in vitro fertilized embryos. Fertility and Sterility 49: 479–482

Porter R N, Smith W, Craft I L, Abdulwahid N A, Jacobs H S 1984 Induction of ovulation for in vitro fertilization using buserelin and gonadotrophins. Lancet ii: 1284

Ronnberg L 1980 The effect of clomiphene citrate on different sperm parameters and serum hormone levels in preselected infertile men: a controlled double blind crossover study. International Journal of Andrology 3: 479–486

Rowland M 1980 Infertility therapy: effects of innovations and increasing experience. Journal of Reproductive Medicine 25: 42–46

Rutherford A J, Subak-Sharpe R J, Dawson K J et al 1988 Improvement of in vitro fertilization after treatment with buserelin, an agonist of luteinizing hormone releasing hormone. British Medical Journal 296: 1765–1768

Schulman J F, Schulman S 1982 Methyl prednisolone treatment of immunological infertility in males. Fertility and Sterility 38: 591–599

Smith D H, Picker R H, Sinosich M, Saunders D M 1980 Assessment of ovulation by ultrasound and oestradiol levels during spontaneous and induced cycles. Fertility and Sterility 33: 387–390

Smith W, Porter R, Ahuja K, Craft I 1984 Ultrasonic assessment of endometrial changes in stimulated cycles in an in vitro fertilisation and embryo transfer programme. Journal of In Vitro Fertilisation & Embryo transfer 1: 233–234

Stanger J D, Yovich J L 1984 Failure of human oocyte release at ovulation. Fertility and Sterility 41: 827–832

Stanger J D, Yovich D L 1985 Reduced in vitro fertilization of human oocytes from patients with raised basal luteinising hormone levels during the follicular phase. British Journal of Obstetrics and Gynaecology 92: 385–393

Steptoe P C, Edwards R G, Walters D E 1986 Observations on 767 pregnancies and 500 births after human in vitro fertilization. Human Reproduction: 89–94

Templeton A, Van Look P, Lumsden M A et al 1984 The recovery of pre-ovulatory oocytes using fixed schedule of ovulation induction and follicle aspiration. British Journal of Obstetrics and Gynaecology 91: 148–154

Trounson A, Mohr L 1983 Human pregnancy following cryopreservation thawing and transfer of an 8-cell embryo. Nature 305: 707–709

Vermesh M, Kletzky O A, Davajan V, Israel R 1987 Monitoring techniques to predict and detect ovulation. Fertility and Sterility 47: 259–264

Verstoppen G R, Steeno O P 1977 Varicocele and the pathogenesis of the associated subfertility: a review of various theories II: results of surgery. Andrologia 9: 133–140

The Voluntary Licensing Authority For Human In-Vitro Fertilisation and Embryology: the second report 1987

Wardle P, Foster P A, Mitchell J D et al 1986 Norethisterone treatment to control timing of the IVF cycle. Human Reproduction i: 455–457

Warnock Dame M 1984 Report of the committee of inquiry into human fertilization and embryology. H M Stationery Office, London

Whittingham D G, Leibo S P, Mazur P 1972 Survival of mouse embryos frozen to −196 & −269°C. Science 178: 411–412

Wiltbank M C, Kosasa T S, Rogers B J 1985 Treatment of infertile patients by intrauterine insemination of washed spermatoza. Andrologia 17: 22–30

18. Anorexia nervosa

Janet Treasure   Laurence Mynors-Wallis

HISTORICAL INTRODUCTION

The classical form of anorexia nervosa was recognized as a disease caused by psychological factors in 1873 by Sir William Gull in England and concurrently by Charles Lasegue in France. In 1979 Russell wrote a seminal paper discussing the clinical features of bulimia nervosa. He described this as a 'ominous variant' of anorexia nervosa as many cases had a prior history of anorexia nervosa and the psychopathology was similar but bulimia nervosa was distinguished by episodes of massive overeating interspersed with the rigid dieting. Extreme fears about weight-gain and fatness led to vomiting, laxative abuse and diuretic abuse in an attempt to counteract the effects of these binges.

EPIDEMIOLOGY

The classical form of anorexia nervosa is rare with an incidence of 4 per 100 000 of young women in an area of North-East Scotland (Szmukler et al 1986) or about 7 per 100 000 population in Rochester, Minnesota (Lucas et al 1988). The higher incidence in the Rochester study probably results from their method as they scrutinized the records of a total of 17 other diagnostic categories for missed cases. Cases of anorexia nervosa were found which had been classified as amenorrhoea, oligomenorrhoea, ovarian dysfunction and delayed puberty. The corresponding incidence figures for bulimia nervosa are unavailable. This is partly because the illness has only been recognized as a distinct entity for less than 10 years and also because this behaviour elicits great shame and has been termed 'the secret illness' by the lay press and so only a few cases will present for medical treatment.

Prevalence studies, however, have been undertaken. The prevalence of bulimia nervosa in schoolgirls and in GPs' practice populations is approximately 1% (Johnson–Sabine et al 1988, King 1986, Meadows et al 1986, Mumford & Whitehouse 1988). No cases of anorexia nervosa were identified in any of these studies and the prevalence of anorexia nervosa is probably between one-tenth and one hundred-fold less common than that of bulimia nervosa. Bulimia nervosa is becoming more common in the ethnic minorities (Mumford & Whitehouse 1988, Holden & Robinson 1988, Lacey & Dolan 1988). Unlike anorexia nervosa it does not appear to be more common in the upper social classes.

AETIOLOGY

Although the eating disorders are often considered to lie on a spectrum, it is premature to assume that they share common aetiological factors.

Biological factors

Genetic

Eating disorders and affective disorders appear to be more common in the relatives of patients with anorexia nervosa and bulimia nervosa (Strober et al 1985). Twin studies suggest that an inherited predisposition to anorexia nervosa would account for this increased incidence (Holland et al 1984, Holland et al 1988), whereas common life-style factors rather than any inherited vulnerability appear to predispose to bulimia nervosa.

Central nervous system dysfunction

The clinical features have suggested to some that anorexia nervosa might represent an abnormality in hypothalamic function (Russell 1970). The arguments recruited to support this thesis are firstly that the hypothalamus is the site of the control of feeding behaviour and also controls reproductive behaviour. Amenorrhoea is an invariable feature of anorexia nervosa and many authors have noted that it occasionally develops prior to weight loss (Kay & Leigh 1954, Halmi 1974, Fries 1977). The illness usually develops at around the time of puberty when hypothalamic function in females is in a state of flux with the emergence of a cyclical pattern. A recently proposed model of anorexia nervosa by Morley and Blundell (1988) suggests that stress releases corticotrophin-releasing hormone which disrupts feeding, increasing satiety. In spite of these imaginative and tantalizing suggestions there is little empirical evidence to support the idea that anorexia nervosa represents a dysfunction in hypothalamic centres.

Biological models of bulimia nervosa

Evidence from epidemiological studies (Johnson–Sabine et al 1988), naturalistic studies of eating behaviour (Davis et al 1988) and the clinical features of patients with bulimia nervosa (Holden & Robinson 1988, Cooper & Taylor 1988) all suggest that bulimia nervosa arises when an attempt is made to keep weight below its constitutional level. This is usually achieved by dieting. Dieting results in changes in central neurotransmitter function (Goodwin et al 1987) and such a change in central neurotransmitters may underpin the overpowering craving to eat, the behaviour which distinguishes this condition (editorial, Lancet 1988). Chronic dieting has been found experimentally to result in overeating, especially under conditions of stress (Polivy & Herman 1987).

Sociocultural factors

One of the central tenets used to suggest that sociocultural factors are important in the aetiology of the eating disorders is the suggestion that the eating disorders are increasing in frequency (Szmukler et al 1986, Willi et al 1983). Bulimia nervosa is indisputably increasing. However, the arguments which suggest that the classical form of anorexia nervosa has not increased in incidence over the last 40 years are impressive (Lucas et al 1988, Williams & King 1987). It is salutory to note that members of the Clinical Society discussing anorexia nervosa one hundred years ago commented on the 'increasing frequency of this illness'. In the section above we argued that dieting appears to be a strong aetiological factor in bulimia nervosa and sociocultural factors have fostered this type of behaviour (Garner & Garfinkel 1980, Garner et al 1985, Brumberg 1988). Groups in which dieting behaviour is common such as models and ballet dancers have a higher prevalence of eating disorder (Garner et al 1980, Szmukler et al 1985b).

Psychological factors

There are several psychological formulations to the aetiology of anorexia nervosa but unfortunately most of them are difficult to test and so verify. One of the oldest of these theories is that anorexia nervosa develops as an attempt to avoid the consequences of adult sexuality. This was initially proposed by Freud in 1895, was later elaborated by psychoanalysts (Waller et al 1940) and has been further refined and elaborated by Crisp (1967).

More recent formulations incorporate the family and suggest that anorexia nervosa forms some sort of function within the family (either to keep the parents together or in some cases to split them apart), and that anorexia develops because of difficulties in separating from such families (Minuchin 1975, Selvini-Palazzoli 1978).

CLINICAL FEATURES

The clinical features which are used to diagnose anorexia nervosa are profound emaciation which results in the physiological and psychological sequelae of starvation. Symptoms include amenorrhoea, poor sleep, nocturia, alteration in hair distribution (loss of head hair, increased bodily hair), susceptibility to the cold, bloating sensation after eating, constipation and occasionally oedema. Bradycardia, hypotension and laguno hair are present on examination. Investigation may reveal a moderate degree of anaemia and leukopenia and, more rarely, thrombocytopenia (with purpura) as a result of marrow suppression. The ESR is reduced. Hypoglycaemia and hypoproteinaemia occasionally develop in severe cases.

A concise detailed review of the medical aspects of anorexia nervosa have been given in Bhanji and Mattingly (1988). The psychological consequences of emaciation result in heightened interest in food and cooking, hoarding of food and non-food items, social isolation, depression and obsessional rituals.

The clinical features of bulimia nervosa vary as the diagnosis can be present in association with the diagnosis of anorexia nervosa (i.e. the patient is emaciated) or it can be present in the obese. The common signs and symptoms relate to the methods of weight loss. These include enlargement of the salivary glands, abrasions inside the mouth, scarring on the back of the second metacarpal phalangeal joint (Russell's sign), tetany (secondary to alkalosis) and cardiac irregularities (secondary to hypokalaemia in those who self-induce vomiting). Rebound oedema, an atonic colon and even rectal prolapse can occur as a result of laxative abuse.

Clinical presentation of patients with eating disorders to obstetricians and gynaecologists

Anorexia nervosa

Primary amenorrhoea. Anorexia nervosa can develop prior to menarche and women may present to gynaecologists with primary amenorrhoea who have had an abnormal eating pattern for many years. Russell in 1985 presented a series of 20 such women. At the time of follow-up which ranged from 4–27 years, only 2 of the 20 patients were above the 50th percentile for height and 7 were below the 2nd percentile suggesting that pre-menarchal anorexia nervosa may result in stunting of growth. Breast development was also severely affected and in 6 patients no breast tissue developed even following weight gain. Figure 18.1 shows the changes in breast development of a 24-year-old woman who gained weight when she eventually presented for treatment. The illness commenced at age 11. So there is evidence that even after such a delay the menarche can occur.

Secondary amenorrhoea. One of the commonest ways anorexia nervosa presents to gynaecologists is as a case of unexplained secondary amenorrhoea (Lucas et al 1988) and it is important that a detailed weight history and eating history is taken in all such patients. The amenorrhoea in anorexia nervosa is a consequence of impaired gonadal hormone secretion caused by a hypothalamic dysfunction. In many ways the hypothalamic

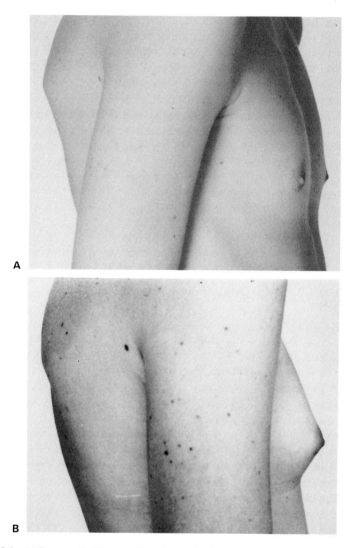

Fig. 18.1 (a) Breasts of a 24-year-old patient at the time of referral when she weighed 41.3 kg (height 163 cm). She developed anorexia nervosa at 14 years of age and had primary amenorrhoea. Ultrasonography at the time of referral showed small ovaries 1.6 cm³ (normal range 4–10 cm³): her uterus was also small at 6.7 cm² (normal range 15–30 cm²); (b) she gained 6 kg in weight during treatment over 5 months and her breasts began to develop. At the time of this photograph her ovaries were 2.7 cm³ and contained multiple small cysts up to 0.9 cm in diameter; her uterine cross-sectional area had increased to 12.8 cm². Two months later she began to menstruate.

pituitary gonadal axis in these patients resembles that of a pre-pubertal girl. Boyar et al (1974) showed that in underweight patients the pattern of LH secretion was infantile with diminished pulsatile release of LH throughout the day. Partial restoration of weight resulted in increased nocturnal secretion of LH. Finally the normal fluctuating pattern of LH secretion throughout the day resumed. These changes appear to be related to weight. The nocturnal increase in LH (the pubertal pattern) only emerged above 69% of ideal body weight and the adult pattern of LH secretion developed above 80% of ideal body weight (Pirke et al 1979).

The pituitary gland reserve in anorexia nervosa has been tested by injection of gonadotrophin-releasing hormone (GNRH). Again this shows weight-related changes. When the patient is severely emaciated, the response of both LH and FSH is diminished. At 70% of the standard weight an exaggerated FSH response was observed but the LH response was again suboptimal. At 80% of standard weight the LH response became greater, exceeding the normal response in adult subjects and with further weight gain, the sensitivity of the pituitary gland was normalized (Beumont et al 1976). A parallel with normal puberty is again seen since during normal puberty there is a transient supersensitivity of gonadotrophin release (Roth et al 1972).

The response of the hypothalamus also shows sequential changes with weight change. Partial weight gain restores the negative feedback response to oestrogen but the return of positive feedback to oestrogen is delayed (Wakeling et al 1977).

Frisch (1977) reported that patients with anorexia nervosa had to attain at least 87% of ideal body weight before normal cycles resumed and she based this on her theory that the onset of menstruation was determined by a critical body composition in terms of its proportion of stored fat (Frisch & Revelle 1971, Frisch & McArthur 1974).

Pelvic ultrasonography also reveals regression in the hypothalamic pituitary axis in anorexics (see Fig. 18.2). At the time of presentation at low weight the ovaries are small (less than 1 cm^3 in volume; normal range $6–10 \text{ cm}^3$) and the uterus is also small with a cross-sectional area of about $5–6 \text{ cm}^2$ (normal range $15–25 \text{ cm}^2$). The ovaries increase in size and become cystic in appearance, a structure which has been termed 'multifollicular ovaries' (Treasure et al 1985) after weight gain. These are analogous to the cystic ovaries seen in pre-pubertal girls (Stanhope et al 1985). In expert hands the ultrasonographic appearance of multifollicular ovaries can be distinguished from that of polycystic ovaries but there are also hormonal differences (Adams et al 1985). The classical hormonal profile in polycystic ovaries is that of high levels of LH, a LH/FSH ratio greater than 3 and raised oestrogen levels. Multifollicular ovaries are associated with a restoration of normal levels of FSH whereas LH levels remain low so the LH:FSH ratio is diminished. Oestrogen levels are also suppressed. Further weight gain leads to the ovaries increasing to normal size or even slightly above normal and one follicle becomes dominant. An increase in uterine size follows. The emergence of a dominant follicle appears to occur in response to an increase in LH secretion with the LH:FSH ratio increasing above 2. Oestrogen secretion from the dominant follicle promotes uterine

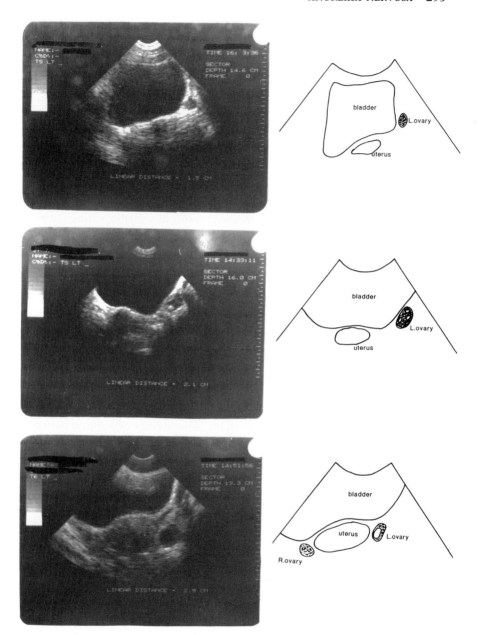

Fig. 18.2 (a) Pelvic ultrasonography in a patient with anorexia nervosa at low weight (34 kg). The ovarian volume was 1.8 cm³ and the ovarian structure was amorphous. The uterine cross-sectional area was 6.9 cm²; (b) the same patient at 44 kg. The ovarian volume had increased to 5.7 cm³ and the ovary contained several small cysts 0.6 cm in diameter. The uterine cross-sectional area had increased to 10.3 cm²; (c) the same patient at 57 kg. The ovaries had a mean volume of 7.2 cm³ and contained a dominant follicle 2.2 cm in diameter. The uterine cross-sectional area had increased to 18.3 cm². The patient menstruated 2 weeks after this scan.

growth (Treasure et al 1988, Treasure 1988). The morphological and hormonal profile in one patient during weight gain is shown in Figure 18.3.

This sequence does not relate to an index of body fatness (the body mass index) very tightly but a closer relationship is seen if weight is expressed as a percentage of the pre-morbid weight. This suggests that the resumption of menses might be related to constitutional factors rather than absolute weight or fat levels. Pelvic ultrasonography offers an efficient and quick method of establishing whether weight gain is sufficient to allow normal menstruation to occur.

There has been much debate whether the return of menstruation relates entirely to body weight changes. Amenorrhoea can persist for several months in spite of weight-gain and it is possible that this is due to persisting anorexic behaviour which might result in a chaotic eating pattern or excessive exercise (Falk & Halmi 1982, Wakeling et al 1979).

Menstrual irregularities in bulimia nervosa

Menstrual irregularities occur commonly in bulimia nervosa. Approximately 60% of patients with bulimia nervosa have had a previous episode of amenorrhoea (Pyle et al 1981, Fairburn & Cooper 1984, Treasure 1988). In addition, 50% of the clinical population also have some degree of menstrual irregularity, either amenorrhoea or oligomenorrhoea (Cantopher et al 1988, Pirke et al 1987, Treasure 1988). The ultrasonographic picture of women with amenorrhoea and bulimia nervosa is similar to that seen in patients with anorexia nervosa; the ovaries are small, containing multiple small follicles and the uterus also is small. The ovaries of bulimic patients with oligomenorrhoea (see Fig. 18.4) are of normal size but have the multifollicular pattern with no follicle becoming dominant during a cycle. Progesterone levels remain low. The uterine area is normal, reflecting a degree of oestradiol secretion (Treasure 1988). Inadequate follicular development occurs in 50% of bulimic patients (Pirke et al 1987). These findings are of interest as they indicate that poor follicular function can occur in women whose eating problems may not be readily apparent, for example patients with bulimia nervosa are often at normal weight and will

Fig. 18.3   Sequential morphological and hormonal measurements in a patient with anorexia nervosa during weight-gain in hospital and during follow-up. The bottom third of the figure shows the patient's weight expressed in terms of percentage of premorbid weight. The ovaries and follicles are drawn to scale in the upper third of the figure. Menstruation is depicted as the black rectangle. The ovaries were initially small with no internal structure. They became multifollicular at about 78% of premorbid weight. A dominant follicle 1.2 cm in diameter appeared at 92% of premorbid weight. The dominant follicle was associated with an increase in the ratio of LH to FSH (upper third of the figure). Oestradiol secretion and uterine area (middle third of the figure) also increased at this time. The patient menstruated 2 weeks after the appearance of a dominant follicle. During the next cycle the patient gradually lost weight, the dominant follicle failed to grow and the ovaries became multifollicular once more. (Reproduced with permission from Treasure 1988).

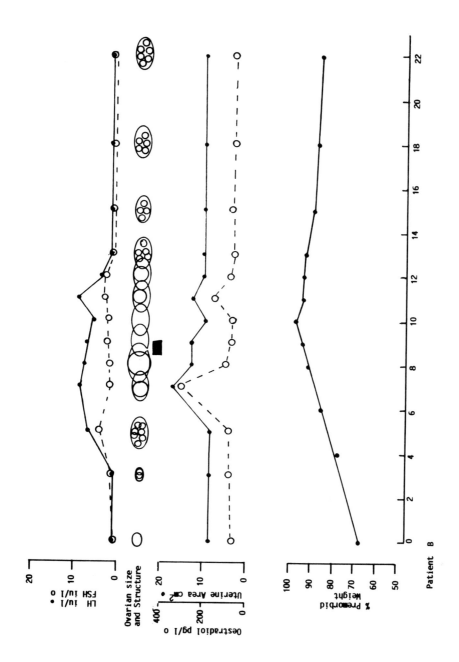

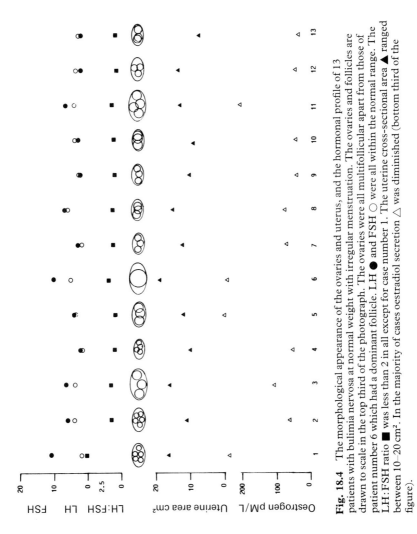

Fig. 18.4   The morphological appearance of the ovaries and uterus, and the hormonal profile of 13 patients with bulimia nervosa at normal weight with irregular menstruation. The ovaries and follicles are drawn to scale in the top third of the photograph. The ovaries were all multifollicular apart from those of patient number 6 which had a dominant follicle. LH ● and FSH ○ were all within the normal range. The LH:FSH ratio ■ was less than 2 in all except for case number 1. The uterine cross-sectional area ▲ ranged between 10–20 cm². In the majority of cases oestradiol secretion △ was diminished (bottom third of the figure).

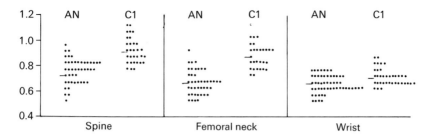

Fig. 18.5   Bone mineral density (BMD) in the spine, femoral neck and wrist measured by dual photon absorptiometry. 45 patients with anorexia nervosa (A.N.) and 31 age-matched controls (C1) were tested: each point represents a measurement for one person.

be secretive about their abnormal eating behaviour. Thus bulimia nervosa must be considered as one cause of poor corpus luteum function and should be enquired about systematically.

OSTEOPOROSIS

The amenorrhoea of anorexia nervosa is associated with osteopenia (see Fig. 18.5). If the illness becomes chronic the osteopenia becomes so severe that pathological fractures develop (Szmukler et al 1985a, Rigotti et al 1984). The osteopenia does not appear to be related to vitamin D or calcium metabolism but it is probably related to the protein calorie malnutrition associated with oestrogen deficiency. There is some indirect evidence that this osteopenia is, however, reversible. In a follow-up study of women who had had anorexia nervosa during their adolescence and early womanhood but who had recovered with normal weight and menstruation, bone density did not differ from that of age-matched controls. However, in those women who had not recovered the osteopenia had continued to develop reaching its maximum severity after 12 years' duration at which time pathological fractures began to develop (Treasure et al 1987).

ANOREXIA AND PREGNANCY

Although it is unusual for pregnancy to occur in anorexia nervosa, there have been reports from specialist centres of patients with a chronic illness who gain sufficient weight to become pregnant or who have received treatment to induce fertility. A small proportion of women who have had anorexia in their teenage years relapse following the birth of the child. There have been several case reports documenting the difficulty in ensuring that adequate weight-gain occurs during the pregnancy in women who have anorexia nervosa and this may result in poor fetal growth (Treasure & Russell 1988; see Fig. 18.6). Weight at conception appears to be the most important variable affecting fetal outcome and those women who develop

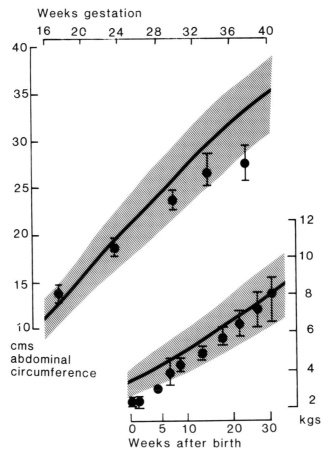

Fig. 18.6 Top left hand corner: intrauterine growth represented by median abdominal circumference (and range) in five fetuses as measured by ultrasonography. Bottom corner: postnatal growth represented by weights from birth to 6 months (median and ranges refer to seven babies, except at 4 weeks [one baby] and after 20 weeks [three babies]). Heavy lines and shaded areas indicate mean (2SD) values in normal populations. (Reproduced with permission from Treasure & Russell 1988).

anorexia during their pregnancy and lose weight, can nevertheless deliver babies of a normal weight. Low birth-weight babies of women with anorexia nervosa show evidence of catch-up growth in the postnatal period when bottle feeding is started. However, such patients need to be followed-up carefully as there have been a few disturbing case reports of children of women with anorexia nervosa who have failed to thrive or who have been severely neglected (Smith & Hanson 1972).

It is much more common for women with bulimia nervosa either to have children or to be pregnant during the course of their illness. Lacey and Smith (1987) have described a series of 20 cases from their clinic. In many cases the bulimic behaviour was attenuated during pregnancy as the mothers feared that their abnormal eating behaviour would damage their unborn child. One baby had a cleft palate, another a cleft lip, and one, whose mother abused alcohol and soft drugs, was born prematurely and died shortly after birth. The authors point out that the series is too small to draw inferences about fetal abnormality in bulimia but suggest that this is an area worthy of further investigation.

TREATMENT

Treatments offered for eating disorders vary according to the diagnosis and the severity of the presentation. For the severely underweight patient a period of supervised inpatient care to facilitate weight-gain is usually required. For most patients with bulimia nervosa treatment can occur on an outpatient basis.

Despite much research that has been done into the role of drug treatments for eating disorders (see below), psychological treatments remain the treatments of choice.

Psychological treatments for anorexia nervosa

It is generally accepted that weight restoration must occur prior to or at least concurrent with any psychotherapeutic work (Goodsitt 1985). This usually requires hospital admission and the provision of a structured, supervised eating programme. For early onset cases it may be possible for weight restoration to occur at home, in conjunction with the family. There is no evidence that different hospital regimes result in different outcome (Hsu 1980).

Whilst the short-term aim of treatment is to reverse potentially dangerous weight loss, the longer term aim is for this to be maintained by the patient outside hospital. It is to this task that any psychological treatment needs to be directed.

Dynamic Psychotherapy

The model on which dynamic psychotherapy is based views the presenting illness as stemming from often unconscious emotional conflicts. It is a time-consuming and lengthy treatment which may well offer a framework within which to understand the patient but there is little evidence that it is an effective treatment option.

Family therapy

Family therapy seeks to help the individual patient with an eating disorder by looking at how the illness is affecting the whole family. It looks at the role the illness has within the family, how individual family members react and how their behaviour might unwittingly be resulting in the persistence of abnormal eating patterns. Therapy consists of engaging as many members of the family as are felt to be important, usually parents, siblings and spouses. In a series of family meetings their ways of interacting are observed and ideas for change gradually instilled. Anorexia is not seen as an individual symptom by some therapists (Minuchin 1978; Selvini-Palazzoli 1978) but as behaviour bound up in family dynamics.

There is one controlled trial of family therapy in eating-disorder patients (Russell et al 1987) in which patients were randomly allocated to either family or individual therapy, after inpatient admission to restore their weights to normal. At 1-year follow-up, family therapy was only more effective than individual therapy in one group: patients with anorexia nervosa whose illnesses had started before the age of 19 and was of less than 3 years' duration.

Cognitive and behaviour therapy

Behaviour therapy defines the patients' abnormal behaviour and seeks to change it directly, rather than hoping behaviour will change once underlying conflicts and difficulties have resolved. It is often combined with cognitive therapy which delineates negative and abnormal attitudes and attempts to alter them.

Behavioural techniques are used to a greater or lesser extent in all inpatient regimes that aim at facilitating weight-gain in anorexia (Halmi 1985). Some hospitals demand strict bed rest until a pre-agreed target weight is achieved. Good eating behaviour is encouraged by having certain privileges such as telephone calls, letters, visits, etc. contingent on a certain amount of weight gain.

Group therapy

Treating patients with eating disorders in groups has certain advantages over individual therapy. The most obvious advantage is that of cost but other advantages include mutual support and socialization and the strengthening of peer relationships (Hendren et al 1987).

Patients with anorexia nervosa have long been acknowledged as difficult to treat in groups (Inbody 1985, Hall 1985). Even when weight is restored, the anorexic remains very preoccupied with her weight and body-image and finds it difficult to identify and express her feelings. She has a low self-esteem (Leon et al 1985) and finds it difficult both to accept the support of others and to provide support in turn.

The value of self-help groups such as Anorexic Aid has not been evaluated. Such groups should not be an alternative to professional treatment but an adjunct to it (Baker et al 1985).

Psychological treatments of bulimia nervosa

Unlike anorexia nervosa there is no need for weight restoration to occur prior to psychological treatment. The vast majority of patients with bulimia nervosa can be managed as outpatients.

Dynamic psychotherapy

There are few reports in the literature concerning the treatment of bulimia nervosa with dynamic psychotherapy (Sugaman & Kurash 1982, Swift & Letvin 1984), and it has as yet no empirical support.

Family therapy

The one controlled trial of family therapy in eating-disorder patients (Russell et al 1987) did not show it to be effective in the subgroup with bulimia. Schwartz et al (1985) showed that it was effective in 66% (19) patients. The place of family therapy in these patients remains uncertain, and although present trends would suggest that family therapy is most effective in young people still living at home, patients with bulimia nervosa often do not fall into this group.

Cognitive and behaviour therapy

Leitenberg et al (1984) report on five patients treated using the technique of exposure and response prevention. The patient is allowed to binge eat and exposed to the anxiety that this engenders but is prevented from relieving this anxiety by vomiting. Their hypothesis is that it is vomiting which reinforces bulimic behaviour and if this is prevented, not only will vomiting stop but so will binge eating. Wilson et al (1986) reported that the technique of exposure and vomit prevention is more successsful when combined with a form of cognitive therapy than with the cognitive therapy alone.

Freeman et al (1988) randomly allocated 92 outpatients with bulimia nervosa to cognitive behaviour therapy, behaviour therapy and group therapy together with a waiting-list control group. They found that behaviour therapy had the lowest dropout rate and modified symptoms earlier than the other two treatments.

Fairburn et al (1986) compared individual cognitive behaviour therapy with short-term focal therapy in a group of 24 outpatients with bulimia nervosa. In the cognitive-behaviour group, therapy was initially directed at getting eating under control using behaviour techniques, for example weight records, diet plans and food diaries, but went on to use cognitive techniques to modify attitudes about food and weight and provide alternative techniques for problem solving. At 1-year follow-up both groups showed substantial improvement, with the cognitive-behaviour group doing slightly better on some outcome measures.

At present behavioural techniques appear to offer an effective treatment for bulimia nervosa. It is not yet known which particular techniques are necessary. There is no clear evidence that the addition of cognitive therapy offers an advantage over simpler measures.

Group therapy

Group therapy combined with individual therapy has been shown to be a successful treatment (Lacey 1983, Connors et al 1984). Cognitive therapy can also be provided in a group setting (Kirkley et al 1985).

The conclusion of Freeman's 1988 study with outpatient bulimics was that a supportive and educational group was as effective as other treatments for those who continued with it. However, there was a high dropout rate (37%).

It is clear that many patients with bulimia nervosa can be treated within groups and that this is the most cost-effective method. The exact components of the group therapy which are important have yet to be clearly shown.

Pharmacological treatments for anorexia nervosa

Neuroleptics

Chlorpromazine has been used in the treatment of anorexia since the 1960s. There are three main reasons why neuroleptics were considered for use in anorexia nervosa:
1. Appetite stimulation: although it must be emphasized that some anorexics have a normal appetite and are indeed hungry;
2. Antipsychotic action: body-image disturbance may be of such delusional intensity that the patient is felt to be psychotic;
3. Anxiolytic and sedative action: for patients who would otherwise be unable to tolerate the weight-gain desired.

Selective dopamine antagonists pimozide (Vandereycken & Pierloot 1983) and sulpiride (Vandereycken 1984) have been used in conjunction with inpatient behavioural therapy. They may facilitate weight-gain but there is no evidence that they alter attitudes or alter outcome. It must be remembered that neuroleptic medication does have side-effects as a case report of tardive dyskinesia in an anorexic shows (Condon 1986).

The present status of neuroleptics is that they might have an anxiolytic role during inpatient weight-gain (Crisp 1983) and be used to treat the rare psychotic episodes (Grounds 1982).

Antidepressants

Depressive symptoms are frequent in anorexic patients and are found in a high proportion of their first-degree relatives (Cantwell et al 1977). Amitriptyline was, however, not superior to placebo on measures of eating and depression in double-blind controlled studies of patients with eating disorders (Bierderman et al 1985, Halmi et al 1986). When used as an adjunct to a behavioural regime clomipramine increased hunger and appetite in the early stages of weight-gain but did not affect ultimate outcome (Crisp et al 1987).

Lithium used in conjunction with a behavioural regime resulted in increased weight-gain at weeks 3 and 4 (Gross et al 1981). Only 16 patients entered the trial and there was no follow-up.

On current evidence antidepressants may have a role as an anxiolytic and may be used to treat coexisting depressive illness that is not responding to weight-gain. There is no evidence that they improve outcome and little evidence that they stimulate weight gain.

Other drugs

Cyproheptadine, a serotonin antagonist, was shown to increase weight-gain and decrease depressed mood in a study of 72 inpatient anorexics (Halmi et al 1986). The drug was tested under double-blind conditions and compared with amitriptyline and placebo. The benefit was confined to non-bulimic patients only. Two other studies combining cyproheptadine with a behavioural inpatient regime did not show significant differences in weight-gain compared with placebo (Vigersky & Loriaux 1977, Goldberg et al 1979).

Case reports exist attesting to the value of zinc in the treatment of anorexia nervosa (Bryce-Smith & Simpson 1984).

Drugs used in the treatment of bulimia nervosa

Antidepressants

There are now several double-blind placebo controlled studies looking at the value of antidepressants in the treatment of bulimia nervosa. Many of them suffer from several flaws which limit the conclusions that can be drawn, including:

1. Numbers enrolled in the trial are often very small, usually only 20–30;
2. Subjects are often recruited from advertisements and as such may be different from those who are treated in hospital clinics;
3. Follow-up is often short, inadequate or non-existent;
4. Serum drug levels are rarely assessed either to check compliance or to check whether the dose is achieving therapeutic serum levels;
5. No consideration is given as to the actual blindness of raters or patients, given that the active drug often has clear side-effects that are not found in the placebo.

The first study published used imipramine (Pope et al 1983). The rate of binge eating and depression were significantly improved in the treated compared with the control group at 6 weeks. In a separate 2-year follow-up (Pope et al 1985) 95% of those assessed were moderately improved or better.

Hughes et al (1986) looked at desipramine, the active metabolite of imipramine. At 6 weeks they reported a 91% reduction in the weekly binge frequency, compared with a 19% increase for those taking placebo. In a study of 32 patients amitriptyline did not prove superior to placebo on measures of eating behaviour (Mitchell & Groat 1984).

A negative result was also obtained using mianserin (Sabine et al 1983). Uncontrolled trials of newer antidepressants trazodone (Damlouji & Ferguson 1985, Pope et al 1983) and fluoxetine (Freeman & Hampson 1987) suggest they may be effective in treating bulimia nervosa, but controlled data is awaited.

Monoamine oxidase inhibitors (MAOIs) have been used in the treatment of bulimia nervosa despite the risk of dietary indiscretion in patients who are known to lack control over-eating. Two studies of phenelzine (Walsh et al 1985, Walsh et al 1987) suggest that the phenelzine group do better on measures of binge eating and depression than controls.

In a preliminary report of 13 patients, treated with lithium or placebo used in conjunction with dietary advice and counselling, lithium had no additional effect on measures of bingeing and vomiting (Hsu et al 1987). As with MAOIs lithium can only be used with great caution in those patients because of its potential toxicity.

Anorexic drugs

Patients with bulimia nervosa by definition suffer from powerful urges to overeat. Studies have been undertaken using two appetite suppressing drugs: methylamphetamine and fenfluramine.

Amphetamines have been known to result in a reduction of food intake since 1937 (Carruba et al 1986). Ong et al (1983) showed that methyl-amphetamine given to bulimic patients after an overnight fast stopped them from binge eating. The potential for abuse limits the clinical usefulness of amphetamines. Fenfluramine is a compound with a similar structure to amphetamine, retaining its anorexic properties but having a central depressant rather than stimulant action. Robinson et al (1985) showed that fenfluramine given to bulimic patients after an overnight fast resulted in significantly less food being eaten and less bulimic symptoms being reported than patients given placebo. A double-blind placebo-controlled trial of fenfluramine has been conducted among outpatient bulimics, the drug being given in conjunction with dietary advice, education and supportive psychotherapy (Russell et al 1988). Of those who completed the trial there was no difference between those who had received fenfluramine or placebo. The clinical place for fenfluramine remains undecided.

OUTCOME

The majority of the studies of outcome have referred only to subjects with anorexia nervosa. Up to half of the patients, who have received specialist care, recover completely although the illness may last 3 or more years (Morgan & Russell 1975, Hsu et al 1979, Hall et al 1984). A further quarter will have residual minor problems while the remainder will have chronic disability with serious weight-loss and disabling psychological and social handicaps. The mortality rate in these studies is approximately 6% which is similar to the standard mortality ratio of 6.1 found in a large outcome study (Patton 1988). Suicide was the most common cause of death. Two variables predicted a fatal outcome, the number of admissions and low weight at presentation. The mortality rate increases in studies with a period of follow-up over 20 years (Theander 1985).

REFERENCES

Adams J, Franks S, Polson D W et al 1985 Multifollicular ovaries: clinical and endocrine features and response to pulsatile gonadotrophin-releasing hormone. Lancet *ii*: 1375–1378

Baker Enright A, Butterfield P, Berkowitz D 1985 Self-help and support groups in the management of eating disorders. In: Garner D M, Garfinkel P E (eds) Handbook of psychotherapy for anorexia nervosa and bulimia. The Guilford Press, New York, pp 491–512

Beumont P J V, George G C W, Pimstone B L, Vinik A I 1976 Body weight and the pituitary response to hypothalamic-releasing hormones in patients with anorexia nervosa. Journal of Clinical Endocrinology and Metabolism 43: 487–496

Bhanji S, Mattingly D 1988 Medical aspects of anorexia nervosa. Wright, London

Bierderman J, Herzog D B, Rivinus T M, Ferber R A 1985 Amitriptyline in the treatment of anorexia nervosa. Journal of Clinical Psychopharmacology 5: 10–16

Boyar R M, Katz J, Finkelstein J W et al 1974 Anorexia nervosa: immaturity of the 24-hour luteinizing hormone secretory pattern. New England Journal of Medicine 291: 861–865

Brumberg J J 1988 Fasting girls: the emergence of anorexia nervosa as a modern disease. Harvard University Press, Cambridge, Massachusetts

Bryce-Smith D, Simpson R I D 1984 Anorexia, depression and zinc deficiency. Lancet *ii*: 350

Cantopher T, Evans C J H, Lacey J H, Pearce J M 1988 Menstrual and ovulatory disturbance in bulimia. British Medical Journal 297: 836–837

Cantwell D P, Sturzenburger S, Burroughs J 1977 Anorexia nervosa: an affective disorder? Archives of General Psychiatry 34: 1087–1093

Carruba M, Coen E, Pizzi M et al 1986 Mechanism of action of anorectic drugs. In: Carruba M, Blundell J E (eds) Pharmacology of eating disorders. Raven Press, New York, pp 1–27

Condon J T 1986 Long-term neuroleptic therapy in chronic anorexia nervosa complicated by tardive dyskinesia. Acta Psychiatrica Scandinavia 73: 203–206

Connors M E, Johnson C L, Stukey M K 1984 Treatment of bulimia with brief psychoeducational group therapy. American Journal of Psychiatry 141: 1512–1516

Cooper P J, Taylor M J 1988 Body-image disturbance in bulimia nervosa. British Journal of Psychiatry Supplement 152: 32–36

Crisp A H 1967 The possible significance of some behavioural correlates of weight and carbohydrate intake. Journal of Psychosomatic Research 11: 117–131

Crisp A H 1983 Anorexia nervosa. British Medical Journal 287: 855–858

Crisp A H, Lacey J H, Crutchfield M 1987 Clomipramine and 'drive' in people with anorexia nervosa. British Journal of Psychiatry 150: 355–359

Dalmouji N F, Ferguson J M 1985 Three cases of post traumatic anorexia nervosa. American Journal of Psychiatry 142: 362–363

Davis R, Freeman R J, Garner D M 1988 A naturalistic investigation of eating behaviour in bulimia nervosa. Journal of Consulting and Clinical Psychology 56: 273–279

Editorial 1988 Lancet *i*: 629

Fairburn C G, Cooper P J 1984 The clinical features of bulimia nervosa. British Journal of Psychiatry 144: 238–246

Fairburn C G, Kirk J, O'Connor M, Cooper P J 1986 A comparison of two psychological treatments for bulimia nervosa. Behaviour Research Therapy 24: 629–643

Falk J R, Halmi K A 1982 Amenorrhoea in anorexia nervosa: examination of the critical body weight hypothesis. Biological Psychiatry 17: 799–806

Freeman C L P, Barry F, Dunkeld-Turnbull J, Henderson A 1988 Controlled trial of psychotherapy for bulimia nervosa. British Medical Journal 296: 521–525

Freeman C P L, Hampson M 1987 Fluoxetine as a treatment for bulimia nervosa. International Journal of Obesity 11(3): 171–178

Fries H 1977 Studies on secondary amenorrhoea, anorectic behaviour and body-image perception: importance for the early recognition of anorexia nervosa. In: Vigersky R A (ed) Anorexia nervosa. Raven Press, New York, pp 163–176

Frisch R E 1977 Food intake and reproductive ability. In: Vigersky R A (ed) Anorexia nervosa. Raven Press, New York, pp 149–162

Frisch R E, McArthur J W 1974 Menstrual cycles: fatness as a determinant of minimum weight for height necessary for their maintenance or onset. Science 185: 949–951

Frisch R E, Revelle R 1971 Height and weight at menarche and a hypothesis of menarche. Archives of Diseases in Childhood 46: 695–701

Garner D M, Garfinkel P E 1980 Sociocultural factors in the development of anorexia nervosa. Psychological Medicine 10: 647–656

Garner D M, Garfinkel P E, Schwartz D, Thompson M 1980 Cultural expectations of thinness in women. Psychological Report 47: 483–491

Garner D M, Rockert W, Olmsted M P, Johnson C, Coscina D V 1985 Psychoeducation and principles in the treatment of bulimia and anorexia nervosa. In: Garner D M, Garfinkel P E (eds) Handbook of psychotherapy for anorexia nervosa and bulimia. Guilford Press, New York, pp 513–572

Goldberg S G, Eckert E D, Halmi K A 1979 Cyproheptadine in anorexia nervosa. British Journal of Psychiatry 134: 67–70

Goodsitt A 1985 Self psychology and the treatment of anorexia nervosa. In: Garner D, Garfinkel P (eds) Handbook of psychotherapy for anorexia and bulimia. Guilford Press, New York pp 107–147

Goodwin G M, Fairburn C G, Cowen P J 1987 Dieting changes serotonergic function in women, not men: implications for the aetiology of anorexia nervosa. Psychological Medicine 17: 839–842

Gross H A, Ebert M H, Faden V B 1981 A double-blind controlled trial of lithium carbonate in primary anorexia nervosa. Journal of Clinical Psychopharmacology 1: 376–381

Grounds A 1982 Transient psychosis in anorexia nervosa: a report of seven cases. Psychological Medicine 12: 107–115

Gull W W 1873 Proceedings of the Clinical Society of London. British Medical Journal 1: 527–529

Gull W W 1874 Anorexia nervosa (apepsia hysterica, anorexia hysterica) Transactions of the Clinical Society of London 7: 22–28

Hall A 1985 Group therapy for anorexia nervosa. In: Garner D M, Garfinkel P E (eds) Handbook of psychotherapy for anorexia nervosa and bulimia. Guilford Press, New York, pp 213–240

Hall A, Slim E, Hawker F, Salmond C 1984 Anorexia nervosa: long-term outcome in 50 female patients. British Journal of Psychiatry 145: 407–413

Halmi K A 1974 Anorexia nervosa: demographic and clinical features in 94 cases. Psychosomatic Medicine 36: 18–26

Halmi K A 1985 Behavioural management for anorexia nervosa. In: Garner D, Garfinkel P (eds) Handbook of psychotherapy for anorexia and bulimia. Guilford Press, New York, pp 147–160

Halmi K A, Eckert E, LaDu T J, Cohen J 1986 Anorexia nervosa: treatment efficacy of cyproheptadine and amitriptyline. Archives of General Psychiatry 43: 177–181

Halmi K A, Goldberg S C, Eckert E, Casper R, Davis J M 1977 Pretreatment evaluation in anorexia nervosa. In: Vigersky R A (ed) Anorexia nervosa. Raven Press, New York, pp 43–54

Hendren R L, Atkins D M, Sumner C R, Barber J K 1987 Model for the group treatment of eating disorders. International Journal of Group Psychotherapy 37: 4–8

Holden N L, Robinson P H 1988 Anorexia nervosa and bulimia nervosa in British blacks. British Journal of Psychiatry 152: 544–549

Holland A J, Hall A, Murray R, Russell G F M, Crisp A H 1984 Anorexia nervosa: a study of 34 twin pairs and one set of triplets. British Journal of Psychiatry 145: 414–419

Holland A J, Sicotte N, Treasure J L 1988 Anorexia nervosa: evidence for a genetic basis. Journal of Psychosomatic Research 32: 561–571

Hsu L K G 1980 Outcome of anorexia nervosa. Archives of General Psychiatry 37: 1041–1046

Hsu L K G, Clement L, Santhouse R 1987 Treatment of bulimia with lithium: a preliminary study. Psychopharmacology Bulletin 23: 45–48

Hsu L K G, Crisp A H, Harding B 1979 Outcome of anorexia nervosa. Lancet i: 61–65

Hughes P L, Wells L A, Cunningham C J, Ilstrup D M 1986 Treating bulimia with desipramine. Archives of General Psychiatry 43: 182–186

Inbody D R, Ellis J J 1985 Group therapy with anorexic and bulimic patients. American Journal of Psychotherapy 39: 411–419

Johnson-Sabine E, Wood K, Patton G, Mann A, Wakeling A 1988 Abnormal eating attitudes in London schoolgirls—a prospective epidemiological study: factors associated with abnormal response on screening questionnaires. Psychological Medicine 18: 615–622

Kay D W K, Leigh D 1954 The natural history, treatment and prognosis of anorexia nervosa, based on a study of 38 patients. Journal of Mental Science 100: 411–431

King M B 1986 Eating disorders in general practice. British Medical Journal 293: 1412–1414

Kirkley B G, Schneider J A, Agras S, Backman J A 1985 Comparison of two group treatments for bulimia. Journal of Consulting and Clinical Psychology 53: 43–48

Lacey J H 1983 Bulimia nervosa, binge eating and psychogenic vomiting. British Medical Journal 286: 1609–1613

Lacey J H, Dolan B M 1988 Bulimia in British blacks and Asians: a catchment area study. British Journal of Psychiatry 152: 73–79

Lacey J H, Smith G 1987 Bulimia nervosa: the impact of pregnancy on mother and baby. British Journal of Psychiatry 150: 771–781

Lasegue E C 1873 On hysterical anorexia. Medical Times Gazette 2: 265–269

Lasegue E C 1873 De l'anorexie hysterique. Archives Generales de Medecine 21: 385–403

Leitenberg H, Gross J, Peterson J, Rosen J L 1984 Analysis of an anxiety model and the process of change during exposure plus response prevention treatment of bulimia nervosa. Behaviour Therapy 15: 3–20

Leon G R, Lucas A R, Colligan R C, Ferdinande R J, Kamp J 1985 Sexual, body-image, and personality attitudes in anorexia nervosa. Journal of Abnormal Child Psychology 13: 245–258

Lucas A R, Beard C M, O'Fallon W M, Kurland L T 1988 Anorexia nervosa in Rochester, Minnesota: a 45-year study. Mayo Clinical Proceedings 63: 433–442

Meadows G N, Palmer R L, Newball E V M, Kenrick J M T 1986 Eating attitudes and disorders in young women: a general practice survey. Psychological Medicine 16: 351–357

Minuchin S, Rosman B, Baker L 1978 Psychosomatic families: anorexia nervosa in context. Harvard University Press, Cambridge

Mitchell J E, Groat R 1984 A placebo-controlled double-blind study of amitriptyline in bulimia. Journal of Clinical Psychopharmacology 4: 186–193

Morgan H G, Russell G F M 1975 Value of family background and clinical features as predictors of long-term outcome in anorexia nervosa: four-year follow-up study of 41 patients. Psychological Medicine 5: 355–371

Morley J E, Blundell V E 1988 The neurobiological basis of eating disorders: some formulations. Biological Psychiatry 23: 53–78

Mumford D B, Whitehouse A M 1988 Increased prevalence of bulimia nervosa among Asian schoolgirls. British Medical Journal 297: 78

Ong Y L, Checkley S A, Russell G F M 1983 Suppression of bulimic symptoms with methyl amphetamine. British Journal of Psychiatry 143: 288–293

Patton G 1988 Mortality and eating disorders. Psychological Medicine 18: 947–951

Pirke K M, Fichter M M, Lund R, Doerr P 1979 Twenty-four hour sleep–wake pattern of plasma LH in patients with anorexia nervosa. Acta Endocrinologica 92: 193–204

Pirke K M, Fichter M M, Chlond C et al 1987 Disturbances of the menstrual cycle in bulimia nervosa. Journal of Clinical Endocrinology 27: 245–251

Polivy J, Herman C P 1987 Diagnosis and treatment of normal eating. Journal of Consulting and Clinical Psychology 55: 635–644

Pope H G, Hudson J I, Jonas J M 1983 Antidepressant treatment of bulimia. Journal of Clinical Psychopharmacology 3: 274–281

Pope H G, Hudson J I, Jonas J M, Yurgelin-Todd D 1985 Antidepressant treatment of bulimia: a two-year follow up study. Journal of Clinical Psychopharmacology 5: 320–327

Pyle R L, Mitchell J E, Eckert E D 1981 Bulimia: a report of 34 cases. Journal of Clinical Psychiatry 42: 60–64

Rigotti N A, Nussbaum S R, Herzog D B, Neer R M 1984 Osteoporosis in women with anorexia nervosa. New England Journal of Medicine 311: 1601–1606

Robinson P H, Checkley S A, Russell G F M 1985 Suppression of eating by fenfluramine in patients with bulimia nervosa. British Journal of Psychiatry 146: 169–176

Roth J C, Kelch R P, Kaplan S L, Grumback M M 1972 FSH and LH response to luteinizing hormone-releasing factor in prepubertal and pubertal children. Journal of Clinical Endocrinology 35: 926–930

Russell G F M 1970 Anorexia nervosa: its identity as an illness and treatment. In: Price J (ed) Modern trends in psychological medicine. Butterworth, London, pp 131–164

Russell G F M 1979 Bulimia nervosa: an ominous variant of anorexia nervosa. Psychological Medicine 9: 429–448

Russell G F M 1985 Premenarchal anorexia nervosa and its sequelae. Journal of Psychiatric Research 19: 363–369

Russell G F M, Checkley S A, Feldman J, Eisler I 1988 A controlled trial of d-fenfluramine in bulimia nervosa. Clinical Neuropharmacology 11(1): S146–S159

Russell G F M, Szmukler G I, Dare C, Eisler I 1987 An evaluation of family therapy in anorexia nervosa and bulimia nervosa. Archives of General Psychiatry 44: 1047–1056

Sabine E J, Yonace A, Farington A J, Barratt K H, Wakeling A 1983 Bulimia nervosa: a placebo-controlled double-blind therapeutic trial of mianserin. British Journal of Clinical Pharmacology 15: 195S–202S

Schwartz R C, Barrett M J, Saba G 1985 Family therapy for bulimia. In: Garner D M, Garfinkel P E (eds) Handbook of psychotherapy for anorexia nervosa and bulimia. Guilford Press, New York, pp 280–310

Selvini-Palazzoli M 1978 Self-starvation: from individual to family therapy in the treatment of anorexia nervosa. Pomerans A (trans). Jason Aronson, New York

Selvini-Palazzoli M, Boscolo L, Cecchin G, Prata G 1978 Paradox and counterparadox. Jason Aronson, New York

Smith S M, Hanson R 1972 Failure to thrive and anorexia nervosa. Postgraduate Medical Journal 48: 382–384

Stanhope R, Adams J, Jacobs H S, Brook C G D 1985 Ovarian ultrasound assessment in normal children, idiopathic precocious puberty, and during low-dose pulsatile gonadotrophin-releasing hormone treatment of hypogonadotrophic hypogonadism. Archives of Diseases in Childhood 60: 116–119

Strober M, Morrell W, Bulrough S, Salkin B, Jacobs C 1985 A controlled family study of anorexia nervosa. Journal of Psychiatric Research 19: 239–246

Sugaman A, Kurash C 1982 The body as a transitional object in bulimia. International Journal of Eating Disorders 1: 57–67

Swift W J, Letvin R 1984 Bulimia and the basic fault: a psychoanalytic interpretation of the bingeing-vomiting syndrome. Journal of the American Academy of Child Psychiatry 23: 489–497

Szmukler G I, Eisler I, Gillies C, Hayward M E 1985a The implications of anorexia nervosa in a ballet school. Journal of Psychiatric Research 19: 177–182

Szmukler G I, Brown S W, Parsons V, Darby A 1985b Premature loss of bone in chronic anorexia nervosa. British Medical Journal 290: 26–27

Szmukler G I, McCance C, McCrone L, Hunter D 1986 Anorexia nervosa: a psychiatric case register study from Aberdeen. Psychological Medicine 16: 49–58

Theander S 1985 Outcome and prognosis in anorexia nervosa and bulimia: some results of previous investigations compared with those of a Swedish long-term study. Journal of Psychiatric Research 19: 493–508

Treasure J L 1988 The ultrasonographic features in anorexia nervosa and bulimia nervosa: a simplified method of monitoring hormonal state during weight-gain. Journal of Psychosomatic Research 32: 623–634

Treasure J L, Russell G F M 1988 Intrauterine growth and neonatal weight-gain in babies of women with anorexia nervosa. British Medical Journal 296: 1038

Treasure J, Gordon P A L, King E A, Wheeler M, Russell G F M 1985 Cystic ovaries: a phase of anorexia nervosa. Lancet *ii*: 1379–1381

Treasure J L, Fogelman I, Russell G F M, Murby B 1987 Reversible bone loss in anorexia nervosa. British Medical Journal 295: 474–475

Treasure J L, Wheeler M, Gordon P, King E, Russell G F M 1988 The ultrasound features in anorexia nervosa: a simplified method of monitoring hormonal states during weight gain. Clinical Endocrinology 29: 607–616

Vandereycken W 1984 Neuroleptics in the short-term treatment of anorexia nervosa. British Journal of Psychiatry 144: 288–292

Vandereycken W, Pierloot R 1983 Combining drugs and behaviour therapy in anorexia nervosa. In: Darby P L, Garfinkel P E, Garner D M, Coscina D V (eds) Anorexia nervosa: recent developments in research. Alan Liss, New York, pp 365–375

Vigersky R A, Loriaux D L 1977 The effect of cyproheptadine in anorexia nervosa. In: Vigersky R A (ed) Anorexia nervosa. Raven Press, New York, pp 349–356

Wakeling A, De Souza V F A, Beardwood C J 1977 Assessment of the negative and positive feedback effects of administered oestrogen on gonadotrophin release in patients with anorexia nervosa. Psychological Medicine 7: 371–380

Wakeling A, De Souza V F A, Gore M B R, Sabur M, Kingstone D, Boss A M 1979 Amenorrhoea, body weight and serum-hormone concentrations with particular reference to prolactin and thyroid hormones in anorexia nervosa. Psychological Medicine 9: 265–272

Waller J V, Kaufman M R, Deutsch F 1940 Anorexia nervosa. A psychosomatic entity. Psychosomatic Medicine 2: 3–16

Walsh T B, Gladis M, Roose S P, Steward J W, Glassman A H 1987 A controlled trial of phenelzine in bulimia. Psychopharmacology Bulletin 23: 49–51

Walsh B T, Steward J W, Roose S P, Gladis M, Glassman A H 1985 A double-blind trial of phenelzine in bulimia. Journal of Psychiatric Research 19: 485–489

Willi J, Grossmann S 1983 Epidemiology of anorexia nervosa in a defined region of Switzerland. American Journal of Psychiatry 140: 564–567

Williams P, King M 1987 The 'epidemic' of anorexia nervosa: another medical myth? Lancet *i*: 205–207

Wilson G T, Rossiter E, Kleinfeld E I, Lindholm L 1986 Cognitive-behavioural treatment of bulimia nervosa: a controlled evaluation. Behaviour Research Therapy 24: 277–288

19. Hormone implants in gynaecology

Adam L. Magos   John Studd

INTRODUCTION

Implants can be considered as a pharmacological delivery system designed to release a controlled amount of a drug into the systemic circulation over a long period. Several formulations have been developed, but it is the biodegradable fused crystalline pellet that is the most widely available and which is the subject of this review.

The literature concerning hormone implants is actually relatively scanty. While this mode of therapy is popular in the UK, it is not so in the rest of Europe and the USA where there are only 200 or so licensed users, its use being incomprehensibly limited by the Federal Drug Administration. Yet hormone implantation offers definite advantages over the oral route of hormone replacement in terms of duration of action, convenience, metabolic effects, potency and a more physiological action, properties that deserve to be better exploited. Whether the newer and pharmacologically similar vaginal and percutaneous preparations such as creams, rings, and particularly transdermal patches of oestradiol (Powers et al 1985) and more recently testosterone (Bals-Pratsch et al 1986) will supplant implants remains to be seen. At present, mainly thanks to a handful of enthusiasts, our knowledge of implants is considerable and the method already has several proven indications in gynaecological practice.

HISTORICAL PERSPECTIVE

Following earlier work in animals (Deanesly & Parkes 1937), the first record of an implant given for medical reasons appeared in the British Medical Journal in 1938. Bishop, an endocrinologist working at Guy's Hospital in London, described the case of a 20 year-old-girl who, having undergone bilateral oophorectomy for ovarian cysts, developed hot flushes 9 days after the operation (Bishop 1938). She was successfully treated over a 2-year period with oestrone, initially orally, subsequently by intramuscular injections, and finally by pure crystalline tablets implanted under the skin of the anterior abdominal wall. Using a dose of 14 mg oestrone, Bishop reported that vasomotor symptoms began to improve

313

about 1 week after insertion of the tablet and were controlled for 4–5 weeks. He further commented that this mode of treatment compared favourably with the other routes of administration.

Eleven years later, Greenblatt and Suran (1949) published on the use of not only crystalline pellets of oestradiol, but also testosterone, progesterone and desoxycorticosterone in the management of a number of endocrine and gynaecological disorders. They referred to conditions such as the climacteric syndrome and uterine hypoplasia (responding to oestradiol), dysmenorrhea, endometriosis, fibroids, reduced libido, menopausal symptoms and the prevention of oestrogen-induced endometrial proliferation (responding to testosterone), 'nervous tension', nymphomania, habitual abortion and pubertal breast hypertrophy (responding to progesterone), and Addison's disease and panhypopituitarism (responding to desoxycorticosterone).

Several articles followed confirming the efficacy of oestradiol implants for the treatment of symptoms associated with both a natural (Perloff 1949 & 1950) and particularly a surgical menopause (Soule 1951; Brown et al 1951, Kupperman et al 1951, Delaplaine et al 1952). The other preparations never gained the same popularity although Greenblatt, unarguably the premier champion of implant therapy, further advocated the use of testosterone implants for dysmenorrhoea (Greenblatt et al 1954). Several years later, he extended the indication for oestradiol implants by describing their anovulatory, and thereby contraceptive properties (Emperaire & Greenblatt 1969).

However, despite the absence of major side-effects and the repeated commendations of Schleyer-Saunders (1974), Greenblatt (1970) in the USA, and Studd in the UK (1976, 1979a), the technique fell from general favour. Isolated reports did appear in the medical press, once more describing the effects of oestradiol implant supplementation in castrated women (Hunter et al 1973, Lobo et al 1980).

More recently, following the realization that endometrial hyperplasia and irregular uterine bleeding can be prevented by the concurrent administration of cyclical oral progestogens (Sturdee et al 1978, Paterson et al 1980), renewed interest has been shown on both sides of the Atlantic as evidenced by extensive biochemical and symptomatic studies in pre- and post-menopausal women.

TYPES OF IMPLANTS

Long-acting implants are available in a number of formulations including steroid-containing permeable silastic capsules and rods, fused crystalline pellets, and the newer polymer systems. The former suffer from the inconvenience of not being biodegradable, thus necessitating their removal once all the hormone has been released, while the latter have predominantly been developed to deliver progestogens for contraceptive purposes.

Crystalline implants, being biodegradable and available as an oestrogen from the earliest days, have always been the most popular method for gynaecological therapy.

Preparations include fused white crystalline pellets of the three major sex steroids, oestradiol-17 beta, testosterone, progesterone (manufactured in the UK by Organon Laboratories), which are chemically identical to the respective endogenous hormones, and the progestogens norethisterone and levonorgestrel. The implants are small, cylindrically shaped, 3–6 mm in length and 2.2–4.5 mm in diameter depending on the dosage, and made up of the hormone in a cholesterol base. They are individually packaged in pre-sterilized glass vials.

Oestradiol-17 beta

The major advantage of subcutaneous oestradiol pellets over oral equivalents is the avoidance of the first-pass liver effect and their physiological action as represented by plasma oestrogen levels comparable to the follicular phase of the ovarian cycle (Studd 1979a). Implants are available in 25, 50 and 100 mg sizes. The typical menopausal replacement dose is 50 mg every 6 months (Studd et al 1977a); for anovulation a step-down regimen starting at 100 mg and reducing to a maintenance dose of 25 mg every 6 months has been described (Greenblatt et al 1977); for the treatment of complaints linked to cyclical ovarian activity such as the premenstrual syndrome and menstrual migraine, the usual dose is 50–100 mg 6-monthly (Magos et al 1983, 1984).

Testosterone

Unlike the 17-alkylated oral methyltestosterone which is hepatotoxic and icterogenic, the implant of the pure hormone is safe and is the route of choice for repeated administration. Doses include 50, 100 and 200 mg, 100 mg being the usual adjunct to oestradiol replacement particularly when reduced libido and other psychosexual problems are present (Studd et al 1977b). The original indication for the androgen, that of amelioration of menorrhagia, has been superceded by oral progestogens. Treatment is rarely complicated by significant virilization.

Progesterone and progestogens

Both natural progesterone and the 19-norsteroid derivatives norethisterone and levonorgestrel are available as subdermal implants. In addition to the gynaecological indications listed by Greenblatt and Suran (1949), both the natural and synthetic hormones have been advocated for contraception (Odlind et al 1979, Croxatto et al 1982). Pellets of the pure hormone, available at a dose of 100 mg, are now never used by us as they are often complicated by expulsion and result in irregular break-through bleeding when combined with oestradiol. For this reason, these implants will not be considered further.

TECHNIQUE OF HORMONE IMPLANTATION

The procedure of hormone implantation has been described in detail by several authors including Greenblatt and Suran (1949) and Thom and Studd (1980). It is an easy, quick and safe office procedure carried out under local anaesthesia. A no-touch technique is used with sterile instruments, but scrubbing up is not required.

Implants are usually inserted either into the subcutaneous fat of the abdominal wall 5 cm above and parallel to the inguinal ligament or into the fat of the buttocks. A small area of skin is cleansed with an antiseptic and a track of underlying tissue is anaesthetized with 1% lignocaine solution, with or without added epinephrine. Once effective, a superficial 5 mm incision is generally made in the skin using a pointed scalpel blade, but this step is optional. Trocars and cannulae, specially designed for implantation of hormone pellets (manufactured in the UK by Organon Laboratories), are available in two sizes depending on the diameter of the implant(s) to be inserted; the appropriate cannula, loaded with the sharp trocar, is pushed through the incision up to the hilt and into the subcutaneous fat. The rectus sheath, muscle and any scar tissue should be avoided.

Once in position, the trocar is withdrawn, and the pellets are loaded into the barrel of the cannula by means of forceps. Care should be taken not to drop any of the implants, an easy accident due to their small size, as they cannot be re-sterilized; precautions can be taken by first emptying the glass vials into a small gallipot and holding this under the cannula. Up to 12 pellets can be inserted, but the usual number is one or two. The blunt trocar (or obturator) is inserted fully into the cannula thereby gently forcing the pellets into the subcutaneous tissues medial to the insertion site. The instrument is then withdrawn and using dry dressing, pressure is applied over the wound for about 1 minute to prevent bleeding. When haemostasis is complete, the incision is covered with a sticky plaster and the patient is advised to keep the area dry for 24 hours. The whole procedure takes 2–3 minutes and is painless.

Complications are unusual. If insertion of the trocar is difficult, the skin incision should be enlarged with the scalpel. Prolonged bleeding after implantation usually responds to manual pressure, but on rare occasions the skin has to be sutured as well. Bruising may follow such cases but it is never extensive. A possible later complication is a wound infection which usually responds to antibiotics, although the pellets may first be extruded; there is then no reason why an identical implant should not be inserted at a different site.

PHARMACOKINETICS OF IMPLANTS

Absorption

The rate of absorption of sex steroid implants in humans has been described by Greenblatt and Hair (1942, 1945). They showed that for compressed crystalline pellets for which the dose is proportional to size, absorption follows an exponential pattern being fast early on and progressively slowing. Thus, for a 100 mg implant, the initial rate of absorption is 1 mg/day, falling to 0.5 mg/day by 3 months and 0.35 mg/day by 6 months (Greenblatt & Hair 1942).

The total rate of absorption appears to depend primarily on the surface area of the pellets, that is, on the number of pellets implanted rather than their size or weight. For instance, Greenblatt and Hair (1942) found that a 100 mg implant gave off only 50% more material per day than a 50 mg implant, and that three 50 mg implants were the equivalent to two 100 mg pellets. Secondary factors that they identified as affecting absorption included the density of the pellets, the size of the particles (crystals) that comprise the pellet and the site of implantation.

Metabolism

Subcutaneous administration has important differences from the oral route. Firstly, the gastrointestinal tract is by-passed where oral oestradiol is preferentially converted to oestrone (Ryan & Engel 1953). Secondly, as intestinal absorption is rapid, oral therapy delivers a large bolus of the steroids into the portal circulation (Lyrenas et al 1981). Thirdly, the 'first pass' effect on liver metabolism is avoided whereby the oral hormones are largely metabolized and inactivated before reaching the systemic circulation (Campbell & Whitehead 1982). Neither is implant action affected to the same extent by drugs that induce liver enzymes.

Once absorbed, oestradiol and testosterone implants are handled by the body as the endogenous hormones and are largely inactivated in the liver. A tiny proportion of the androgen is also converted to oestrogens, chiefly oestriol and oestrone. It has recently been shown that the metabolic clearance rate of both sex steroids, a function of tissue blood flow and tissue extraction, does not change significantly with age (Longcope et al 1980).

Excretion

Both hormones are chiefly excreted in urine in the form of water-soluble glucuronides or sulphates of oestradiol, oestrone, and oestriol (after oestradiol), and androsterone and etiocholanolone (after testosterone).

METABOLIC EFFECTS

Relatively few publications have provided metabolic data about oestradiol implants specifically, and even fewer have reported on testosterone. Considerably more information is available concerning percutaneous oestradiol-17 beta, metabolically similar to the implant equivalent, and these will be referred to where necessary.

Ovarian and pituitary hormones

The acute and chronic effects of subcutaneous implants on plasma oestrogens, testosterone and gonadotrophins have been determined by several investigators, mostly in postmenopausal women. Greenblatt et al (1980) showed in three postmenopausal subjects that after a 25 mg oestradiol pellet an increase in plasma oestradiol concentrations can be detected by 6 hours, levels rising by a factor of three within 24 hours and a factor of four after 48 hours. Plasma oestrone levels remained unchanged during the study period. In contrast, the oral administration of micronized oestradiol-17 was followed by a rise predominantly in plasma oestrone levels. Lobo et al (1980), studying 22 pre-menopausal women immediately after hysterectomy and bilateral salpingo-oophorectomy, reported that plasma oestradiol remained unchanged during the first 7 days of implantation, a discrepancy probably explained by the younger age of their study group.

The later effects of oestradiol implants on previously untreated menopausal patients have also been studied in detail, with a broad concensus of results (Hunter et al 1973, Lobo et al 1980, Thom et al 1981, Burger et al 1984) Table 19.1). The only study to report on a variety of dosage combinations, that of Thom et al (1981), showed that plasma oestradiol and oestrone concentrations came to a peak after 1–2 months of 50 or 100 mg pellets, and began to decline thereafter. Both steroids remained within the normal reproductive range, but there was a differential effect with respect to the two major plasma oestrogens, oestradiol and oestrone. The maximum increase in plasma oestradiol was five-fold after a

Table 19.1 Effects of different routes of natural oestrogen administration on pituitary and ovarian hormones

Variable	Route of administration	
	non-oral	oral
Oestrone	+ +	+ +
Oestradiol	+ +	+
Oestradiol: oestrone ratio	+ +	− −
LH	− −	−
FSH	− −	−
Prolactin	nc	+

+ + Considerably increased; + Slightly increased; nc No change; − Slightly decreased; − − Considerably decreased.

50 mg implant and ten-fold after 100 mg, whereas the figures for oestrone were two- and four-fold respectively. Thus, independent of the dose of oestradiol, the pre-menopausal ratio of the two oestrogens (1–2:1) was recreated, an important relationship for it highlights the physiological nature of hormone replacement with implants, and contrasts with the effects of oral therapy (Strecker et al 1979). Although the transdermal route also by-passes the gut and first-pass effect in the liver, plasma oestradiol concentrations and the ratio of oestradiol to oestrone fluctuate widely at least during the first 24 weeks of treatment (Stanczyk et al 1988).

The increase in plasma oestrogens after implants is paralleled by opposite changes in the concentrations of the gonadotrophins FSH and LH (Thom et al 1981). Levels fall to the pre-menopausal range within 2 weeks of implantation, reaching a minimum at 2–3 months (Table 19.1). Thereafter, the concentration of both gonadotrophins slowly rise but remain in the pre-menopausal range even after 6 months, particularly after the higher dose of oestradiol. These changes also contrast with the effects of oral and trans-dermal replacement which do not suppress gonadotrophins into the pre-menopausal range (Lind et al 1979, Selby & Peacock 1986). There is scant information about other pituitary hormones, Holst et al (1983a) finding that unlike oral oestrogens, percutaneous replacement does not increase plasma prolactin.

As to the duration of action of oestradiol implants, Thom et al (1981) were able to detect an effect at 12 months, the duration of their follow-up. Hunter et al (1973), reporting on a study of almost 3 years, found that oestrogen release was in fact maintained for up to 2 years after 100 mg oestradiol implants.

The hormonal effects of chronic implant administration in the menopause have received less attention. Cardozo et al (1984), studying patients from the Dulwich Hospital Menopause Clinic reported on the symptomatic and hormonal effects of regular, 6-monthly oestradiol and testosterone implants. Their results suggested an accumulative effect with a progressive rise in oestrone and oestradiol concentrations, and a fall in gonadotrophins. Despite this pattern, the mean oestrogen levels were within the pre-menopausal range even after six successive implants such that regular monitoring after each implant is unnecessary provided the therapeutic guidelines are adhered to (Studd et al 1987). From the same clinic, Brincat et al (1984) showed that the symptoms responded to active implants and not placebo in spite of normal oestradiol concentrations.

Biochemical data concerning testosterone pellets in post-menopausal women have been presented by Thom et al (1981), Burger et al (1984) and Cardozo et al (1984), although only the first team looked at the hormone on its own as well as in combination with oestradiol. Using a large dose of 200 mg testosterone, Thom et al found that the androgen alone had minimal effect on gonadotrophins or oestrogens (or vasomotor symptoms), but did lead to a three-fold elevation of plasma testosterone concentrations by the second month of treatment. A similar but lesser increase was noted when 100 mg of the androgen was given with 50 mg oestradiol, although with this regimen plasma levels of oestrogens and gonadotrophins were comparable with those seen when the oestrogen was administered on its own. In contrast to the effects of oestradiol pellets, Cardozo et al (1984) did not find the same degree of accumulation of testosterone on prolonged therapy, an observation that is probably explained by the shorter half-life of these implants.

Ovarian function

As indicated earlier in the text, the application of oestradiol implants has been extended to pre-menopausal women. Hormonal data from this group have been presented by Greenblatt et al (1977) and Asch et al (1978) in the USA, and Magos et al (1983, 1987) in the UK. The first publication (Greenblatt et al 1977) reported on the immediate effects of 100 mg oestradiol and suggested that ovulation can be immediately suppressed by this dose provided the pellet is inserted early in the cycle. While this may be the case for the majority, we found that follicular development continued in almost half the cases studied during the first three cycles after the initial implant, with evidence of follicular rupture and luteinization in a small proportion up to that time (Figs 19.1, 19.2) (Magos et al 1987). No

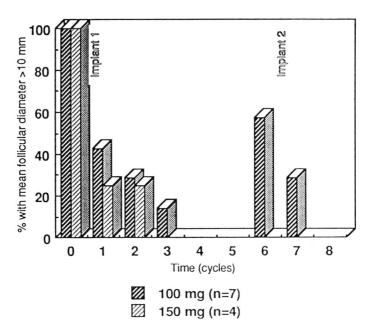

Fig. 19.1   Follicular growth before and after treatment with oestradiol implants in pre-menopausal women.

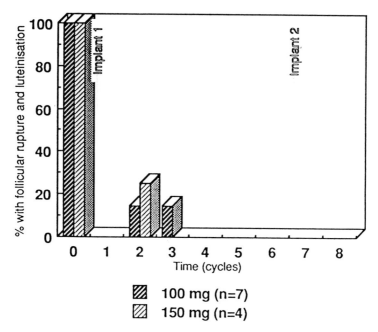

Fig. 19.2 Follicular rupture and luteinization before and after treatment with oestradiol implants in pre-menopausal women.

advantage was gained by using a higher dose of 150 mg oestradiol. Once more, the potency of this route of therapy is evidenced by the observation that up to 7.5 mg daily of oral equine oestrogens would be required to suppress ovarian function (Greenblatt et al 1954), a dose that is 6–12 times larger than the standard menopausal replacement dose.

The effects of regular therapy in this age group depends on dosage. With regular 6-monthly implants of 50 mg oestradiol the same trend of gradual accumulation is apparent as found in post-menopausal women. In our study, 13% of women who had been treated for longer than 3–4 years had supraphysiological plasma levels of oestradiol but not of oestrone (Magos et al 1983). Pertinent to this finding, Greenblatt et al (1977) had earlier showed that the dose of oestradiol can be reduced every 6 months to a maintenance dose of 25 mg without any loss of contraceptive effect. This regimen avoided any accumulation of plasma oestradiol, although interestingly oestrone levels did increase slightly (Asch et al 1978).

Serum biochemistry

Irrespective of the mode of administration, natural oestrogens have no significant influence on general biochemical variables (Sharf et al 1985) (Table 19.2). The effect on glucose tolerance and insulin metabolism is more controversial, but the two studies reporting on oestradiol implants

Table 19.2 Effects of different routes of natural oestrogen administration on biochemical variables

Variable	Route of administration	
	non-oral	oral
Glucose	nc	nc
Glucose tolerance	nc	nc
Urea	nc	nc
Sodium	nc	nc
Potassium	nc	nc
Chloride	nc	nc
Total protein	nc	nc
Albumin	nc	nc
Uric acid	nc	nc

+ + Considerably increased; + Slightly increased;
nc No change; − Slightly decreased;
− − Considerably decreased.

specifically reported no change (Greenblatt et al 1977, Notelovitz et al 1987).

Hepatic metabolism

The important differences in the body's handling of exogenous oestrogens is demonstrated by the differential effects of subcutaneous and oral routes of administration on the hepatic synthesis of proteins. It is evident from the results of subcutaneous or the metabolically similar percutaneous therapies that these routes are associated with minimal induction of protein synthesis in contrast to oral natural oestrogens (Lind et al 1979, Holst et al 1983b, Elkik et al 1982, Sharf et al 1985, Hassager et al 1987, Alkjaersig et al 1988) (Table 19.3). Although in theory oral treatment should be avoided in patients with high blood pressure as the increased production of renin substrate may aggravate the hypertension, in practice there seems to be no

Table 19.3 Effects of different routes of natural oestrogen administration on hepatic metabolism

Variable	Route of administration	
	non-oral	oral
Liver enzymes (LDH, GOT)	nc	nc
Alpha2 macroglobulin	nc	nc
Sex hormone binding globulin	+	+ +
Corticosteroid binding globulin	nc	
Pregnancy-zone protein (PZP)	nc	+ +
Alpha1-antitrypsin	nc	+ +
Caeruloplasmin	nc	+ +
Renin substrate	nc	+ +

+ + Considerably increased; + Slightly increased; nc No change;
− Slightly decreased; − − Considerably decreased.

Table 19.4 Effects of different routes of natural oestrogen administration on lipid metabolism

Variable	Route of administration	
	non-oral	oral
Cholesterol	nc	+
Triglycerides	nc	+
Phospholipids	+ +	+ +
Low density lipoprotein (LDL)	− −	− −
Very low density lipoprotein (VLDL)	− −	nc
High density lipoprotein (HDL)	+	+ +
HDL subfraction 1	−	
HDL subfraction 2	+	+ +
HDL subfraction 3	+	+

+ + Considerably increased; + Slightly increased; nc No change;
− Slightly decreased; − − Considerably decreased.

correlation between either systolic or diastolic blood pressure and circulating concentrations of renin substrate, and indeed both oral or percutaneous routes prevent the age-related rise in diastolic blood pressure (Hassager et al 1987).

Lipid metabolism

This is an area of prolific research because of the link between lipids and cardiovascular disease. The consensus is that both subcutaneous/percutaneous and oral therapies result in favourable changes in the various lipid and lipoprotein factions even with doses as low as 25 mg subcutaneous oestradiol (Brook et al 1982, Sharf et al 1985, Sherwin et al 1987, Notelovitz et al 1987) (Table 19.4). For instance, the ratio of HDL:LDL cholesterol is increased, particularly the HDL2 faction as shown by studies in our clinic (Cook et al 1986), and the ratio of HDL:LDL cholesterol is elevated. Interestingly, it has recently been noted that smoking reduces the lipid and lipoprotein 'benefits' following oral oestrogen replacement but has no effect after non-oral routes (Jensen & Christiansen 1988), this being further evidence of the anti-oestrogenic effect of cigarette smoking (Editorial 1986).

Changes in lipid metabolism with oestrogen replacement has been interpreted as being protective against ischaemic heart disease (Miller & Miller 1975), a view supported by much of the epidemiological data concerning oestrogen use (Henderson et al 1988, Beaglehole 1988). Of similar importance, a recent prospective study has extended the protective benefits of post-menopausal oestrogens to strokes (Paganini-Hill et al 1988).

Bone metabolism

Oestrogen inhibits bone resorption and improves calcium balance, changes

Table 19.5 Effects of different routes of natural oestrogen administration on bone metabolism

Variable	Route of administration	
	non-oral	oral
Calcium	− −	− −
Renal calcium excretion	− −	− −
Phosphate	− −	− −
Renal phosphate threshold	− −	− −
Alkaline phosphatase	nc	nc
Parathyroid hormone	+ +	+
Calcitonin	+	+
25 hydroxyvitamin D	−	−
1,25 dihydroxyvitamin D	−	−
Collagen (in skin)	+ +	

+ + Considerably increased; + Slightly increased; nc No change; − Slightly decreased; − − Considerably decreased.

that have been proposed as the explanation for the prevention of post-menopausal osteoporosis by replacement therapy (Whitehead et al 1982, Ralston et al 1984, Notelovitz et al 1987) (Table 19.5). Until recently it was thought that there was little difference between the various routes of administration, but a recent study found that a combination of subcutaneous oestradiol and testosterone implants is more effective than oral oestrogen in preventing osteoporosis (Savvas et al 1988). An earlier study showed that testosterone itself, although anabolic, does not augment the benefits secondary to oestradiol implants (Ralston et al 1984). As with the lipid changes noted above, Jensen and Christiansen (1988) also found that smoking reduced the beneficial effects of oral oestrogen replacement on bone-mineral content in contrast to percutaneous hormones.

An alternative line of research has shown that post-menopausal women receiving oestradiol and testosterone implants had significantly greater skin collagen content and thickness compared with untreated controls (Brincat et al 1985). This observation suggests that increased bone resorption may not be as important in post-menopausal bone loss as decreased collagen formation by osteoblasts. Brincat (1986) has shown that post-menopausal women with thin skin and reduced skin collagen will replace virtually all the skin collagen after 9 months of therapy with 50 mg pellets of oestradiol. The same mechanism may well be relevant in corticosteroid induced osteoporosis (Studd et al 1989).

Haemostasis

Platelet count and function are unaffected by natural oestrogen administration by whatever route (Studd et al 1978). Adverse changes in the clotting and fibrinolytic systems are well-known effects of synthetic oestrogens such as ethinyloestradiol. Although the data concerning oral

Table 19.6 Effects of different routes of natural oestrogen administration on haematological variables

Variable	Route of administration	
	non-oral	oral
Platelet count	nc	nc
Platelet aggregation	nc	nc
Plasminogen activation	nc	nc
Fibrin degradation products	nc	nc
Fibrinopeptide A	nc	nc
Fibrinogen turnover	nc	nc
Kaolin-cephalin clotting time	nc	nc
Factor XIII	nc	nc
Anti-thrombin III	nc	− −
Plasminogen	nc	+ +

+ + Considerably increased; + Slightly increased; nc No change; − Slightly decreased; − − Considerably decreased.

natural oestrogens is somewhat contradictory, our studies comparing this route with subcutaneous oestradiol implants did not report any significant alterations in haemostatic variables (Studd et al 1978, Thom et al 1978) (Table 19.6). Although confirmation is awaited, Elkik et al (1982) found that oral conjugated equine oestrogens reduced the plasma concentrations of anti-thrombin III, a natural coagulation inhibitor, unlike percutaneous oestradiol-17 beta, while Alkjaersig et al (1988) reported increased plasminogen with higher doses of oral oestrogen. If a genuine effect, modes of therapy that have minimal effects on hepatic protein synthesis would appear preferable.

ENDOMETRIAL EFFECTS

Oestrogens cause endometrial proliferation, and oestradiol implants are no exception. Indeed, because pellets are associated with predominantly an increase in the circulating concentration of oestradiol, shown to be the major intracellular oestrogen (King et al 1980), they are all the more potent. Despite this, and the link between prolonged, unopposed oestrogen therapy and endometrial carcinoma (Studd & Thom 1981), treatment with oestradiol implants has been shown to be safe provided it is combined with cyclical oral progestogen in both pre- (Greenblatt et al 1977, Magos et al 1983) and post-menopausal women (Sturdee et al 1978, Paterson et al 1980, Studd et al 1980). The latter investigators showed that, just as with oral replacement therapy, the degree of endometrial protection afforded by progestogens was duration-dependent rather than dose-dependent, the risk of hyperplasia being negligible if the tablets are taken for 10 or more days of each calendar month. Simultaneously in the USA, Gambrell (1978) showed that women receiving oestrogen/progestogen hormone replacement therapy are at a reduced risk of developing endometrial carcinoma compared with untreated controls.

As progestogens are often associated with minor symptomatic side-effects similar to the pre-menstrual syndrome (Magos et al 1986a), non-compliance is always a potential problem with combined hormone therapy, and this is especially so with implants. Unless the progestogen is reliably taken for more than 10 days per calendar month, regular outpatient endometrial biopsies are indicated and any endometrial hyperplasia should be treated with an extended course of progestogen for two or three cycles (Studd et al 1980).

As discussed above, progestogens are traditionally given cyclically. We have investigated continuous low-dose progestogen therapy in combination with oestradiol and testosterone implants in an attempt to avoid the necessity of monthly withdrawal periods (Magos et al 1985a). Starting with doses of norethisterone ranging from 0.35–5 mg daily, it was found that unacceptable breakthrough bleeding affected the majority of women and only 8 of the 71 women (11%) in the study group achieved long-term amenorrhoea of over 12 months. This was in direct contrast to oral continuous combined therapy, where irregular bleeding early on tended to be slight and eventual amenorrhoea was the norm (Magos et al 1985b).

Although testosterone has been used to treat menorrhagia (Greenblatt et al 1954), it does not prevent endometrial stimulation caused by concurrent therapy with oestrogens. Whether androgen augments the antiproliferative actions of progestogens to any significant degree remains to be determined.

BREAST DISEASE

Apart from the putative thrombotic, cardiovascular and endometrial risks of hormone replacement therapy, now more apparent than real, the other major concern has been over a possible link with breast cancer, the commonest malignancy in women. It is not the purpose of this article to review the available evidence, particularly as there is no data concerning oestradiol or testosterone implants with the exception of the palliative use of testosterone pellets in advanced carcinoma as listed, for instance, by Greenblatt and Suran (1949). Suffice it to say that a recent review of the literature by Gambrell (1986) concluded that there is no evidence that oestrogens truly increase the risk of breast cancer, while the addition of progestogen seems to reduce the incidence.

IMPLANTS AND THE MENOPAUSE

Undoubtedly, the major indication for oestradiol implants at present is in the management of the complications of the menopause, be it for the symptomatic relief of vasomotor instability, vaginal atrophy or other climacteric complaints, or as prophylaxis against osteoporosis. Most commonly, as originally described by Bishop in 1938, pellets are given to pre-menopausal women who have undergone hysterectomy and bilateral oophorectomy for non-malignant indications, when it represents a convenient method of hormone replacement. As already indicated, the effectiveness of oestrogen pellets under these circumstances has been repeatedly confirmed (Soule 1951, Brown et al 1951, Delaplaine et al 1952, Hunter et al 1973, Studd et al 1977a, Lobo et al 1980).

Implants are less often given to women with intact uteri, oral therapy generally being chosen, although their efficacy has been well documented (Cardozo et al 1984). This preference stems from the fear of uncontrolled uterine bleeding with oestradiol pellets, an irrational worry if treatment is combined with cyclical oral progestogens (Sturdee et al 1978, Paterson et al 1980). It should also be apparent from the preceding discussion that subcutaneous therapy offers definite metabolic advantages over the oral route. A direct symptomatic comparison of the two modes of treatment is however still awaited.

While there can be little doubt that oestradiol pellets are an effective therapy for the climacteric, implants have only now been subjected to placebo-controlled studies. The earlier study from our clinic showed that a combination of oestradiol and testosterone pellets were statistically superior to placebo with respect to both physical and psychological symptoms (Brincat et al 1984). More recently, Montgomery et al (1987), concentrating on the psychological rather than somatic effects of such treatment in 70 peri- and post-menopausal women, reported significant benefits of both oestradiol and a combination of oestradiol and testosterone over placebo, particularly in the younger age group.

Related to these results, there is increasing evidence of the benefits of testosterone supplementation in menopausal therapy. Androgens have been advocated for the treatment of reduced libido for many years by Greenblatt (Greenblatt et al 1942), a common problem at the menopause. Although oestrogens themselves have been shown to improve sexual functioning (Maoz & Durst 1980), possibly because of relief of vaginal dryness and dyspareunia, uncontrolled data has been presented that a combination of the two sex hormones results in a superior response (Studd et al 1977b, Burger et al 1984). These impressions have been confirmed by two controlled studies (Sherwin et al 1985, Burger et al 1987) and challenged by one (Dow et al 1983). Differences in patient groups may explain the apparent discrepancy. While Dow et al monitored women who had undergone a natural menopause, the former studies included either surgically castrated women or patients most of whom had undergone hysterectomy. It has been shown that the post-menopausal ovary is an important source of androgens, secreting 50% of plasma testosterone and 30% of androstenedione (Vermeulen 1976). While a direct relationship between testosterone levels and libido has never been shown, it may be that oophorectomized 'hypoandrogenic' women would gain more benefit from such therapy. Certainly, Sherwin and Gelfand (1985) have demonstrated, once more in castrates, that combined oral oestrogen/testosterone treatment is statistically superior to oestrogen alone with respect to energy, well-being and appetite. The same investigators had already made the observation that the androgen on its own failed to alleviate vasomotor symptoms despite elevated plasma oestrogen levels (Sherwin & Gelfand 1984). It is therefore possible that some type of synergy, perhaps mediated by alterations in the metabolism of the major sex hormone carrier protein, sex hormone-binding globulin, occurs with combined therapy.

Whatever the ultimate truth concerning testosterone supplementation, in the absence of percutaneous preparations, there can be little argument that the optimum route of administration of this hormone is not oral but subcutaneous.

IMPLANTS AND THE PRE-MENOPAUSE

The finding by Emperaire and Greenblatt in 1969 that oestradiol pellets can suppress ovulation in premenopausal women opened the door on a totally new set of applications. This, and the later updates by the same investigators describing a step-down regimen of 6-monthly implants combined with cyclical oral progestogen showed the contraceptive efficacy of this approach (Greenblatt et al 1977, Greenblatt et al 1979). During their entire series of over 7000 cycles there were only five pregnancies, four within the first 6 months of the first 100 mg implant and one with the maintenance dose of 25 mg. As rightly pointed out by the authors, this method of birth control has several advantages over conventional techniques for the middle-aged woman.

The potential of such anovulatory therapy for the management of cyclical disorders such as the pre-menstrual syndrome (PMS) was realized by Studd (1979b). From the mass of essentially negative data concerning this nebulous condition it was apparent that cyclical ovarian activity was of primary importance in pathogenesis (Magos & Studd 1984). That this should be the case is not unexpected when one realizes that well over 200 physical, psychological and behavioural changes normally accompany ovulation (Magos & Studd 1985). In the absence of a specific biochemical abnormality in women suffering from the PMS, it seemed that the syndrome represented an exaggerated response to these many bodily fluctuations.

The corollary of considering cyclical ovarian activity as fundamental in the aetiology of the PMS is that suppression of ovulation should abolish symptoms (Studd 1979b). This hypothesis was initially tested in a pilot uncontrolled study of 92 women, treated for up to 7 years with regular anovulatory doses of oestradiol pellets and cyclical oral progestogen. Testosterone implants were also given in 87% of cases, for those who complained of a severe loss of libido in addition to their pre-menstrual problems. Retrospective analysis showed that implant treatment was associated with complete or almost complete relief of PMS in 84% of cases, with only three women failing to respond (Magos et al 1984).

The treatment, this time without the androgen, was subsequently tested under placebo-controlled conditions on 68 women over a 10 month-period. The results of this prospective study confirmed the efficacy of oestradiol implants, even in the face of an initial response to placebo pellets of 94% (Magos et al 1986b). Using a technique of trend analysis to assess the daily symptom records (Magos & Studd 1986), active treatment proved to be superior to placebo for all six adverse symptoms clusters of a modified Moos Menstrual Distress Questionnaire after the first 2 months, a differential response that was maintained for the duration of the follow up (Fig. 19.3). Compared with other anovulatory measures, such treatment is

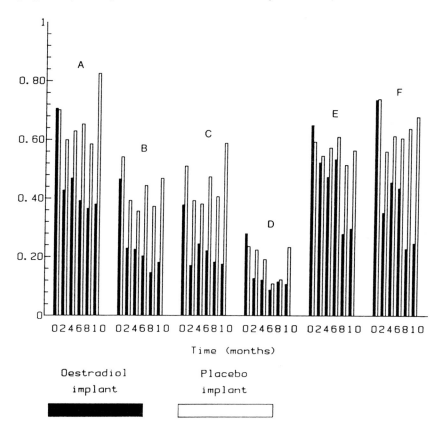

Fig. 19.3   Effect of 100 mg oestradiol implant and cyclical oral norethisterone on the mean daily symptom scores of women with pre-menstrual syndrome. Symptoms of a modified Menstrual Distress Questionnaire scored on a scale of 0–3 (no symptoms to severe symptoms).
A = Pain, B = Concentration, C = Behavioural change, D = Autonomic reactions, E = Water retention, F = Negative effect.

not only effective but is safe for the age group typically affected by this disorder (unlike the combined contraceptive pill), is well tolerated (unlike danazol) and is suitable for long-term therapy (unlike LHRH agonists).

The PMS is by no means the only condition with a close link with cyclical ovarian activity. A recent review of the literature revealed that over 70 other medical disorders are precipitated or aggravated by ovulation (Magos & Studd 1985). One, menstrual migraine, has already been shown by us to respond to oestradiol pellets (Magos et al 1983) and more recently to oestradiol gel (de Lignieres et al 1986). Many more, including common ailments such as diabetes, rheumatoid arthritis, asthma and epilepsy await investigation along these lines. Our understanding of the therapeutic indications for implants, particularly oestradiol, is clearly still in its infancy.

CONCLUSIONS

Sex hormone implants have been available for almost 50 years, yet only a few doctors administer them regularly. They represent a physiological mode of therapy with many metabolic advantages over other routes, yet they are relatively ignored by physicians. This may well reflect their surgical nature, yet the technique of hormone implantation is simple and fast, and obviates daily oral medication. As the list of indications for hormone pellets grows, hopefully more of us will take advantage of the benefits on offer.

REFERENCES

Alkjaersig N, Fletcher A P, De Ziegler D et al 1988 Blood coagulation in postmenopausal women given estrogen treatment: comparison of transdermal and oral administration. Journal of Laboratory and Clinical Medicine 111: 224
Asch R H, Greenblatt R B, Mahesh V B 1978 Pure crystalline estradiol pellet implantation for contraception. International Journal of Fertility 23: 100
Bals-Pratsch M, Knuth U A, Yoon Y-D et al 1986 Transdermal testosterone substitution therapy for male hypogonadism. Lancet *ii*: 943
Beaglehole R 1988 Oestrogens and cardiovascular disease. British Medical Journal ii: 571
Bishop P M F 1938 A clinical experiment in oestrin therapy. British Medical Journal i: 939
Brincat M 1986 Skin and the menopause. In: Greenblatt R B (ed) A modern approach to the perimenopausal years. New Developments in Biosciences 2, Walter de Gruyter, Berlin, p 57
Brincat M, Magos A L, Studd J W W et al 1984 Subcutaneous hormone implants for the control of climacteric symptoms. Lancet *i*: 16
Brincat M, Moniz C F, Studd J W W, Darby A J et al 1985 Long term effects of the menopause and sex hormones on skin thickness. British Journal of Obstetrics and Gynaecology 92: 256
Brook J G, Aviram M, Oettinger M et al 1982 The effect of oestrogen implants on high density lipoproteins and its subfractions in women in their premature menopause. Maturitas 4: 257
Brown M L, Lucente E R, Alesbury J M et al 1951 Treatment of the surgical menopause with estradiol pellets at the time of operation. American Journal of Obstetrics and Gynecology 61: 200

Burger H G, Hailes J, Menelaus M et al 1984 The management of persistent menopausal symptoms with oestradiol-testosterone implants: clinical, lipid and hormonal results. Maturitas 6: 351

Burger H, Hailes J, Nelson Y et al 1987 Effect of combined implants of oestradiol and testosterone on libido in postmenopausal women. British Medical Journal i: 936

Campbell S, Whitehead M I 1982 Potency and hepato-cellular effects of oestrogens after oral, percutaneous and subcutaneous administration. In: van Keep P A, Utian W, Vermeulen A (eds) The controversial climacteric. M.T.P. Press, Lancaster, p 103

Cardozo L, Gibb D M F, Tuck S M et al 1984 The effects of subcutaneous hormone implants during the climacteric. Maturitas 5: 177

Cook D, Godsland I, Montgomery J C et al 1986 Gonadal steroids and hormone antagonists. Presented at the 9th Symposium on Drugs affecting Lipid Metabolism, Florence, Italy

Croxatto H B, Diaz S, Peralta O et al 1982 Fertility regulation in nursing women. II. Comparative performance of progesterone implants versus placebo and copper T. American Journal of Obstetrics and Gynecology 144: 201

Deanesly R, Parkes A S 1937 Biological properties of some new derivatives of testosterone. Biochemistry Journal 9: 1161

Delaplaine R W, Bottomy J R, Blatt M et al 1952 Effective control of the surgical menopause by estradiol pellet implantation at the time of surgery. Surgery, Gynecology and Obstetrics 94: 323

Dow M G T, Hart D M, Forrest C A 1983 Hormonal treatment of sexual unresponsiveness in post-menopausal women: a comparative study. British Journal of Obstetrics and Gynaecology 90: 361

Editorial 1986 Anti-oestrogenic effect of cigarette smoking. Lancet ii: 1433

Elkik F, Gompel A, Mauvais-Jarvis P 1982 Cited by Campbell S, Whitehead M I in Potency and hepato-cellular effects of oestrogens after oral, percutaneous and subcutaneous administration. In: van Keep U A, Utian W, Vermeulen A (eds) The controversial climacteric. M.T.P. Press, Lancaster, p 103

Emperaire J C, Greenblatt R B 1969 L'implantation de pellets d'oestradiol dans la contraception. Gynecologie Pratique 20: 327

Gambrell R D Jr 1978 The prevention of endometrial cancer in post-menopausal women with progestogens. Maturitas 1: 107

Gambrell R D Jr 1986 Hormonal replacement therapy and breast cancer. In: Greenblatt R B (ed) A modern approach to the perimenopausal years. New Developments in Biosciences 2. Walter de Gruyter, Berlin, p 177

Greenblatt R B 1970 In: Conn H F (ed) The Menopause in Current Therapy. W B Saunders, London, p 757

Greenblatt R B, Hair L Q 1942 Testosterone propionate pellet absorption in the female. Journal of Clinical Endocrinology 2: 315

Greenblatt R B, Hair L Q 1945 Absorption of pellets of progesterone. Journal of Clinical Endocrinology 5: 38

Greenblatt R B, Suran R R 1949 Indications for hormone pellets in the therapy of endocrine and gynecological disorders. American Journal of Obstetrics and Gynecology 57: 294

Greenblatt R B, Hammond D O, Clark S L 1954 Membranous dysmenorrhea: studies in etiology and treatment. American Journal of Obstetrics and Gynecology 68: 835

Greenblatt R B, Mortara F, Torpin R 1942 Sexual libido in the female. American Journal of Obstetrics and Gynecology 44: 658

Greenblatt R B, Nezhat C, McNamara P V 1979 Appropriate contraception for middle-aged women. Journal of Biosocial Science 6: 119

Greenblatt R B, Asch R H, Mahesh V B et al 1977 Implantation of pure crystalline pellets of estradiol for conception control. American Journal of Obstetrics and Gynecology 127: 520

Greenblatt R B, Natrajan P K, Aksu M F et al 1980 The fate of a large bolus of exogenous estrogen administered to postmenopausal women. Maturitas 2: 29

Hassager C, Riis B J, Strom V, Guyene T T, Christiansen C 1987 The long-term effect of oral and percutaneous estradiol on plasma renin substrate and blood pressure. Circulation 76: 753

Henderson B E, Paganini-Hill A, Ross R K 1988 Estrogen replacement therapy and protection from acute myocardial infarction. American Journal of Obstetrics and Gynecology 159: 312

Holst J, Cajander S, Carlstrom K et al 1983a Percutaneous estrogen replacement therapy.

Effects on circulating estrogens, gonadotropins and prolactin. Acta Obstetrica et Gynecologica Scandinavica 62: 49

Holst J, Cajander S, Carlstrom K et al 1983b A comparison of liver protein induction in postmenopausal women during oral and percutaneous oestrogen replacement therapy. British Journal of Obstetrics and Gynaecology 90: 355

Hunter D J S, Akande E O, Carr P et al 1973 Clinical and endocrinological effect of oestradiol implants at the time of hysterectomy and bilateral salpingo-oophorectomy. Journal of Obstetrics and Gynaecology of the British Commonwealth 80: 827

Jensen J, Christiansen C 1988 Effects of smoking on serum lipoproteins and bone mineral content during postmenopausal hormone replacement therapy. American Journal of Obstetrics and Gynecology 159: 820

King R J B, Dyer G, Collins W P et al 1980 Intracellular estradiol, estrone and estrogen receptor levels in endometria from postmenopausal women receiving estrogens and progestins. Journal of Steroid Biochemistry 13: 377

Kupperman H S, Delaplaine R W, Bottomy D 1959 Effective control of the surgical menopause by estradiol implantation at the time of oophorectomy and total hysterectomy. Journal of Clinical Endocrinology 11: 788

Lignieres B de, Vincens M, Mauvais-Jarvis P, Mas S L, Touboul P J, Bousser M G 1986 Prevention of menstrual migraine by percutaneous oestradiol. British Medical Journal ii: 1540

Lind T, Cameron E C, Hunter W M et al 1979 A prospective, controlled trial of six forms of hormone replacement given to postmenopausal women. British Journal of Obstetrics and Gynaecology (suppl) 3: 1

Lobo R A, March C M, Goebelsmann U et al 1980 Subdermal estradiol pellets following hysterectomy and oophorectomy. Effects upon serum estrone, estradiol, luteinizing hormone, follicle-stimulating hormone, corticosteroid binding globulin-binding capacity, testosterone-estradiol binding globulin-binding capacity, lipids, and hot flushes. American Journal of Obstetrics and Gynecology 138: 714

Longcope C, Jaffe W, Griffing G 1980 Metabolic clearance rates of androgens and oestrogens in ageing women. Maturitas 2: 283

Lyrenas S, Carstrom K, Backstrom T et al 1981 A comparison of serum oestrogen levels after percutaneous and oral administration of oestradiol-17 beta. British Journal of Obstetrics and Gynaecology 88: 181

Magos A L, Studd J W W 1984 The premenstrual syndrome. In: Studd J W W (ed) Progress in obstetrics and gynaecology vol. 4. Churchill Livingstone, Edinburgh, p 334

Magos A L, Studd J W W 1985 Effects of the menstrual cycle on medical disorders. British Journal of Hospital Medicine 33: 68

Magos A L, Studd J W W 1986 Assessment of menstrual cycle symptoms by trend analysis. American Journal of Obstetrics and Gynecology 155: 271

Magos A L, Zilkha K J, Studd J W W 1983 Treatment of menstrual migraine by oestradiol implants. Journal of Neurology, Neurosurgery and Psychiatry 46: 1044

Magos A L, Collins W P, Studd J W W 1984 Management of the premenstrual syndrome by subcutaneous implants of oestradiol. Journal of Psychosomatic Obstetrics and Gynaecology 3: 93

Magos A L, Brincat M, O'Dowd T et al 1985a Endometrial and menstrual response to subcutaneous and testosterone implants and continuous oral progestogen therapy in postmenopausal women. Maturitas 7: 297

Magos A L, Brincat M, Studd J W W et al 1985b Amenorrhea and endometrial atrophy following continuous oral estrogen and progestogen therapy in post-menopausal women. Obstetrics and Gynecology 65: 496

Magos A L, Brewster E, Singh R et al 1986a The effects of norethisterone in post-menopausal women on oestrogen replacement therapy: a model for the pre-menstrual syndrome. British Journal of Obstetrics and Gynaecology 93: 1290

Magos A L, Brincat M, Studd J W W 1986b Treatment of the pre-menstrual syndrome by subcutaneous oestradiol implants and cyclical oral norethisterone: placebo controlled study. British Medical Journal i: 1629

Magos A L, Collins W P, Studd J W W 1987 Effects of subcutaneous oestradiol implants on ovarian activity. British Journal of Obstetrics and Gynaecology 94: 1192

Maoz B, Durst N 1980 The effects of oestrogen therapy on the sex life of post-menopausal women. Maturitas 2: 327

Miller G J, Miller N E 1975 Plasma high-density lipoprotein concentration and development of ischaemic heart-disease. Lancet *i*: 16

Montgomery J C, Appleby L, Brincat M et al 1987 A placebo-controlled study of the effect of oestrogen and testosterone upon psychological disorders in the climacteric. Lancet *i*: 297

Notelovitz M, Johnston M, Smith S et al 1987 Metabolic and hormonal effects of 25 mg and 50 mg 17-beta-estradiol implants in surgically menopausal women. Obstetrics and Gynecology 70: 749

Odlind V, Moo-Young A J, Gupta G N et al 1979 Subdermal norethindrone pellets—a method for contraception? Contraception 19: 636

Paganini-Hill A, Koss R K, Henderson B E 1988 Postmenopausal oestrogen treatment and stroke: a prospective study. British Medical Journal ii: 519

Paterson M E L, Wade-Evans T, Sturdee D W et al 1980 Endometrial disease after treatment with oestrogens and progestogens in the climacteric. British Medical Journal i: 822

Perloff W H 1949 Treatment of menopause. American Journal of Obstetrics and Gynecology 58: 684

Perloff W H 1950 Treatment of estrogen deficiency with estradiol pellets. Journal of Clinical Endocrinology 47: 447

Powers M S, Schenkel L, Darley P E et al 1985 Pharmacokinetics and pharmacodynamics of transdermal dosage forms of 17-beta-estradiol: comparison with conventional oral estrogens used for hormone replacement. American Journal of Obstetrics and Gynecology 152: 1099

Ralston S H, Fogelman I, Leggate J et al 1984 Effect of subdermal oestrogen and oestrogen/testosterone implants on calcium and phosphorus homeostasis after oophorectomy. Maturitas 6: 341

Ryan K J, Engel L L 1953 The interconversion of estrone and estradiol by human tissue slices. Endocrinology 52: 287

Savvas M, Studd J W W, Fogelman I et al 1988 Skeletal effects of oral oestrogen compared with oestrogen and testosterone in post-menopausal women. British Medical Journal ii: 331

Schleyer-Saunders E 1974 Social and gerontological problems of the menopause. Hormonal implant. In: Greenblatt R B, Makesh V, McDonogh P G (eds) The Menopausal Syndrome. Medcom Press, New York, p 88

Selby P L, Peacock M 1986 Dose dependent response of symptoms, pituitary, and bone to transdermal oestrogen in postmenopausal women. British Medical Journal ii: 1337

Sharf M, Oettinger M, Lanir A et al 1985 Lipid and lipoprotein levels following pure estradiol implantation in post-menopausal women. Gynecological and Obstetrical Investigations 19: 207

Sherwin B B, Gelfand M M 1984 Effects of parenteral administration of estrogen and androgen on plasma hormone levels and hot flushes in the surgical menopause. American Journal of Obstetrics and Gynecology 148: 552

Sherwin B B, Gelfand M M 1985 Differential symptom response to parenteral estrogen and/or androgen administration in the surgical menopause. American Journal of Obstetrics and Gynecology 151: 153

Sherwin B B, Gelfand M M, Brender W 1985 Androgen enhances sexual motivation in females: a prospective, crossover study of sex steroid administration in the surgical menopause. Psychosomatic Medicine 47: 339

Sherwin B B, Gelfand M M, Schucher R et al 1987 Postmenopausal estrogen and androgen replacement and lipoprotein lipid concentrations. American Journal of Obstetrics and Gynecology 156: 414

Soule S D 1951 Treatment of the post surgical menopause by implantation of oestradiol pellets. Journal of the International College of Surgeons 16: 622

Stanczyk F Z, Shoupe D, Nunez V et al 1988 A randomized comparison of nonoral estradiol delivery in postmenopausal women. American Journal of Obstetrics and Gynecology 159: 1540

Strecker J R, Lauritzen Ch, Goessens L 1979 Plasma concentrations of unconjugated and conjugated estrogens and gonadotrophins following application of various estrogen preparations after oophorectomy. Maturitas 1: 183

Studd J W W 1976 Hormone implants in the climacteric. In: Campbell S (ed) The management of the menopause & post-menopausal years. M.T.P. Press, Lancaster, p 383

Studd J W W 1979a The climacteric syndrome. In: van Keep P A, Serr D M, Greenblatt R B (eds) Female and male climacteric. M.T.P. Press, Lancaster, p 23

Studd J W W 1979b Premenstrual tension syndrome. British Medical Journal i: 410

Studd J W W, Thom M H 1981 Oestrogens and endometrial cancer. In: Studd J W W (ed)
  Progress in obstetrics and gynaecology vol. 1. Churchill Livingstone, Edinburgh, p 182

Studd J W W, Chakravarti S, Oram D 1977a The climacteric. Clinics in Obstetrics and
  Gynaecology 4: 3

Studd J W W, Collins W P, Newton J R et al 1977b Oestradiol and testosterone implants in
  the treatment of psychosexual problems in the post-menopausal woman. British Journal of
  Obstetrics and Gynaecology 84: 314

Studd J W W, Dubiel M, Kakkar V V et al 1978 The effect of hormone replacement therapy
  on glucose tolerance, clotting factors, fibrinolysis and platelet behaviour in post-
  menopausal women. In: Cooke I D (ed) The role of oestrogen/progestogen in the
  management of the menopause. M.T.P. Press, Lancaster, p 41

Studd J W W, Savvas M, Johnson M 1989 Correction of corticosteroid-induced osteoporosis
  by percutaneous hormone implants. Lancet i: 339

Studd J W W, Savvas M, Watson N R et al 1987 Monitoring oestradiol implantation. Lancet
  ii: 1404

Studd J W W, Thom M H, Paterson M E L et al 1980 The prevention and treatment of
  endometrial pathology in post-menopausal women receiving exogenous oestrogens. In:
  Pasetto N, Paoletti R, Ambrus J L (eds) The menopause and post-menopause. M.T.P.
  Press, Lancaster, p 127

Sturdee D W, Wade-Evans T, Paterson M E L et al 1978 Relations between bleeding
  pattern, endometrial histology, and oestrogen treatment in menopausal women. British
  Medical Journal i: 1575

Thom M H, Studd J W W 1980 Procedures in practice: hormone implantation. British
  Medical Journal i: 848

Thom M H, Collins W P, Studd J W W 1981 Hormone implantation in postmenopausal
  women after therapy with subcutaneous implants. British Journal of Obstetrics and
  Gynaecology 88: 426

Thom M H, Dubiel M, Kakkar V V et al 1978 The effect of different regimens of oestrogens
  on the clotting and fibrinolytic system of the post-menopausal woman. Frontiers of
  Hormone Research 5: 192

Vermeulen A 1976 The hormonal activity of the post-menopausal ovary. Journal of Clinical
  Endocrinology and Metabolism 42: 247

Whitehead M I, Lane G, Townsend P T et al 1982 Effects in postmenopausal women of
  natural and synthetic estrogens on calcitonin and calcium-regulating hormone secretion.
  Acta Obstetrica et Gynecologica Scandinavica (suppl) 106: 27

20. Reproductive endocrinology in Africa

R. J. Norman   Z. M. van der Spuy

INTRODUCTION

Africa is a continent which exhibits stark contrasts in the sociopolitical and economic lives of its 500 million people. A burgeoning population and food shortages combine with political factors to produce severe stresses in individuals and communities relating to health care needs. There are, as a result, major discrepancies in health delivery ranging from large teaching hospitals capable of maintaining sophisticated transplantation programmes through to small community clinics where basic medical supplies are difficult to obtain.

These contrasts are particularly marked in the field of reproduction. While privately funded patients throughout Africa can obtain treatment equivalent to that offered in the best centres of Europe, the patient dependent on State-run health services often receives little help for diseases such as infertility which understandably have a low priority in a continent with the highest population growth in the world.

In this chapter we shall discuss the role of nutrition on the reproductive patterns in Africa—where the study of reproductive endocrinology is all too often the study of undernutrition—and we shall highlight diseases that are either unique to the developing world or are far more prevalent than in North America or Europe.

NUTRITION AND EFFECTS ON REPRODUCTION

Adequate nutrition is essential for the development of optimal reproductive capability and every aspect of reproductive function may be adversely affected by malnutrition. Many countries in Africa struggle with the problem of chronic undernutrition in large sections of their population and the devastation of famine conditions has once again been highlighted by the tragedies in Ethiopia and Mozambique. An understanding of the impact of undernutrition on normal reproductive function is therefore essential both in the practice of gynaecological endocrinology and the planning of community health strategies together with the allocation of resources. In this section we briefly review the impact of nutrition on puberty and reproduction.

Nutrition and puberty

The physiology of normal pubertal development has been well characterized in several studies (Boyar et al 1972, 1973, Wildt et al 1980). Pulsatile secretion of gonadotrophin-releasing hormone (GnRH) results in sequential changes in gonadotrophin secretion with subsequent development of secondary sexual characteristics, the adolescent growth spurt and the eventual attainment of reproductive competence. Secondary sexual characteristics develop in a fixed sequence with growth acceleration occurring at the time of menarche in girls and later in puberty in boys.

These external physical features can be scored using the system devised by Tanner (1962). Menarche is a relatively late event in puberty and is followed by a period of subfertility before regular ovulation occurs (Marshall & Tanner 1969, 1970, Apter et al 1978). Any major insult during childhood or puberty which alters hypothalamic-pituitary function will therefore result in delayed or arrested puberty and a delay in attaining reproductive maturity. It is against the background of this physiology that the influence of undernutrition needs consideration.

Frisch and Revelle (1970, 1971) postulated a direct relationship between body weight and the onset of pubertal events. This 'critical weight' hypothesis was subsequently reviewed and body composition and percentage body fat rather than absolute weight was found to correlate with pubertal development and reproductive competence—a hypothesis that has been substantially supported both by human studies and animal experimentation (Frisch 1984, Crawford & Osler 1975, Osler & Crawford 1973, Kennedy & Mitra 1963).

According to Frisch and her co-workers, fat should comprise 17% of the total body weight for menarche to occur and 22% for the maintenance of ovulatory cycles (Frisch et al 1973, Frisch 1980). It has been shown that the mean age of menarche has decreased over the past century with improved socioeconomic conditions. Delay in growth and pubertal development with subsequent delay in fertility therefore represent an adaptive phenomenon since pregnancy in the undernourished woman may compromise both mother and baby (Wyshak & Frisch 1982, Tanner 1973, Warren 1983).

Puberty in Africa

The mean age of menarche in well-nourished girls in the UK was reported to be 13.5 ± 1.0 years with puberty commencing at 8–9 years in girls and slightly later in boys (Tanner 1962, Marshall & Tanner 1969, 1970). Information on puberty in Africa is less well documented; Table 24.1 shows the results of a number of studies of menarchal age in African communities.

Kark, as described in 1953, demonstrated an earlier menarche in the higher socioeconomic classes in the Durban immigrant Asian community compared with less affluent groups—a difference which may be attributed to improved nutrition (Kark 1953, 1956).

Kulin's study from Kenya also demonstrates the impact of nutrition on puberty. He compared rural and urban school children who had different nutritional backgrounds and demonstrated a marked delay in development in rural children after chronic childhood malnutrition (Kulin et al, 1982). There appeared to be full 'catch-up' growth during puberty, an observation noted in other studies which may present as accelerated growth if adequate food is available (Prader et al 1963, Dreizen et al 1967, Ashworth 1969).

Data on pubertal progress and final growth patterns are not currently available from areas such as Ethiopia where the population has been affected by starvation for many years. This deprivation has been gross and prolonged and these children may never reflect the same catch-up growth since the later the nutritional compensation, the less the final growth achievement.

Direct comparisons between the African studies (Table 20.1) and Tanner's work are difficult because many of these studies were performed more than 20 years ago. However, there is little doubt that pubertal development reflects the nutritional well-being of a community and there are still wide variations throughout Africa reflecting the differing nutritional status of various communities in the continent.

Table 20.1   Average age of menarche in 9 African studies

Population	Region	Age (years)	Authors
Rural Xhosa 'poor' 'not poor'	Transkei	15.42 ± 0.04 15.02 ± 0.02	Burrell et al (1961)
Urban Black	Johannesburg	14.89 ± 1.66	Oettle & Higginson (1961)
'Coloured' (mixed ethnic origin)	Johannesburg	13.2 ± 0.04	Margolius (1970)
Urban Black 'Average nutrition' 'Poor nutrition'	Johannesburg	14.74 ± 0.04 14.76 ± 0.04	Frere (1971)
White	Cape Town	14.6	Benjamin (1960)
Indian	Durban	13.6 ± 1.13	Kark (1956)
Nigeria (social class I & II)	Onitsha and Owerri	14.07 ± 0.16	Tanner & O'Keeffe (1962)
Uganda (upper social classes)	Kampala	13.4 ± 0.165	Burgess & Burgess (1964)
Kenya	Rural Urban	15.3 ± 2.3 13.2 ± 1.5	Kulin et al (1982)

Fertility and nutrition

Weight loss (10–15% of normal weight for height) and the subsequent alteration in fat stores and body composition will eventually result in impaired reproductive function. In childhood, undernutrition causes retarded growth and pubertal development while in the post-menarchal woman anovulation, infertility and eventually amenorrhoea may develop. Should fertility be maintained, pregnancy outcome may be compromised. The effects of malnutrition are less marked in the male but in severe cases may result in hypogonadism and Leydig-cell deficiency (Smith et al 1975, Brasel 1978). The causes of undernutrition may be classified broadly into three main groups: abstinence, increased energy demands and altered metabolism. Some of the main causes are listed in Table 20.2.

The various syndromes of undernutrition have different aetiologies but the endocrinology resulting in impaired reproduction is the same with the disorder being mainly hypothalamic in origin (Warren 1983, van der Spuy 1985). The major endocrine abnormality is impaired gonadotrophin secretion with resultant failure in ovarian steroidogenesis, folliculogenesis and ovulation (Warren & van de Wiele 1973, Boyar et al 1974). The inadequate ovarian steroidogenesis is further compounded by decreased extragonadal production of estrogen with the loss of body fat (Fishman et al 1975). Besides these changes, there are other endocrine abnormalities such as alterations in adrenal and thyroid function and growth hormone secretion. Since gonadal steroids are also essential for the full expression of the growth spurt, nutritionally compromised peripubertal children will demonstrate retarded growth. The endocrine abnormalities of undernutrition are usually reversible with appropriate and adequate refeeding.

Abstinence

Self-imposed dietary restriction is the commonest cause of secondary amenorrhoea in gynaecology in Western countries (Jacobs et al 1975, Nillius 1978). In contrast, in developing countries the impact of chronic

Table 20.2 Causes of undernutrition

Abstinence	(a) Self-imposed	Anorexia nervosa
		Dietary restrictions
	(b) Involuntary	Starvation
		Chronic food shortage
Increased energy demands	(a) Self-imposed	Intensive exercise, training programs, e.g. ballet, athletics
	(b) Involuntary	Physical labour
Altered metabolism	(a) Self-imposed	Vegans
		'Fad' diets
	(b) Involuntary	Malabsorption syndrome
		Intestinal parasites
		Debilitating illness, e.g. TB

malnutrition is of far greater importance. Reduced income, rapid population growth, inadequate food supplies and the additional problem of tropical infections all contribute to the nutritional depreciation. The effects of chronic moderate malnutrition on the fecundity of a population is probably minimal with fertility rates being more affected by the longer period of adolescent subfertility and the contraceptive effects of prolonged breast feeding (Bongaarts 1980). Unfortunately, the major cost of this undernutrition is the increased pregnancy wastage, and greater infant and maternal morbidity (Venkatachalam et al 1960, Gopalan & Nadamuni Naidu 1972, Yach et al 1987). In contrast, the experience of the Dutch 'hunger winter' of 1944 demonstrates that the acute nutritional deprivation of famine has a profound effect on fertility. The severity and rapidity of the impact of famine is determined by the nutritional health of a community and when acute deprivation is superimposed upon chronic undernutrition, the effects can be rapid and disastrous (Antonov 1947, Stein & Susser 1978).

Increased energy demand

The impact of intensive exercise and the resultant energy drain on reproduction has excited much interest in recent years when related to Western populations involved in athletics, ballet and other sports (Warren 1980, Baker 1981). A far more important aspect of exercise in many of our disadvantaged communities is the effect of physical labour on pregnancy outcome. Intrauterine growth retardation and placental infarction are more common in women engaged in physical activity during pregnancy, particularly when they conceive in a suboptimal state of nutrition (Naeye 1977, 1979, Naeye and Peters 1982).

PREGNANCY AND NUTRITION

Delayed pubertal development and compromised fertility are obviously important but the most significant effect of undernutrition on reproductive performance is on the outcome of pregnancy.

Low pre-pregnancy weight and poor weight-gain during pregnancy are known to result in an increased prevalence of low birthweight infants (Lechtig et al 1975a, Tafari et al 1980, Luke et al 1981, van der Spuy et al 1988). Besides an increased prevalence of pre-term and growth-retarded infants, women with suboptimal nutrition have higher rates of other pregnancy complications such as pre-term rupture of membranes, anemia, endometritis, and cardiovascular and respiratory complications (Niswander & Jackson 1974, Edwards et al 1979).

The impact of nutritional deprivation depends upon the phase of growth at which it occurs. An insult in early pregnancy impedes cell division resulting in a cell deficit and growth retardation which does not respond to subsequent improvement in nutrition. In contrast, later deprivation causes reduced cell size and this growth restriction responds to refeeding with growth 'catch-up' (Winick & Noble 1966, Widdowson & McCance 1975, Widdowson et al 1972).

Clinical studies support this experimental data and infants born to mothers who were acutely starved during pregnancy but who conceived in a state of good nutrition exhibited only a small reduction in birth-weights with no excess in fetal abnormality or long-term adverse sequelae (Smith 1947, Stein & Susser 1978). When the nutritional insult occurs very early in pregnancy or pre-conception, the fetus is at risk from long-term damage and developmental abnormalities (McCance & Widdowson 1974, Fancourt et al 1976, Wynn & Wynn 1981, Smithells et al 1983).

In their study of Cape Town primigravida with poor socioeconomic circumstances, Woods et al (1979) found that low maternal weight and poor weight-gain correlated with an excess of growth-retarded infants. These babies tended to be proportionally light and short suggesting that growth had been affected from early pregnancy. Maternal 'fatness' rather than muscle volume was the main determinant of the fetal outcome and Woods suggests that slowing of growth early in the compromised pregnancy is an adaptive phenomenon which protects mother and fetus from severe nutritional stress in late pregnancy (Woods 1984).

A subsequent study of a group of Black women who usually had normal or elevated body mass indices but whose home circumstances were often markedly disadvantaged has confirmed that 'fatness' is one of the main determinants of fetal growth. In this group 8.8% of the infants were of low birthweight and 7.6% were pre-term—findings very similar to those in well nourished, more affluent communities (Rip et al 1988a, van der Spuy 1988). The poor socioeconomic background was reflected in subsequent infant mortality which was particularly high in a squatter settlement (Rip et al 1988a, 1988b).

Pregnancy outcome can be improved by good weight-gain during pregnancy, and dietary supplementation in undernourished communities will reduce the incidence of low-weight infants (Naeye 1979, Lechtig et al 1975b, Prentice et al 1983). Ideally, the nutritional state of the mother should be improved before conception to have maximum impact but this will involve major alterations in the allocation of resources for health care and most developing countries are still far from achieving this. Finally, it must be remembered that the short- and long-term sequelae of growth retardation may be considerable and these assume greater significance when pediatric facilities are limited.

LACTATION AND EFFECTS ON REPRODUCTION

More births are prevented world-wide by lactation than by all other forms of contraception combined. Lactation results in anovulation and amenorrhoea in a considerable number of women due to increased prolactin levels and altered GnRH pulsatility. High basal levels of prolactin are maintained by frequent suckling episodes and suppress endogenous gonadotrophin concentrations (McNeilly 1979).

For millions of impoverished women prolonged lactation is the norm, providing both 'natural' contraception and infant nutrition. Widespread abandonment of this practice without adequate contraceptive and nutritional support results in both higher birth-rates and an increased infant mortality (Knodel 1977). Ross and his colleagues (1983a 1983b) have shown that breast-feeding is maintained longer in a rural environment than in the city and that supplementary feeding leads to earlier abandonment of breast-feeding.

In communities with a high prevalence of undernutrition, lactation enhances child survival and promotes longer birth intervals. Combined with customs encouraging abstinence from sexual intercourse until weaning, lactation and undernutrition are important regulators of fertility in Africa.

Perhaps the outstanding example of this effect on reproduction is the example of the Kung tribesmen of the Kalahari. These nomadic hunter-gatherers have an average birth-interval of 4 years and infants are demand breast-fed for 3–4 years. Menarche occurs at an average of 15.5 years and adolescent subfertility leads to a delay of first conception for about 4 years. Conception peaks during the wet season when food is most plentiful and nutrition therefore optimal and prolonged lactation is essential because soft food for weaning is not available.

As in other parts of Africa, urbanization has had negative effects on breast-feeding. Supplementary feeding leads to earlier weaning and return to fertility and reduced birth intervals with a consequent increase in population growth (Kolata 1974, Short 1976, van der Walt et al 1978). These changes serve to underline the need for education, contraception and paediatric services to accompany any major nutritional programme. No single aspect of this vast problem can be addressed in isolation.

PATTERNS OF INFERTILITY IN AFRICA

While the common endocrine causes of infertility (e.g. anovulation, hyper-prolactinemia, polycystic ovarian disease) undoubtedly occur frequently in Africans, their importance is totally overshadowed by the presence of tubal disease, usually resulting from infection. Cates et al (1985) in a report from a WHO multicentre study have highlighted the fact that up to 85% of women have a cause of infertility directly attributable to infection (Table 20.3). This figure is nearly two-and-a-half times the prevalence seen in developed countries. There are several other important features highlighted by this study, including the fact that women seeking assistance were much younger than those in developed countries as well as the

Table 20.3 Causes of infertility among women in 4 African centres contrasted with that in developed countries (Cates et al, 1985)

	Developed	Africa	
Tubal factor	35%	85%	
Bilateral occlusion	11		49
Pelvic adhesions	13		24
Acquired tubal abnormality	12		12
Endocrine related	39%	27%	
Anovulation	19		17
Ovulating oligomenorrhoea	7		4
Hyperprolactinemia	7		5
Endometriosis	6		1
No demonstrable cause	40%	16%	

prevalence of secondary (as opposed to primary) infertility being far more common. The reason for these figures is almost certainly due to the high occurrence of pelvic inflammatory disease caused by *Neisseria gonococcus* and other sexually transmitted pathogens (Muir and Belsey 1980). All accounts from Africa emphasize the common occurrence of acute and chronic salpingitis and puerperal sepsis. The young age of first sexual intercourse (Grech et al 1973), repeated infections and inadequate therapy combine to produce a marked adverse effect on the fallopian tube with respect to infertility and ectopic pregnancy. Not all pelvic infection is necessarily sexually transmitted; some is undoubtedly due to post-abortal and post-partum infections. Tuberculosis of the tube is relatively uncommon in Southern Africa but may be more prevalent elsewhere.

UNUSUAL ASPECTS OF REPRODUCTIVE ENDOCRINOLOGY

Sheehan's syndrome

There have been many histological and clinical studies of Sheehan's syndrome in developed countries since the first description in 1937. However, improved obstetric care has led to a decrease in the incidence of this condition over the past decades and there is relatively little modern endocrine information on these patients. Sheehan's syndrome is still seen in Africa, probably as a result of poor obstetric care, and two groups have published comprehensive work in this area.

In Durban, our group initially studied 10 patients and showed that the symptoms of hypothyroidism and amenorrhoea were the commonest presenting features (Jialal et al 1984). The most striking endocrine abnormality was the lack of a prolactin response to thyrotropin-releasing hormone TRH. No patient had an increase above $12\,\mu g/l$ at 20 minutes confirming the initial demonstration by Shahmanesh et al (1980) in Tehran. While growth hormone deficiency was common, our initial screening test for Sheehan's syndrome in the appropriate clinical setting of post-partum amenorrhoea has been to do a thyrotrophin-releasing hormone test with a 20-minute prolactin, or alternatively, to use 10 mg metochlopramide intravenously (Jialal et al 1986) (chlorpromazine is an inexpensive alternative). Table 20.4 shows some of the important features of the Durban studies.

In Algiers, Bakiri and co-workers have clearly defined the common prevalence of improved antidiuretic hormone (ADH) secretion in 20 patients with the characteristic clinical picture of panhypopituitarism of slow onset after delivery. Partial ADH deficiency was common when evaluated by maximum urine concentrating ability following water deprivation (Bakiri & Benmiloud 1984). However, the maximum urinary arginine vasopressin (AVP) excretion was markedly diminished compared to controls despite the fact that all subjects reached a urine osmolality of at least 500 mOsmol/kg (Bakiri et al 1984). Jialal et al (1987) in Durban confirmed these observations and added three patients with frank diabetes insipidus (urine osmolality < 600 mOsm per kg after water deprivation with an increase in osmolality of greater than 9% on AVP administration). From these results, it is obvious that a variety of endocrine manifestations may lead to presentation of a woman with Sheehan's syndrome.

While the condition is not uncommon in Africa the exact prevalence is not known. In a study of post-partum patients following massive *abruptio placentae*, haemorrhage and shock, we were unable to detect any abnormality of pituitary function in the first 7 days following delivery (Norman et al 1987).

Table 20.4 Characteristics of Sheehan's syndrome from two African centres. Percentages refer to proportion of patients with a hormonal response in the reference range for premenopausal patients in the follicular phase of the cycle. Date from Jialal et al (1984, Durban 1), Jialal et al (1986, Durban 2), Bakiri & Benmiloud; Bakiri et al 1984, Algiers

	Durban 1	Durban 2	Algiers
	n = 10	n = 16	n = 20
Age (mean & range years)	41.1 (30–56)	41.4 (29–56)	35.3 (21–44)
Duration of disease (years)	7.7	8.7	7.5
Response of			
FSH to GnRH	80%	60%	5%
LH to GnRH	90%	63%	5%
TSH to TRH	20%	13%	5%
Prolactin to TRH	0%	0%	0%
Cortisol to insulin	10%	6%	0%
HGH to insulin	0%	0%	0%
Maximal urine osmodality on water deprivation (mOsm/kg)	—	633	688
Number with frank diabetes insipidus (< 600 mOsm/kg on water deprivation)	—	3	?4*

* 0 Less than 500 mOsm/kg, ?4 under 600 mOsm/kg from Figure 1, Bakiri & Benmiloud.

A further unusual observation is that Sheehan's syndrome is more common among patients of Asian extraction in Durban than in Africans, despite a better obstetric service for the former group. Clearly, post-partum haemorrhage and shock alone are not the only predisposing factors for Sheehan's syndrome; some other factor must be operating in the aetiology of the condition. What is of interest, however, is the observation that Sheehan's syndrome is the second-most common cause of hypo-pituitarism seen in our population in Durban.

Pseudocyesis

Pseudocyesis manifests a 'phantom' pregnancy with clinical and emotional features of pregnancy, amenorrhoea, galactorrhoea and fetal movements (Drife 1985). The virtual disappearance of this condition from developed countries has not been paralleled in Africa where the strong cultural pressure on women to be fertile is reflected by a high incidence of pseudocyesis. At King Edward VIII Hospital, Durban, between 25 and 30 patients are seen annually; in Western countries most case reports indicate that the majority of the patients are immigrants from the developing world.

Brenner in Johannesburg (Brenner 1976) studied 21 patients he saw in 4 months in Soweto. Amenorrhoea, a firm belief in their pregnant state and abdominal enlargement were present in all patients. Fetal movements were felt in 38% and breast secretion in 14%. Similar findings have been reported by Osotimehin et al (1981) in Nigeria, while Padayachi et al (unpublished observations) noted that the majority of patients were multiparous, with amenorrhoea present for 8 months and fetal movements for 7 months on average. Galactorrhoea was present in 8 of 10 patients studied. Not all patients were desirous of pregnancy.

While a few reports have concentrated on the endocrinology of this condition from Mexico and North America (Zarate et al 1974, Tulandi et al 1982, 1983, Yen et al 1976) only Osotimelin et al (1981) and Padayachi et al (unpublished observations) have studied these findings in Africans. The Nigerians showed increased prolactin levels in patients with galactorrhoea and raised LH levels in patients without galactorrhoea. The Durban study of 10 Zulu women with pseudocyesis showed normal fasting levels of serum prolactin, LH and FSH with no abnormality of the pituitary-adrenal axis (as assessed by insulin-induced hypoglycaemia) or pituitary-thyroid axis (TRH test). Administration of gonadotropin-releasing hormone (GnRH 0.1 mg) resulted in exaggerated stimulation of LH and FSH in four and two patients respectively. Impaired growth-hormone secretion was frequent, probably due to oestrogen deficiency, and two patients had progesterone values suggestive of a luteal phase defect. There has been little investigation of the hypothalamic cause of pseudocyesis but preliminary results in our laboratory suggest a disturbance of pulsatile GnRH release which is partially corrected by an infusion of naloxone (Norman & Padayachi, unpublished data).

While therapy is directed towards convincing patients that they are not pregnant, some patients may continue with the delusion of pregnancy even to the extent of going into labour with painful intermittent contractions.

Intersex and true hermaphroditism

Congenital adrenal hyperplasia and androgen insensitivity occur reasonably commonly in Black patients in cities in Africa where adequate facilities for laboratory diagnosis exist. However, in outlying areas many of these patients will go unrecognized and in the case of salt-losing congenital adrenal hyperplasia, most of the neonates would die without a diagnosis being made. In the past 7 years approximately 7 patients with congenital adrenal hyperplasia have been seen at King Edward VIII Hospital in Durban. Complete androgen insensitivity (testicular feminization) is found relatively frequently because primary amenorrhoea is a symptom that leads patients to seek medical advice.

By far the commonest cause of intersex in Black patients in Southern Africa is true hermaphroditism (van Niekerk 1974, 1976). Ovarian as well as testicular tissue should be present to make the diagnosis. Presentation in our population is of two categories:

1. Indeterminite genitalia or hypospadias in a neonate or young child,
2. Pubertal occurrence of breast development in a child brought up as a male with ambiguous genitalia.

Despite the genital ambiguity, 75% of children are assigned the male gender by their parents on the basis of an enlarged phallus and a degree of scrotalization. The genitalia usually have the following features: phallus in chordee with urogenital sinus opening between the labia, scrotal folds, occasionally palpable gonads, usually on the right side of the scrotum or inguinal canal. The most common gonad is an ovotestis usually occurring intra-abdominally in the position of a normal ovary. The more testicular tissue present, the more likely the ovotestis to be located in the scrotum or inguinal canal. In 409 cases of true hermaphroditism reviewed by van Niekerk (1976) lateral true hermaphroditism (ovary on one side and testis on the other) occurred in 29.6% of cases, unilateral true hermaphroditism (ovotestis on one side and ovary on the other) in 29.1% and bilateral true hermaphroditism (ovotestis both sides) in 20.8%. A combination of ovotestis on the one side with a testis on the other is much less common (11%). The ovary is more commonly found on the left (62.8%) and the testis on the right (59.5%). When an ovotestis is present, the right side is a more common site than is the left (57.7% vs 42.3%). These figures, based on a worldwide literature survey, were reinforced by Aaronson (1985) in Cape Town who found the right gonad to be either predominantly or entirely testicular in 39 of 41 patients.

Endocrine studies of this condition are limited. Most adult patients have testosterone levels intermediate between male and female values; the testicular tissue is LH-dependent as shown by hCG induction of testosterone production (Aaronson 1985, Norman et al unpublished observations). Oestradiol levels are also in the intermediate range but are sufficiently raised to lead to gynaecomastia. In neonates, the hormonal profile differs little between those with male and female phenotypes.

The aetiology of true hermaphroditism remains a mystery. Most patients have a 46XX chromosomal complement in Africa and mosaicism is rare. Studies of the HY antigen and testis-determining gene have not been performed on a large series of patients.

Premature menopause

Although apparently not documented before, there is little doubt that premature menopause is extremely common in the African population of Southern Africa. This cannot be attributed to an earlier age of menopause in Black women because the median age of 51 years is similar in Whites and Blacks. In Durban (Naidoo et al 1985) we described clinical and endocrine features of 35 women with premature menopause (defined as amenorrhoea lasting for more than 6 months in woman under the age of 35 years). In all patients, the chromosomes were 46XX, no autoantibodies were detected against smooth muscle, parietal cells, mitochondria or thyroid. Most patients had given birth to at least one child. Basal and stimulated pituitary hormone concentrations were not different from those expected for menopause of normal age of onset. In 10 patients where ovarian biopsy was performed, no follicles were seen. The aetiology of this condition is completely unknown in Africa with none of the usual predisposing causes being seen (autoimmunity, cytotoxic drugs, radiotherapy, surgery etc.). The desire for fertility overrides all other complaints and obviously cannot be treated other than by ovum donation.

Isolated gonadotrophin-releasing hormone deficiency

This also appears to be a common cause of amenorrhoea in African women (Norman et al 1986a, 1986b), presenting as primary amenorrhoea with no secondary sexual development. It is due to a genetic lack of GnRH synthesis and is much more frequent than among males in a Black population (Norman et al 1986a). None of the 17 cases seen in Durban had anosmia or midline defects, unlike the pattern expected in a Caucasian population. The endocrinology of this disease appears to conform to that seen in Whites (Norman et al 1986b).

CONCLUSION

Africa is a continent of mystery and ignorance and this applies as much to our knowledge of reproductive endocrinology as to any other aspect of its fascinating life. Much of the data presented in this chapter is derived by extrapolation from studies in the developed countries. It is hoped that this discussion will stimulate scientists to seek collaboration with their colleagues in Africa to explore the urgent problems and fascinating mysteries in this continent.

REFERENCES

Aaronson I 1985 True hermaphrodatism. A review of 41 cases with observations on testicular histology and function. British Journal of Urology 57: 775–779

Antonov A 1947 Children born during the siege of Leningrad in 1942. Journal of Pediatrics 30: 250–259

Apter D, Viinikka L, Vihko R 1978 Hormonal pattern of adolescent menstrual cycles. Journal of Clinical Endocrinology and Metabolism 47: 944–954

Ashworth A 1969 Growth rates in children recovering from protein-calorie malnutrition. British Journal of Nutrition 23: 835–845

Baker E R 1981 Menstrual dysfunction and hormonal status in athletic women: A review. Fertility and Sterility 36: 691–696

Bakiri F, Benmiloud M 1984 Antidiuretic function in Sheehan's syndrome. British Medical Journal 289: 579–580

Bakiri F, Benmiloud M, Vallotton M B 1984 Arginine-vasopressin in postpartum panhypopituitarism: urinary excretion and kidney response to osmolar load. Journal of Clinical Endocrinology and Metabolism 58: 511–515

Benjamin F 1960 The age of the menarche and of the menopause in white South African women and certain factors influencing these times. South African Medical Journal 34: 316–320

Bongaarts J 1980 Does malnutrition affect fecundity? A summary of evidence. Science 208: 564–569

Boyar R M, Finkelstein J W, David R et al 1973 Twenty-four hour patterns of plasma luteinizing hormone and follicle stimulating hormone in sexual precocity. New England Journal of Medicine 289: 282–286

Boyar R M, Finkelstein J W, Roffwag H, Kapens S, Weitzman E, Hellman L 1972 Synchronization of augmented luteinizing hormone secretion with sleep during puberty. New England Journal of Medicine 281: 582–586

Boyar R M, Katz J, Finkelstein J W et al 1974 Immaturity of the 24-hour luteinizing hormone secretory pattern. New England Journal of Medicine 291: 861–865

Brasel J A 1978 Impact of malnutrition on reproductive endocrinology. In: Mosley W H (ed) Nutrition and human reproduction. Plenum Press, New York, pp 29–60

Brenner B N 1976 Pseudocyesis in blacks. South African Medical Journal 50: 1757–1759

Burgess A P, Burgess H J L 1964 The growth pattern of East African school girls. Human Biology 36(2): 177–193

Burrell R J W, Healy M J R, Tanner J M 1961 Age at menarche in South African Bantu school girls living in the Transkei Reserve. Human Biology 33(2): 250–261

Cates W, Farley T M M, Rowe P J 1985 Worldwide patterns of infertility: is Africa different? Lancet ii: 596–598

Crawford J D, Osler D C 1975 Body composition at menarche: the Frisch-Revelle hypothesis revisited. Pediatrics 56: 449–458

Dreizen S, Spirakis C N, Stone R E 1967 A comparison of skeletal growth and maturation in undernourished and well-nourished girls before and after menarche. Journal of Pediatrics 70: 256–263

Drife J D 1985 Phantom pregnancy. Editorial, British Medical Journal 291: 687–688

Edwards L E, Alton I R, Barrada M I, Hakanson E Y 1979 Pregnancy in the underweight woman. Course, outcome and growth patterns of the infant. American Journal of Obstetrics and Gynecology 135: 297–302

Fancourt R, Campbell S, Harvey D, Norman A P 1976 Follow-up study of small-for-dates babies. British Medical Journal 2: 1435–1437

Fishman J, Boyar R M, Hellman L 1975 Influence of body weight on estradiol metabolism in young women. Journal of Clinical Endocrinology and Metabolism 41: 989–991

Frere G 1971 Mean age at menopause and menarche in South Africa. South African Journal of Medical Science 36: 21–24

Frisch R E 1980 Pubertal adipose tissue: is it necessary for normal sexual maturation? Evidence from the rat and human female. Federation Proceedings 39: 2395–2400

Frisch R E 1984 Body fat, puberty and fertility. Biological Reviews 59: 161–188

Frisch R E, Revelle R 1970 Height and weight at menarche and a hypothesis of critical body weights and adolescent events. Science 169: 397–399

Frisch R E, Revelle R 1971 Height and weight at menarche and a hypothesis of menarche. Archives of Disease in Childhood 46: 695–701

Frisch R E, Revelle R, Cook S 1973 Components of weight at menarche and the initiation of the adolescent growth spurt in girls: estimated total water, lean body weight and fat. Human Biology 45: 469–483

Gopalan C, Nadamuni Naidu A 1972 Nutrition and fertility. Lancet ii: 1077–1079

Grech E S, Everett J V, Mukasa F 1973 Epidemiologic aspects of acute pelvic inflammatory disease in Uganda. Tropical Doctor 3: 123–127

Jacobs H S, Hull M G R, Murray M A F, Franks S 1975 Therapy-orientated diagnosis of secondary amenorrhoea. Hormone Research 6: 268–287

Jialal I, Naidoo C, Normal R J, Rajput M C, Omar M A K, Joubert S M 1984 Pituitary function in Sheehan's Syndrome. Obstetrics & Gynecology 63: 15–19

Jialal I, Desai R K, Rajput M C, Naidoo C, Omar M A K, Joubert S M 1986 Prolactin secretion in Sheehan's Syndrome. Response to thyrotropin-releasing hormone and metochlopramide. Journal of Reproductive Medicine 31: 487–490

Jialal I, Desai R K, Rajput M C 1987 An assessment of posterior pituitary function in patients with Sheehan's syndrome. Clinical Endocrinology 27: 91–95

Kark E 1953 Puberty in South African girls. (i) The menarche in Indian girls of Durban. South African Journal of Clinical Science 4: 23–35

Kark E 1956 Puberty in South African girls. (ii) Social class in relation to the menarche. South African Journal of Laboratory and Clinical Medicine 2: 84–88

Kennedy G C, Mitra J 1963 Body weight and food intake as initiating factors for puberty in the rat. Journal of Physiology 166: 408–418

Knodel J 1977 Breast-feeding and population growth. Science 198: 1111–1115

Kolata G B 1974 Kung hunter-gatherers: feminism, diet and birth control. Science 185: 932–934

Kulin H E, Bwibo N, Mutie D, Santner S J 1982 The effect of chronic childhood malnutrition on pubertal growth and development. American Journal of Clinical Nutrition 36: 527–536

Lechtig A, Yarbrough C, Delgado H, Habicht J P, Martorell R, Klein R E 1975a Influence of maternal nutrition on birth weight. American Journal of Clinical Nutrition 28: 1223–1233

Lechtig A, Habicht J P, Delgado H, Klein R E, Yarbrough C, Martorell R 1975b Effect of food supplementation during pregnancy on birth weight. Pediatrics 56: 508–520

Luke B, Dickinson C, Petrie R H 1981 Intrauterine growth: correlations of maternal nutritional status and rate of gestational weight gain. European Journal of Obstetrics, Gynecology and Reproductive Biology 12: 113–121

Margolius K 1970 The age at menarche in South African Coloured girls. Leech XL i: 19–22

Marshall W A, Tanner J M 1969 Variation in pattern of pubertal changes in girls. Archives of Disease in Childhood 44: 291–303

Marshall W A, Tanner J M 1970 Variation in the pattern of pubertal changes in boys. Archives of Disease in Childhood 45: 13–23

McCance R A, Widdowson E M 1974 Review lecture: The determinants of growth and form. Proceedings of the Royal Society of London. 185: 1–17

McNeilly A S 1979 Effects of lactation on fertility. British Medical Bulletin 35(2): 151–154

Muir D G, Belsey M A 1980 Pelvic inflammatory disease and its consequences in the developing world. American Journal of Obstetrics and Gynecology 138: 913–928

Naeye R L 1977 Placental infarction leading to fetal or neonatal death. Obstetrics and Gynecology 50: 583–588

Naeye R L 1979 Weight-gain and the outcome of pregnancy. American Journal of Obstetrics and Gynecology 135: 3–9

Naeye R L, Peters E C 1982 Working during pregnancy: effects on the fetus. Pediatrics 69: 724–727

Naidoo C, Norman R J, Khatree M, Joubert S M 1985 Idiopathic premature ovarian failure: a clinical and biochemical study. South African Medical Journal 68: 91–94

Nillius S J 1978 Psycho-pathology of weight-related amenorrhoea. In: Jacobs H S (ed) Advances in gynaecological endocrinology. Royal College of Obstetricians and Gynaecologists, London, pp 118–130

Niswander K, Jackson E C 1974 Physical characteristics of the gravida and their association with birth weight and perinatal death. American Journal of Obstetrics and Gynecology 119: 306–313

Norman R J, Mobbs C M, Joubert S M 1987 Effects of severe postpartum haemorrhage on puerperal pituitary function. Journal of Obstetrics and Gynaecology 7: 197–200

Norman R J, Naidoo C, Reddi K, Khatree M, Joubert S M 1986a Clinical studies in black women with isolated gonadotrophin-releasing hormone deficiency. South African Medical Journal 69: 546–548

Norman R J, Naidoo C, Reddi K, Vink G J, Naidoo B N, Joubert S M 1986b Endocrine studies in patients with isolated gonadotrophin-releasing deficiency. South African Medical Journal 70: 152–155

Norman R J, Reddi K, Padayachi T 1987, unpublished data

Oettle A G, Higginson J 1961 'The age of menarche in South African (negro) girls: with a comment on methods of determining mean age at menarche. Human Biology 33: 181–190

Osler D C, Crawford J D 1973 Examination of the hypothesis of a critical weight at menarche in ambulatory and bedridden mentally retarded girls. Pediatrics 51: 675–679

Osotimehin B O, Ladipo O A, Adejuwon C A, Otolorin E O 1981 Pituitary and placental hormone levels in pseudocyesis. Internal Journal of Gynaecology and Obstetrics 19: 399–402

Padayachi T, Moodley J, Norman R J, Jialal I unpublished observations

Prader A, Tanner J M, von Harnack G A 1963 Catch-up growth following illness or starvation. Journal of Pediatrics 62(5): 646–659

Prentice A M, Whitehead R G, Watkinson M, Lamb W H, Cole T J 1983 Prenatal dietary supplementation of African women and birth weight. Lancet i: 489–492

Rip M R, Keen C S, Woods D L, de Groot H van C 1988a Perinatal health in the black peri-urban township of Khayelitsha, Cape Town. I. Mothers and their newborn infants. South African Medical Journal 74: 829–832

Rip M R, Keen C S, Woods D L, de Groot H van C 1988b Perinatal health in the black peri-urban township of Khayelitsha, Cape Town. II. Infant mortality. South African Medical Journal 74: 833–834

Ross S M, van Middlekop A, Khoza N C 1983a Breast feeding practices in a black community. South African Medical Journal 63: 23–25

Ross S M, Loening W E K, van Middlekop A 1983b Breast feeding—evaluation of a health education programme. South African Medical Journal 64: 361–363

Shahmanesh M, Ali Z, Pourmand M, Nourmand I 1980 Pituitary function tests in Sheehan's syndrome. Clinical Endocrinology 12: 303–311

Short R V 1976 Definition of the problem. The evolution of human reproduction. Proceedings of the Royal Society of London 195: 3–24

Smith C A 1947 The effect of wartime starvation in Holland upon pregnancy and its product. American Journal of Obstetrics and Gynecology 53: 599–608

Smith S R, Chhetri M K, Johanson A J, Radfar N, Migeon C J 1975 The pituitary-gonadal axis in men with protein-calorie malnutrition. Journal of Clinical Endocrinology and Metabolism 41: 60–69

Smithells R W, Nevin N C, Seller M J et al 1983 Further experience of vitamin supplementation for prevention of neural tube defect recurrences. Lancet i 1027–1031

Stein Z, Susser M 1978 In: Mosely W H (ed) Nutrition and human reproduction. Plenum Press, New York, pp 123–145

Tafari N, Naeye R L, Gobezie A 1980 Effects of maternal undernutrition and heavy physical work during pregnancy on birth weight. British Journal of Obstetrics and Gynaecology 87: 222–226

Tanner J M 1973 Trend towards earlier menarche in London, Oslo, Copenhagen, the Netherlands and Hungary. Nature 243: 95–96

Tanner J M 1962 Growth at adolescence 2nd edn. Blackwell Scientific Publications, Oxford

Tanner J M, O'Keeffe B 1962 Age at menarche in Nigerian schoolgirls, with a note on their heights and weights from age 12–19. Human Biology 34(3): 187–196

Tulandi T, McInnes R A, Lal S 1983 Altered pituitary hormone secretion in patients with pseudocyesis. Fertility and Sterility 40: 637–641

Tulandi T, McInnes R A, Mehta A, Tolis G 1982 Pseudocyesis: Pituitary function before and after resolution of symptoms. Fertility and Sterility 59: 119–121

van der Spuy Z M 1985 Nutrition and reproduction. Clinics in Obstetrics and Gynaecology 12(3): 579–604

van der Spuy Z M, Steer P J, McCusker M, Steele S J, Jacobs H 1988 Outcome of pregnancy in underweight women after spontaneous and induced ovulation. British Medical Journal 296: 962–965

van der Walt L A, Wilmsen E N, Jenkins T 1978 Unusual sex hormone patterns among desert-dwelling hunter-gatherers. Journal of Clinical Endocrinology and Metabolism 46: 658–663

van Niekerk W A 1974 True hermaphroditism: morphologic and cytogenetic aspects. Harper and Row, New York

van Niekerk W A 1976 True hermaphroditism. American Journal of Obstetrics and Gynecology 126: 890–907

Venkatachalam P S, Shankar K, Gopalan C 1960 Changes in body weight and body composition during pregnancy. Indian Journal of Medical Research 48: 511–517

Warren M P 1983 Effects of undernutrition on reproductive function in the human. Endocrine Reviews 4: 363–377

Warren M P 1980 The effects of exercise on pubertal progression and reproductive function in girls. Journal of Clinical Endocrinology and Metabolism 51: 1150–1157

Warren M P, van de Wiele R L 1973 Clinical and metabolic features of anorexia nervosa. American Journal of Obstetrics and Gynecology 117: 435–449

Widdowson E M, Crabb D E, Milner R D G 1972 Cellular development of some human organs before birth. Archives of Disease in Childhood 47: 652–655

Widdowson E M, McCance R A 1975 A review: new thoughts on growth. Pediatric Research 9: 154–156

Wildt L, Marshall G, Knobil E 1980 Experimental induction of puberty in the infantile female rhesus monkey. Science 207: 1373–1375

Winick M, Noble A 1966 Cellular response in rats during malnutrition at various ages. Journal of Nutrition 89: 300–306

Woods D L 1984 Maternal, infant and placental size at birth. A study of first-born term infants and their mothers in Cape Town. (Dissertation) University of Cape Town

Woods D L, Malan A F, Heese H de V, van Schalkwyk D K 1979 Maternal size and fetal growth. South African Medical Journal 56: 562–564

Wynn M, Wynn A 1981 The prevention of handicap of early pregnancy origin. Foundation for Education and Research in Childbearing, London

Wyshak G, Frisch R E 1982 Evidence for a secular trend in age of menarche. New England Journal of Medicine 306: 1033–1035

Yach D, Klopper J M L, Taylor S P 1987 Use of indicators in achieving 'Health for all' in South Africa, 1987. South African Medical Journal 72: 805–807

Yen S S C, Rebar R W, Quesenberry W 1976 Pituitary function in pseudocyesis. Journal of Clinical Endocrinology and Metabolism 43: 132–136

Zarate A, Canales E S, Soria J et al 1974 Gonadotropin and prolactin secretion in human pseudocyesis: Effect of synthetic luteinizing hormone-releasing hormone (LH-RH) and thyrotropin-releasing hormone (TRH). Annalls d'Endocrinologie 35: 445–450

21. The surgical treatment of gynaecological congenital malformations

N. Johnson   R. J. Lilford

INTRODUCTION

Progress in some aspects of the treatment of obstetrical and gynaecological congenital malformations has been so considerable in the past few years that agonadal females and a Rokitansky sufferer have delivered children (Formigili & Formigili 1986, Singh & Devi 1983). However, these advances have only affected a handful of patients and most conditions are still managed according to long-established principles. Even today we copy Hypocrites' operation of 400 BC to correct an imperforate hymen and we copy the Romans' vaginoplasty techniques of 600 AD.

VAGINAL AGENESIS

Some of the most interesting developments have been in the field of vaginoplasty. From the 6th century onwards the Roman, Arabic, Jewish and Renaissance medical writers made reference to the treatment of vaginal atresia. By the combination of blunt and sharp dissection, they created a vaginal cavity between the rectum and bladder which was then lined with all manner of ingenious stents until epithelization occurred. However, Nature is such that she will try to close any unepithelialized sinus and she does not discriminate in favour of an iatrogenic neovagina. Siriecieke of Prussia in 1892 lined a vagina with a rabbit intestinal graft (Cains & De Villers 1980) but despite his claims, our present-day knowledge of hetero-grafts suggests that his enthusiasm was greater than his objectivity and it is not surprising that subsequent workers have turned to autografts. Abbe in 1898 was the first to line a cavity with split-thickness skin grafts supported on a mould, but it was McIndoe who popularized the procedure after the Second World War. At about the same time Baldwin transposed bowel to create a vagina and then Williams described a posteriorly directed external pouch. Medical techniques were pioneered by Frank (1938), who found that he could achieve success by applying pressure to the rectovesical septum. More recently, elegant full-thickness flaps have been performed, further revolutionizing the life of females who are born without a vagina.

351

Frank's dilators

Frank (1938), Broadbent and Woolf (1977), Dewhurst (1987) and Smith (1983) have all claimed success by applying pressure to the Mullerian pit. In practice the patient is asked to apply manual pressure to the fourchette with a dilator twice a day for 15 minutes. Ingram (1981) has advocated the wearing of a small mould under the pants and sitting aside a special stool designed like a bicycle seat. Gradually the area becomes indented and more of the dilator can be inserted. Although reasonable results have been published suboptimal cases are rarely notified and with few exceptions the final vaginal length is unsatisfactory. Most patients require surgical treatment.

Pre-operative care

Pre-operative counselling, psychological support and gynae-urological investigations are essential (Harkins et al 1981). Genotyping will help to differentiate vaginal agenesis from testicular feminization and ultrasound is superseding the intravenous pyelogram to investigate the 25–40% of upper urinary tract anomalies associated with vaginal agenesis (Hauser & Schreiner 1961, Phelen et al 1953, Miller & Stout 1957). Although most women who are born without a vagina also lack a functioning uterus and may possess ectopic or abnormal gonads, pre-operative laparoscopy is rarely essential (Baramki 1984). Definitive vaginal surgery can be delayed, in cases where there is no obstruction to menstrual flow, until the young woman is psychologically ready and feels the need to have a vagina.

Perineal pouch

Williams's vulvovaginoplasty (Williams 1964, 1970) frees the patient from the routine of using dilators and has the advantage that the pouch created is of full thickness epithelium and significant contraction does not occur. It is safe, simple and provides rapid results but leaves the patient with an abnormal looking perineum and a short vagina at an abnormal angle. In an understanding relationship, this does not present a problem, for the functional results are good, clitoral stimulation at coitus is excellent and the couple can easily adjust to their preferred position by rotating the female pelvis with respect to the male penis. Unfortunately, most teenage virgins will be conscious of their malformation and because of modern society's demands for perfect sex, initial relationships with men may be inhibited.

In this procedure, the labia majora are retracted laterally and a U-shaped incision is made with the apex at the fourchette, extending upwards and forwards internal to the hairline of the labia majora, the upper point being 4 cm lateral to the urethra (any higher and the pouch would obstruct micturition). The two layers of each labia majora are separated by blunt

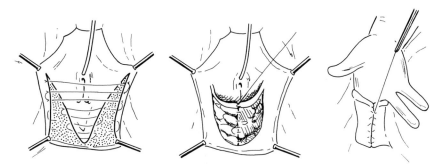

Fig. 21.1 Williams's vulvovaginoplasty (Perineal marsupialized pouch). After a U-shaped perineal incision the two layers of each labia majora are separated. Each layer is then united in the midline to the corresponding layer from the opposite side.

dissection until the superficial perineal muscles are exposed. Each layer is then united in the midline to the fellow of the opposite side (Fig. 21.1). With time, the vagina tends to become re-orientated as penile pressure stretches the rectovesical septum in a mechanism of action not dissimilar to that of Frank's dilators.

McIndoe jayes operation

The McIndoe procedure (McIndoe & Bannister 1938) and its various modifications are aesthetically pleasing and provide a normal-looking perineum and a normal vaginal axis. Following a transverse incision just over the Mullerian pit (a dimple invariably present just behind the urethra), a cavity is surprisingly easily created by a blunt dissection with the fingers between the rectum and bladder during which the pulp of the fingers should be directed away from the rectum. The creation of this cavity, which needs to be larger at the top, is occasionally hampered by a midline sagittal septum which can be divided by scissors. In order to prevent the natural closure of the cavity, it must be lined with epithelium; split-skin graft, amnion (Dhall 1984, Morton & Dewhurst 1986, Ashworth et al 1986), devitalized bowel and peritoneum (Tamaya et al 1984), pulled down from the pouch of Douglas, have all been used. The cavity is kept open with stents and regularly dilated.

Classically, a split-skin graft (amnion has lost favour following the outbreak of AIDS) is taken from the thigh or buttock and moulded around a vaginal obturator containing a sponge. The obturator is placed in the newly created rectovesical space (Fig. 21.2) and then withdrawn, leaving the sponge to support the split-skin graft against the cavity wall. One to two weeks later, under anaesthetic, the sponge is replaced with a mould for a further period (1–12 weeks) and thereafter vaginal dilatation is practised each night until regular intercourse begins. Unless persistent and regular

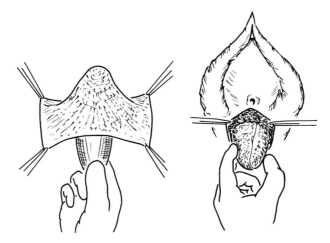

Fig. 21.2   The McIndoe procedure. A split skin graft is moulded around a vaginal obturator and placed in the newly developed rectovesical space.

dilatation is practised, stricture and scarring can occur and the vagina will close, especially in the vault area within a matter of days to weeks.

In uncomplicated cases the functional and cosmetic results are excellent. The neovagina behaves and functions in an almost normal manner; it stores glycogen (Holmstrom et al 1976), responds to the instructions of the ovarian hormones (Willemsen et al 1985) and it may even develop intra-epithelial neoplasia (Imrie et al 1986) and primary vaginal carcinoma (Jackson 1959). Unfortunately, leucorrhoea secondary to granulation tissue and pain/dyspareunia from scar tissue are considerable problems. There is risk of intra-operative damage to the bladder and rectum, and a risk of fistula formation attributable to the solid mould in the post-operative stage. Although this complication may be less likely with the newer soft sponge moulds, Jackson (1965) reported nine rectovaginal fistulas and two vesico-vaginal fistulas from 128 cases using hard moulds.

Full-thickness skin flaps

The solution to most of these problems is to use a full-thickness skin flap because this will not contract, or stenose down, and the need for obturators, moulds and dilators is therefore avoided.

From 1963 onwards, Song (1982) used the labia majora and minora as pedicle flaps. These two bilateral full-thickness flaps on a vascular pedicle (base posteriorly) are created by a Y-shaped incision at the introitus. The labia majora and minora which can be lifted up off the vulva and the skin defect from which they were taken, is then closed. The two labia, on their pedicles, are united to each other in the midline forming a skin tube with a blind end like a condom; the medial aspect of the flap becomes the posterior

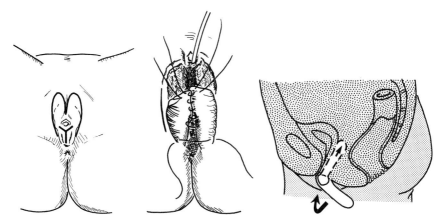

Fig. 21.3 Song's vaginoplasty. A rectovesical space is developed after a Y-shaped perineal incision and pedicle grafts of labia majora and minora are created by incising along the black line (a). The grafts are lifted up off the vulva and united to each other in the midline (b) to form a sheath which is folded inwards, to line the neovaginal cavity (c).

suture line and the lateral edge lies anteriorly. This tube, skin innermost, is then placed to line the vaginal cavity which has been created by blunt dissection. The opening of the tube is then united with the introitus (Fig. 21.3). In cases of intersex with clitoromegaly, where clitoroplasty has been neglected, preputial skin can be incorporated into the neo-vagina during a simultaneous clitoroplasty and vaginoplasty (Parrott et al 1980). As the pedicled skin graft is of full thickness, stenosis is not a problem and stents are not required. Unfortunately, the vulva is mutilated and the vagina tends to be short.

To overcome this skin shortage, McCraw et al (1976) and Lacey et al (1988) advocate using a long gracilis musculocutaneous flap graft. A long narrow pedicle consisting of gracilis and its overlying skin is taken from the thigh with its base at the inguinal ligament. The flap is rotated 180° and dropped into the newly created vaginal cavity. The disadvantage of this musculocutaneous flap is the bulk of tissue used and the possibility that this long narrow flap will lose viability, especially if the vascular pedicle is distally situated. However, preliminary anatomical and clinical studies by Wang et al (1987) suggest that the muscle and its vascular pedicle may be sacrificed and the long narrow flap will still retain its viability even at the distal end.

The much safer, distally based rectus abdominis musculocutaneous paddle flap (Tobin & Day 1988, McCraw & Kurtzman 1988) has been used in cases of pelvic exenteration and Lilford et al (1988) have adapted this to patients with vaginal agenesis. The end of this flap, which is wide like a paddle, is rolled about its axis to form a tube, skin innermost, before being transposed intra-abdominally down into the pelvis between the bladder and rectum. The cranial portion of the flap is united to the introitus by a

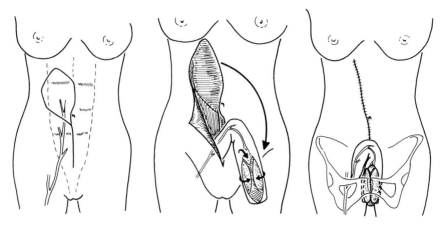

Fig. 21.4 The rectus abdominis musculocutaneous flap vaginoplasty. A cutaneous paddle flap supported by the inferior epigastric vessels from the rectus muscle, is rolled about its axis to form a tube, skin innermost. It is then transposed intra-abdominally down into the pelvis between the bladder and rectum.

surgeon working from below, while flap viability is ensured by the preserving inferior epigastric pedicle (Fig. 21.4). Both gracilis and rectus musculocutaneous flaps procedures are a major undertaking and leave considerable defects and scars at the donor site.

The theoretical solution to these problems is to use local full-thickness skin. In male transsexuals requesting vaginoplasty, the scrota provide the skin. Following orchidectomy and creation of a rectovesical cavity the scrota can be inverted to form a neo-vagina. Lilford et al (1988) have combined this principle with that of tissue expansion, thus converting the labia minora into scrota-like structures (Fig. 21.5). The principle of tissue expansion is simple and a copy of nature. Pregnancy increases the surface

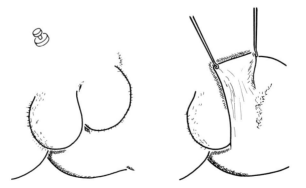

Fig. 21.5 Lilford's tissue expansion vaginoplasty. A balloon placed subcutaneously in the labia minora is slowly inflated (approximately 5 ml/day) (a). This creates sufficient skin (b) to line a cavity which can be made by blunt dissection between the rectum and bladder.

area of the abdominal wall and the breasts and following delivery and lactation both structures are left with excess skin. A balloon placed subcutaneously in the labia minora is slowly inflated via an integral catheter connected to an inflation reservoir and this causes the labia to swell slowly, analogous to slowly developing scrota. Active mitosis occurs in the skin over the tissue expander as it increases in size (Austad et al 1986). Approximately 5 ml of saline per day are added to the expander (depending on patient comfort) until approximately 120 ml is reached bilaterally. As chafing in the midline, infection, ulceration and ischaemia of the underlying skin can occur with all tissue expanders during this first stage, particularly if they are sited too superficially, it is important to inspect the vulva regularly and deflate the device as necessary. This may necessitate prolonged hospitalization. If infection does supervene (10–40% cases) the expanders must be removed and the procedure postponed for 6 months. Once it is considered that ample skin is available the patient is returned to the operating theatre and the expanders are further inflated acutely to 300 ml (to disrupt the pseudocapsule of fibromyoblasts which forms around the expanders). A rectovesical cavity is created by blunt dissection between the rectum and bladder. Two pedicle flaps (based posteriolaterally) are fashioned from the new skin (pseudoscrota) and the edges of these flaps are united to the fellow of the opposite side forming a pouch which can then be inverted to allow the skin to fall innermost. The apex of the flaps form the blind edge of the pouch (the vault of the new vagina). Some of the hair-bearing area may have to be incorporated in the vagina, but this does not seem to matter and leaves the patient with full-thickness vaginal skin which needs no dilatation, and creates very little disturbance of the perineum.

As with all these procedures the vagina tends to be dry. The only technique which leaves the vagina moist is transposition of the intestine.

Intestine grafts

The neovagina is created in the normal manner whilst a second surgeon opens the abdomen. The bowel is interrupted and a segment of either ileum (Baldwin 1904, Hanna 1987), caecum (Morton & Dewhurst 1984) or sigmoid (Goligher 1983), together with its mesentery, is transposed down into the pelvis to line the new vagina. The distal mucosa is sutured to the introitus, the cranial end of the neovagina closed and intestinal continuity restored (Fig. 21.6). It matters little which way round the gut lies it is important to maintain its vascular supply and to fashion the intestino-introital anastomosis in an oval rather than in a circle in the transverse plane thus preventing introital stenosis. This major procedure can leave the patient with an ugly stoma, which looks like a colostomy at the introitus through which mucosa often prolapses. Mucous secretion may be a problem but the patients often reassure their physicians that they do not mind. However, success rates are high. It is a one-stage procedure, and

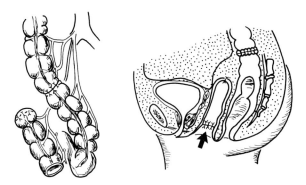

Fig. 21.6   Lining the neovagina with an intestinal graft. The neovagina is created by developing the rectovesical space whilst a second surgeon isolates a segment of bowel and transposes it down into the pelvis to line the new vagina. The distal mucosa is sutured to the introitus and the cranial end of the neovagina is closed.

functional results for the female are excellent (although satisfaction for the male may be poor). It is ideally suited to complex cloacal anomalies (see below), or to patients where previous attempts have failed or even created fistulae. Success is so high that despite the considerable morbidity and potential mortality, many choose it as their procedure of choice.

CLOACAL ABNORMALITIES

The Wolffian duct (mesonephric duct and future trigone, ureter and pelvic calyces), the Mullerian duct (paramesonephric duct and future vagina and uterus) and the hind gut all enter the cloaca. Failure of cloacal development produces a spectrum of abnormalities ranging from bladder exstrophy and a high recto-vaginal fistula to a bifid clitoris or shotgun perineum (Beazley 1974). The diagnosis is made in the early neonatal period.

A sacral radiograph is essential to exclude sacral agenesis, particularly as the associated absence of nervous outflow and subsequent urinary and rectal incontinence, which is not amenable to local treatment, significantly influences the prognosis. As far as the management of the vagina is concerned, the treatment is initially expectant, for the cloaca often enlarges considerably at puberty and is often of sufficient capacity to facilitate coitus.

Defects of the vagina and vulva

Fusion of the posterior vaginal introitus (labioscrotal folds) may be seen as an isolated anomaly or as part of the adrenogenital syndrome. Simple cut-back procedures are suitable for small defects. The skin covering the posterior introitus is divided vertically and posteriorly and repaired in a transverse plane (Fig. 21.7). More extensive defects require a flap-

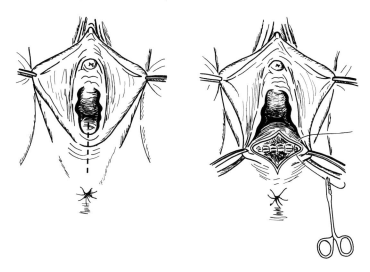

Fig. 21.7   The Heineke-Mikulich procedure. The fused posterior introitus is divided vertically and posteriorly and repaired in a transverse plane.

vaginoplasty; an inverted U-shaped incision in the posterior perineum (requiring a large base and a blunt point) provides a flap which can be folded inwards to cover a defect made by a vertical incision in the posterior vaginal wall (Fig. 21.8). This increases the vaginal diameter and produces a funnel in the posterior perineum, thereby relieving introital constriction.

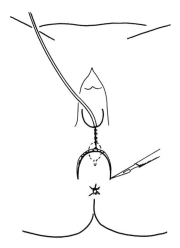

Fig. 21.8   The flap-vaginoplasty. The fused posterior introitus is divided vertically and the raw area is covered by advancing a perineal skin flap which is defined by the inverted U-shaped incision.

These operations are now often carried out with clitoral reduction in infancy but the long-term results of such early operations are not known.

In even more extensive cases, particularly in association with the adreno-genital syndrome, the lower vagina and urethra may share a common opening. This is best treated by a perineal pull-through vaginoplasty which involves fashioning a lower urethra and uniting the upper vaginal cavity with the introitus. The procedure entails placing a balloon catheter in the upper vaginal cavity, either by direct subcutaneous puncture or by passing it via the existing urethrovaginal fistula under direct urethroscopic vision. Anterior and posterior U-shaped skin flaps are created from the perineum with their bases away from the vagina. After a transverse introital incision, the vaginal cavity is created by blunt dissection which is directed to unite with the inflated balloon sited in the patient's existing upper vagina. The distal cuff of the high vagina is united to the posterior and anterior skin flaps which are folded inwards to line the cavity and cover the urethrovaginal fistula. The urethral meatus is transposed anteriorly (Fig. 21.9) (Hendren & Donahoe 1980).

Other abnormalities of the vagina include duplication, septa and a whole host of abnormalities associated with maternal ingestion of Stilboestrol during intrauterine life. Symptomatic vertical septa or those causing obstructed labour are simply divided. Transverse horizontal septa, if obstructing outflow or giving rise to a relative shortening of the vagina, may be excised. As excision of thick septa with vaginal advancement (as advocated by Jeffcoate 1969) may produce a ring of stenosis and vaginal

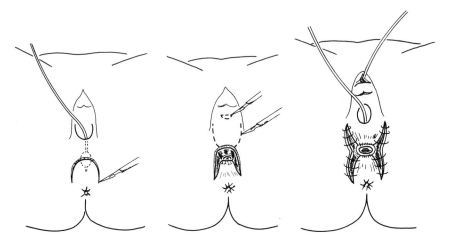

Fig. 21.9 The perineal-pull-through vaginoplasty. A balloon catheter (1) is placed in the upper vaginal cavity via the existing urethro-vaginal fistula. Posterior (a) and anterior (b) U-shaped perineal skin flaps are created and the vaginal block is relieved using blunt dissection after a transverse introital incision. The skin flaps are folded inwards to unite to the existing upper cavity and thus line the new conduit (c). An opening in the anterior flap (2) forms the urethral meatus which is now transposed anteriorly. (This anterior flap covers the urethrovaginal fistula and forms the anterior urethral wall.)

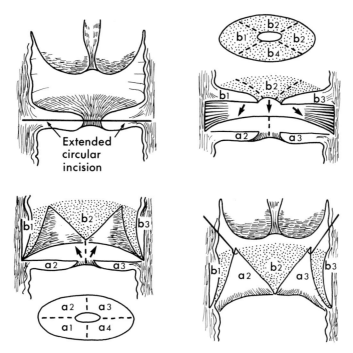

Fig. 21.10   Garcia's Z-plasty for a transverse vaginal septum. The layers of the septa are separated. Four radial incisions are made in the lower flap (at 0°, 90°, 180° and 270°) so as to form triangular tags (a_1, a_2, a_3, a_4). The upper layer is similarly incised but at 45°, 135°, 225° and 315° to form b_1, b_2, b_3, b_4. The upper tags are then transposed down and the lower flaps lifted up thus lining in the wall of the vagina.

shortening, a Z-plasty may be preferable (Garcia 1967). In this operation, the thick septum is perforated centrally, the upper and lower layers are separated and triangular flaps are fashioned by incising the upper and lower layers with alternative radial incisions 45° apart. The upper flaps are then transposed down and the lower flaps lifted up thus lining in the wall of the vagina with a circular saw-shaped suture line (Garcia 1967, Rankin 1973) (Fig. 21.10). An alternative is to leave a post-operative cylindrical stent intravaginally for 3 months (Dewhurst 1981).

Thin septa at the introitus such as an imperforate hymen are simply incised or excised depending on the patient's culture.

Defects of the posterior cloacal wall

Management of the defects of the posterior cloacal wall depend on the level at which the bowel opens into the urogenital sinus. In the majority of cases this is below the levators.

The anus may be ectopic, situated anteriorly, bringing the anal and vaginal orifice into close proximity creating an appearance like a double-barrelled shot gun. This anus is often so constricted that free discharge of faeces is prevented, thus necessitating manual dilatation, with or without a cutback. A cutback is performed by incising the anus in a posterior vertical direction in the sagittal plane and then closing it in a transverse plane. This Heineke–Mikulich manoeuvre widens the orifice and directs the anus and faeces posteriorly (compare with Fig. 21.7) and consequently cosmesis and subsequent soiling of the closely neighboring vaginal area is rarely a problem (Dewhurst 1968, 1981). Other anal abnormalities include a stenosed anus responding to dilatation, a membranous anus analogous to an imperforate hymen, and a covered anus, where the anus is covered by skin but a tract exists, directed towards the perineal raphe.

If the bowel enters the vagina above the levators, the matter is more serious. Depending upon other abnormalities the choice is between (i) an initial colostomy followed later by an anal pull-through; (ii) a one-stage dissection of the recto-vaginal fistulae and anal pull-through, or (iii) a permanent stoma for the serious cloacal abnormalities where the vagina, bladder and rectum enter a common cavity (Hendren & Donahoe 1980, Bennett et al 1972).

Defects of the anterior cloacal wall

Abnormalities of the anterior cloacal wall are due to the failure of the mesodermal structures to fuse. The urorectal fold emerges above the genital tubercles instead of below them and these abnormalities range from epispadais to bladder exstrophy (ectopia vesicae) (Uson et al 1959, Stanton 1974). The characteristic deformities of the severely affected female include a bifid clitoris (often separated as two distinct bodies) lying behind a shortened urethra which may be deficient of the internal and external sphincters. If the patient is continent, treatment is expectant. If the patient is incontinent, the urethra may be elevated from above or below, be lengthened and the bladder may be reconstructed or supported. For example in the Yung Dees operation a urethroplasty is achieved by excising an inverted triangle of mucosa from the trigone. The apex of the triangle is at the bladder neck and the base is at the level just below ureteric orifices. Following closure of this defect the large neo-urethra may be supported by a sling. Alternatively, the disorder may be so severe that the ureters need diversion.

Bladder exstrophy, the most severe defect, is characterized by absence of the infra-abdominal wall which incorporates the posterior wall of the bladder and ureteric orifices as well as a poorly defined bladder neck. An incompetent urethra, clitoral separation, displacement of the anus and umbilicus, separation of the pubic body with deficient anterior attachment of the pelvic floor and consequent rectogenital prolapse are also features. Urological treatment is paramount since without ureteric transplantation and excision of the potentially malignant exteriorized bladder, 50% of sufferers will succumb to recurrent pyelonephrosis before the age of 30. Uterine prolapse, a consequence of the defective pelvic floor, is frequently a serious associated problem even in the very young (Uson 1959, Overstreet & Hinmann 1955, Ramaswamy & Kadambari 1986) and it is often refractory to treatment.

The standard gynaecological procedure for congenital prolapse must be modified according to the patient's anatomy and other malformations. Well's rectopexy is particularly valuable and involves the insertion of a polyvinyl Teflon® sponge which is fixed to the sacrum at a laparotomy and wrapped 270° around the infra-peritoneal rectum (Nauton-Morgan 1962). Ripstein's operation may offer an extremely safe and simple alternative. In this operation the rectosigmoid junction is hitched up by a Teflon® sling in front of the sacrum just below the promontory (Porter 1962).

UTERINE ABNORMALITIES

While most patients with vaginal agenesis do not have a uterus, Mullerian tissue, ranging from primitive cords to a functioning organ, is occasionally present. If both the cervix and corpus uteri are present, then the creation of a new vagina will allow drainage and frequently conserve reproductive potential. However, the cervix is frequently absent and it is generally considered that the reproductive capability of such patients is hopeless. In most cases the rudimentary uterus should be excised, for functional endometriotic tissue which has no access to a healthy cervix is likely to produce cyclical pain, endometriosis (Rosenfeld & Lecher 1981) and chronic pelvic infection. Excision also prevents the occurrence of a future carcinoma in the organ (fortunately rare) and limits infection which usually occurs in a rudimentary uterus complicated by haematosalpinges and inadequate drainage. Despite these problems, a hysteroplasty and vaginal reconstruction has been attempted using a synchronous abdominal and vaginal approach. The hysteroplasty is performed at the time of vaginoplasty by incising the two Mullerian bulbs medially and excising the central oval tissue. The bulbs are then united in the midline over a T-tube and the lower end of the neo-uterus is then united with the upper end of the newly constructed vagina. Singh and Devi's (1983) report of a single pregnancy following such a technique is remarkable but exceptional.

Other uterine abnormalities are treated according to the symptoms they induce. Absence of the Mullerian system in the testicular feminizing syndrome may present as deep dyspareunia in a patient with a short vagina. Continued penetration in itself will increase vaginal length but vaginoplasty is sometimes required. Agenesis or arrested development of one Mullerian duct will result in a unicornate uterus which is quite capable of reproductive function although premature labour and growth retardation will be constant enemies of the obstetrician. A rudimentary horn containing endometrium which is not connected to the uterine cavity

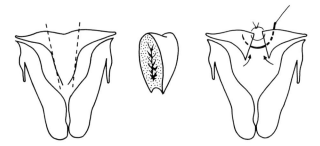

Fig. 21.11 Uteroplasty. The septum of the sub-septate uterus is excised and the myometrium repaired.

is best excised early in life. Not only will this relieve cyclical pain which is secondary to haematometria or retrograde dysmenorrhoea but it will also limit the occurrence of endometriosis.

Occasionally fusion abnormalities are associated with recurrent abortion. Uteroplasty (Strassman 1961, Genell & Sjorval 1959) may be associated with a successful outcome in a future pregnancy. The sub-septate uterus is exposed at laparotomy and incised from left to right with a coronal incision at the fundus exposing each cornu. The septum is divided under direct vision and the uterus repaired so that the scar now lies in an anterior-posterior plane. Alternatively, the septum may be excised (Jones & Jones 1953, Tompkins 1962, Khunda & Al-Juburi 1988) (Fig. 21.11). The post-operative placement of an intrauterine stent should reduce adhesion formation. Recently uterine septa have been vapourized by a laser under direct hysteroscopic vision.

CERVICAL ABNORMALITIES

A double cervix secondary to uterine didelphis needs no treatment. The practitioner only needs to be aware of the need for two intrauterine contraceptive devices and bilateral cervical cytological screening.

Cervical atresia in the presence of a functioning uterus and adequate vagina is rare (Geary & Weed 1973, Zarou et al 1973). Those teenagers who present with periodic pains benefit from a uterovaginal fistula before endometriosis, haematosalpingosis and adenomyosis develop. After pre-operative investigations to establish pelvic and renal anatomy, the uterus is exposed during a laparotomy, opened and the hysterotomy site is anastomozed to an opening in the vaginal vault. Attempts to recanalize a hypoplastic cervix (establishing a communication by passing a probe through the uterine fundus to connect with a synchronous-combined dissection from below) have been associated with one successful pregnancy. More commonly, the fistula closes and repeat surgery is necessary (Zarou et al 1973). The alternative is hysterectomy.

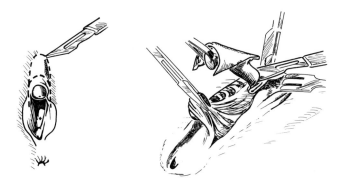

Fig. 21.12   Clitoroplasty. The clitoris is exposed and the corpora cavernosa is isolated from the nervous and vascular supply. The corpora is then excised and the skin defect is closed.

CLITORIS AND LABIA

Female intersex due to the adrenogenital syndrome or intrauterine exposure of androgens frequently results in clitoromegaly and fused labia. These genetically female and potentially fertile infants are incapable of achieving normal sexual and reproductive function as men despite their initial appearances. Cosmetic clitoroplasty is offered during the early neonatal period once any potentially lethal salt-losing ATCH-induced condition is controlled. The skin over the dorsal clitoris is excised, exposing the corpora. The nervous and vascular supply entering the glands from the ventral surface are preserved and isolated from corpora cavernosa which are then removed. The gland is returned to its original site and the skin defect is closed (Goodwin 1969, Randolph & Hugh 1970, Kumar et al 1974, Shaw 1977) (Fig. 21.12). Clitoroplasty is superior to amputation which may (although not invariably) render the patient anorgasmic (Money et al 1955) and it is superior to bending the phallus ventrally (burring it; Lattimer 1961) as this may lead to painful erections.

Providing micturition is unimpeded, fused labial folds may be left until puberty when the tissue is well oestrogenized, when simple manipulation augmented with oestrogen cream will usually achieve separation. Extensive plastic procedures involving labial flaps (Dewhurst & Gordon 1969) are only rarely required. The long-term results of operations performed in infancy, or the time of clitoroplasty, are unknown and subsequent surgery is difficult if the original operation was unsuccessful.

FALLOPIAN TUBES

The common hydatids of Morgagni are remnants of the terminal ends of the Mullerian ducts. They rarely undergo torsion and are best left undisturbed. Atresia and underdeveloped ostia are rare causes of infertility and the treatment for these patients has been revolutionized by in vitro fertilization. Alternatively, salpingostomy, particularly if constructed under the operating microscope, may be attempted but the procedure is associated with little success because the poor development is not always limited solely to the ostia.

UROLOGICAL TRACT REMNANTS

Remnants of the pronephros or mesonephros (either epoophoron, paroophoron or Gartner's cyst) if symptomatic may be marsupialized. Excision is for the brave and uneducated.

GONAD

Absence of function in ovarian mesenchyme, whether due to dysgenesis or aplasia, requires hormone replacement therapy. Many regimes are available (Tscherne 1983, Lucky 1970, McDonaugh 1972) but the cyclical oral contraceptive pill is popular. Unopposed oestrogen can lead to carcinoma of the endometrium (Wilkinson et al 1973) and troublesome endometrial polyps (DeKoos 1974, Dewhurst et al 1975).

Dysgenic gonads containing a Y-chromosome (especially if they are H-Y antigen positive) need excision. Thirty percent of these gonads have malignant potential and these tumours will affect young women (Manuel et al 1976). Some patients who are psychologically adjusted to amenorrhoea may prefer unopposed oestrogen therapy via implants or patches and thus request hysterectomy at the time of the prophylactic oophorectomy. However, a hysterectomy should be avoided because the advent of donor zygote intrafallopian tube transfer, and its success in agonadal females means that they are quite capable of mothering a child even if the genetic material may not be their own.

Those patients afflicted with testicular intersex and ambiguous genitalia have a smaller risk of malignancy but still need orchidectomy.

CONCLUSION

The greatest progress in the field of the treatment of gynaecological congenital malformation has been the advance in physicians' thinking. Acknowledging the need for pre-operative assessment of all patients has avoided many of the disasters of the recent past. Particular care is now taken to investigate the patient's psychology, her aspirations, biochemistry, genotype and full anatomy of her genital tract. It is widely accepted that the first attempt to correct an abnormality is the most valuable one and it is now unacceptable for workers untrained in the field to 'have a go'.

REFERENCES

Abbe R 1898 A new method of creating a vagina in a case of congenital absence. Medical Record of New York 836–838

Ashworth M F, Morton K E, Dewhurst Sir J, Lilford R J, Bates R G 1986 Vaginoplasty using amnion. Obstetrics and Gynecology 67(3): 443–446

Austad E D, Thomas S B, Pasyk K 1986 Tissue expansion: divided or loan? Plastic and Reconstructive Surgery 78(1): 63–67

Baldwin J F 1904 The formation of an artificial vagina by intestinal transplantation. Annals of Surgery 40: 398–403

Baramki T A 1984 Treatment of congenital anomalies in girls and women. Journal of Reproductive Medicine 29(6): 376–384

Beazley J M 1974 Congenital malformations of the genital tract (excluding intersex). Clinics in Obstetrics and Gynaecology 1(3): 571–592

Bennett R C, Hughes E S R, Cuthbertson A M 1972 Long-term review of function following pull-through operations of the rectum. British Journal of Surgery 59(9): 723–725

Broadbent T R, Woolfe R M 1977 Congenital absence of the vagina: reconstruction without operation. British Journal of Plastic Surgery 30: 118–122

Cairns T S, De Villiers W 1980 Vaginoplasty. South African Medical Journal 57: 50–55

DeKoos E B 1974 Oestrogen-induced endometrial hyperplasia in gonadal dysgenesis. Proceedings of the Royal Society of Medicine 67: 590–591

Dewhurst C J 1968 Congenital malformations of the genital tract in childhood. The Journal of Obstetrics and Gynaecology of the British Commonwealth 75(4): 377–391

Dewhurst Sir J 1981 Genital tract obstruction. Pediatric Clinics of North America 28(2): 311–344

Dewhurst Sir J 1987 Intersexuality. In: Whitfield C R (ed) Dewhurst's textbook of obstetrics and gynaecology for postgraduates. Blackwell Scientific Press, Oxford, pp 25–39

Dewhurst C J, DeKoos E B, Haines R M 1975 Replacement-hormone therapy in gonadal dysgenesis. British Journal of Obstetrics and Gynaecology 82: 412–416

Dewhurst C J, Gordon R R 1969 The Intersexual disorders. Baillière Tindall & Cassell, London, pp 82–83

Dhall K 1984 Amnion graft for the treatment of congenital absence of the vagina. British Journal of Obstetrics and Gynaecology 91: 279–282

Formigli L, Formigli G 1986 In vivo fertilized ovum donated successfully to a woman without ovaries. Lancet i: 747

Frank R T 1938 The formation of an artificial vagina without operation. American Journal of Obstetrics and Gynecology 35: 1053–1055

Garcia R F 1967 Z-plasty for correction of congenital transverse vaginal septum. American Journal of Obstetrics and Gynecology 99(8): 1164–1165

Geary W L, Weed J C 1973 Congenital atresia of the uterine cervix. Obstetrics and Gynecology 42: 213–217

Genell S, Sjovall A 1959 The Strassmann operation: results obtained in 58 cases. Acta Obstetrica et Gynecologica Scandinavica 38: 477–486

Goligher J C 1983 The use of pedicled transplants of sigmoid or other parts of the intestinal tract for vaginal construction. Annals of the Royal College of Surgeons of England 65: 353–355

Goodwin W E 1969 Surgical revision of the enlarged clitoris. In: de la Camp H G, Linder F, Trede M (eds) American College Surgeons and Deutsche Gellschaft Fur Chirurgie. Springer, New York, pp 253–269

Hanna M K 1987 Vaginal construction. Urology 29(3): 272–275

Harkins J L, Gysler M, Cowell C A 1981 Anatomical amenorrhea: the problems of congenital vaginal agenesis and its correction. Pediatric Clinics of North America 28(2): 345–354

Hauser G A, Schreiner W E 1961 Das Mayer–Rokitansky–Kuster Syndrome. Schweizerische Medizinische Wochenschrift 12: 281

Hendren W H, Donahoe P K 1980 Correction of congenital abnormalities of the vagina and perineum. Journal of Pediatric Surgery 15(6): 751–763

Holmstrom H, Heyden G, Johanson B 1976 Congenital absence of the vagina: a clinical, histological and histochemical study on 17 patients with graft-constructed vaginas. Scandinavian Journal of Plastic and Reconstitutional Surgery 10(3): 231–236

Imrie J E A, Kennedy J H, Holmes J D, McGrouther D A 1986 Intraepithelial neoplasia arising in an artificial vagina: case report. British Journal of Obstetrics and Gynaecology 93: 886–888

Ingram J M 1981 The bicycle seat-stool and the treatment of vaginal agenesis and stenosis: a preliminary report. American Journal of Obstetrics and Gynecology 140: 867–873

Jackson G W 1959 Primary carcinoma in an artificial vagina—report of a case. British Journal of Plastic Surgery 14: 534–536

Jackson I 1965 The artificial vagina. Journal of Obstetrics and Gynaecology of the British Commonwealth 72: 336–341

Jeffcoate T N A 1969 Advancement of the upper vagina in the treatment of haematocolpos and haematometria caused by vaginal aplasia. Pregnancy following construction of an artificial vagina. Journal of Obstetrics and Gynaecology of the British Commonwealth 76(11): 961–968

Jones H W Jr, Jones G E S 1953 Double uterus as an etiological factor in repeated abortion: indications for surgical repair. American Journal of Obstetrics and Gynecology 65: 325–339

Khunda S, Al-Juburi A 1988 Metroplasty—a new approach. Journal of Obstetrics and Gynaecology 8(4): 343–344

Kumar H, Kiefer J H, Rosenthal I E, Clarke S S 1974 Clitoroplasty: experience during a 19-year period. Journal of Urology 111(1): 81–84

Lattimer J K 1961 Relocation and recession of the enlarged clitoris with preservation of the glans: an alternative to amputation. Journal of Urology 86: 113–116

Lacey C G, Stern J L, Feigenbaum S, Hill E C, Braga C A 1988 Vaginal reconstruction after exenteration with use of gracilis myocutaneous flaps: the University of California, San Francisco experience. American Journal of Obstetrics and Gynecology 158(6): 1278–1284

Lilford R J, Sharpe D T, Thomas D F M 1988 Use of tissue expansion techniques to create skin flaps for vaginoplasty: Case report. British Journal of Obstetrics and Gynaecology 95: 402–407

Lilford R J, Johnson N, Batchelor A 1989 A new operation for vaginal agenisis; construction of a neo-vagina from a rectus abdominus musculocutaneous flap. British Journal of Obstetrics and Gynaecology 96: 1089–1094

Lucky A W, Marynick S P, Rebar R W et al 1970 Replacement of oral ethinyloestridiol therapy for gonadal dysgenesis: growth and androgen studies. Acta Endocrinologica 91(3): 519–528

Manuel M, Katayama K P, Jones H W 1976 The age of occurrence of gonadal tumors in intersex patients with a Y-chromosome. American Journal of Obstetrics and Gynecology 124(3): 293–299

McCraw J B, Kurtzman L 1988 Vaginal and pelvic reconstruction with distally based rectus abdominis myocutaneous flaps: discussion. Plastic and Reconstructive Surgery 81(1): 71–73

McGraw J B, Massey F M, Shanklin K D, Horton C E 1976 Vaginal reconstruction with gracilis myocutaneous flaps. Plastic and Reconstructive Surgery 58(2): 176–183

McDonaugh P H 1972 Gonadal dysgenesis and its variants. Pediatric Clinics of North America 19(3): 631–662

McIndoe A H, Banister J B 1938 An operation for the cure of congenital absence of the vagina. Journal of Obstetrics and Gynecology of the British Commonwealth 45: 490–494

Miller N F, Stout W 1957 Congenital absence of the vagina. Obstetrics and Gynecology 8(1): 48–54

Money J, Hampson J G, Hampson J L 1955 Hermaphroditism: recommendations concerning assignment of sex, change of sex, and psychologic management. Bulletin of the Johns Hopkins Hospital 97: 284–299

Morton K E, Dewhurst Sir J 1984 The use of bowel to create a vagina: a follow-up study. Pediatric and Adolescent Gynaecology 2(1): 51–61

Morton K E, Dewhurst Sir J 1986 Human amnion in the treatment of vaginal malformations. British Journal of Obstetrics and Gynaecology 93(1): 50–54

Naunton-Morgan C 1962 The use of Ivalon® sponge. Proceedings of the Royal Society of Medicine 55: 1084–1086

Overstreet E W, Hinmann F 1955 Some gynecologic aspects of bladder exstrophy. Transactions of the Pacific Coast Obstetrical and Gynecological Society 23: 102–109

Parrott T S, Scheflan M, Hester T R 1980 Reduction clitoroplasty and vaginal construction in a single operation. Urology 16(4): 367–369

Phelan J T, Counsellor V S, Greene L F 1953 Deformities of the urinary tract with congenital absence of the vagina. Surgery Gynecology and Obstetrics 97(1): 1–3

Porter N 1962 Collective results for operations for rectal prolapse. Proceedings of the Royal Society of Medicine 55: 1087–1091

Ramaswamy S, Kadambari 1986 Mullerian agenesis with vaginal prolapse. Case report. British Journal of Obstetrics and Gynaecology 93: 640–641

Randolph J G, Hung W 1970 Relocation clitoroplasty in females with hypertrophied clitoris. Journal of Pediatric Surgery 5: 224–231

Rankin R P 1973 The use of Z-plasty in gynecologic operations: case reports. American Journal of Obstetrics and Gynecology 117(2): 231–232

Rosenfeld D L, Lecher B D 1981 Endometriosis in a patient with Rokitansky–Kuster–Hauser syndrome. American Journal of Obstetrics and Gynecology 139(1): 105

Shaw A 1977 Subcutaneous reduction clitoroplasty. Journal of Pediatric Surgery 12: 331–338

Singh K J, Devi L Y 1983 Pregnancy following surgical correction of nonfused Mullerian bulbs and absent vagina. American Journal of Obstetrics and Gynecology 61(2): 267–269

Smith M R 1983 Vaginal aplasia: therapeutic options. American Journal of Obstetrics and Gynecology 146(5): 488–494

Song R, Wang X, Zhou G 1982 Reconstruction of the vagina with sensory function. Clinics in Plastic Surgery 9(1): 105–108

Stanton S L 1974 Gynecologic complications of epispadias and bladder exstrophy. American Journal of Obstetrics and Gynecology 119(6): 749–754

Strassman E O 1961 Operation for double uterus and endometrial atresia. Clinics in Obstetrics and Gynaecology 4: 240

Tamaya T, Yamamoto T, Nakata Y, Ohno Y, Okada H 1984 The use of pelvic peritoneum in the construction of a vagina: 10 cases. Asia-Oceania Journal of Obstetrics and Gynaecology 10(4): 439–443

Tobin G R, Day T G 1988 Vaginal and pelvic reconstruction with distally based rectus abdominis myocutaneous flaps. Plastic and Reconstructive Surgery 81(1): 62–70

Tompkins P 1962 Comments on the bicornuate uterus and twinning. Surgical Clinics of North America 42: 1049–1061

Tscherne G 1983 Proceedings of the 10th World Congress of Gynecology and Obstetrics, San Francisco, October, Academy professional Information Science (ed.) Newton M

Uson A C, Lattimer J K, Melicow M M 1959 Types of exstrophy of urinary bladder and concomitant malformations. Pediatrics 23: 927–934

Wang T-N, Whetzel T, Mathes S J, Vasconez L O 1987 A fasciocutaneous flap for vaginal and perineal reconstruction. Plastic and Reconstructive Surgery 80(1): 95–102

Wilkinson E J, Friedrich E G Jr, Mattingly R, Regali J A, Garancis J C 1973 Turner's syndrome with endometrial adenocarcinoma and stilboestrol therapy. Obstetrics and Gynecology 42: 193–200

Willemsen W N, Mastboom J L, Thomas C M, Rolland R 1985 Absorption of 17 beta-estradiol in a neovagina constructed from the peritoneum. European Journal of Obstetrics Gynecology and Reproductive Biology 19(4): 247–253

Williams E A 1970 Vulvo-vaginoplasty. Proceedings of the Royal Society of Medicine 63: 1046

Williams E A 1964 Congenital absence of the vagina: a simple operation for its relief. Journal of Obstetrics and Gynaecology of the British Commonwealth 71(4): 511–516

Zarou G S, Esposito J M, Zarou D M 1973 Pregnancy following the surgical correction of congenital atresia of the cervix. International Journal of Obstetrics and Gynecology 4: 143–146

22. Barrier methods of contraception

Yunus Tayob   John Guillebaud

INTRODUCTION

Barrier contraceptives are among the oldest and simplest means by which women and men have attempted to control their fertility. The ancient Chinese, Egyptians, Greeks, Hebrews, Indians, Japanese and Romans knew of an extensive array of barrier preparations for fertility control (Himes 1970). These remained the principal methods of contraception until the 1960s and '70s when widespread availability of the oral contraceptive pill and the intrauterine device was accompanied by a decline in the use of barrier methods.

Recent concern about the side-effects of oral contraceptives and intrauterine contraceptive devices has revived interest in barrier methods. Moreover, the increase in the incidence of pelvic inflammatory disease in the past decade, particularly in women aged 15–20 years (Westrom 1980), has stimulated interest in a 'return to barriers' (Serlin 1981). Since bacteria can be transported to the upper genital tract by spermatozoa (Toth et al 1984) impeding the entry of sperm should theoretically reduce the risk of such infection. There is clear evidence to indicate a reduction in the incidence of pelvic inflammatory disease in users of barrier methods compared to non-users (Harris et al 1980).

Human immunodeficiency virus (HIV) is mainly transmitted by sexual intercourse (Fischl et al 1987) and HIV has been isolated from semen (Zagury et al 1985). Indeed, 4 out of 8 women receiving semen from an infected donor in an infertility clinic in Sydney, Australia, were found to have antibodies to HIV (Stewart et al 1985). In vitro studies have shown that condoms prevent the passage of HIV (Conant et al 1986). The commonly used spermicides nonoxynol-9 (Hicks et al 1985) and benzalkonium chloride (Mills 1988) inactivate the virus in laboratory studies.

After more than two decades of scientific eclipse following the introduction of hormonal methods, research directed towards developing improved barrier methods has only recently been initiated. The main challenge will be to develop methods which as well as being effective contraceptives, will protect against sexually transmitted diseases, with minimal infringement of the spontaneity of sexual intercourse.

371

BACKGROUND

The concept of barrier contraception dates back to the time when a cause and effect relationship between sexual intercourse and pregnancy was first recognized. The ancient Greeks believed that the man provided the seed and that the woman was simply the incubator, providing the place for it to grow. In 1678 Anton van Leeuwenhoek, the inventor of the microscope, was the first person to report the existence of animalcula or sperm in semen. This, probably, was the beginning of the scientific basis of contraception, as van Leeuwenhoek began working on compounds that would inactivate sperm. One of the first substances used successfully was rain water but long before this a wide range of substances and procedures had been tried empirically.

1100 BC. The ancient Chinese suggested that a woman assume complete passivity during intercourse. They advised that 'at the moment of ejaculation draw a deep breath and think of other things.'

1550–1850 BC. Egyptian papyri dating back to these times are the first written instructions on the use of lactic acid, honey, natron (native sodium carbonate) and a variety of other irrigating, plugging and gummy substances to be inserted into the vagina before intercourse. Prescriptions of a mixture containing either elephant or crocodile dung first appear in the ancient papyri and continue to be mentioned by writers in the Mediterranean area over a span of 3000 years.

Avicenna, an Arab physician, proposed that 'the woman rise up when intercourse is finished and take several jumps backwards, sneezing at the same time and endeavouring to jump higher each time.' He warned that 'great care must be taken to jump backwards to dislodge the sperm for jumping forwards would cause the sperm to remain where it is.' Rhazes, who inherited Avicenna's reputation as a great scholar and physician, added that the woman should call out in a loud voice at the same time.

1st century AD. Dioscarides mentions the vaginal use of peppermint in lemon juice mixed with honey in his writings.

2nd century. Soranos, in his classical gynaecological text, lists oil, honey, cedar, gum, various fruit acids, and astringents like alum as vaginal contraceptives. The Talmud advocates the insertion of a moistened sponge into the vagina before intercourse.

4th century. Aristotle recommended the use of a cervical plug made of oil of cedar and frankincense in olive oil.

6th century. Aetios, the Greek physician, produced a pessary partially made of the pulp of pomegranates or figs.

8th century. Indian writers mention the use of rock salt dipped in honey or oil. From ancient Egypt to the present, various substances often highly acidic have been employed as vaginal contraceptives.

BARRIER METHODS

Barrier methods of contraception consist of a mechanical and/or a chemical component.

Diaphragm

Dr C. Hasse, a German physician, is credited with inventing the present-day diaphragm. In 1882, using the pseudonym Wilhelm P. J. Mensinga, he wrote an article (Himes 1970) on an effective contraceptive method called 'facultative sterility' which described the use of the diaphragm. Its use spread in Europe until its introduction to England via Holland, explaining why it came to be called the 'Dutch cap'. The first mention of the device in England is attributed to H.A. Albutt, a Leeds physician who in 1887 wrote a pamphlet called *The Wife's Handbook* in which he gave instructions for use of the diaphragm (Himes 1970). For this he was struck off the Medical Register and because of this kind of opposition diaphragms and other caps only became readily available in the 1920s. The diaphragm reached the peak of its popularity around 1959 when it was reported that the method was used by about 12% of British couples. In 1965 the figure was 10%, usage then declined rapidly with the introduction of the pill and in 1982 only 4% of women used this method in the UK (Guillebaud 1985).

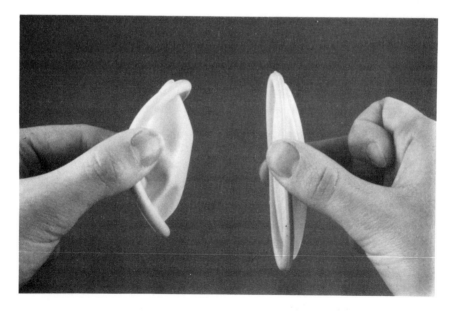

Fig. 22.1   Arcing-spring diaphragm (left) and flat-spring diaphragm (right). Reproduced with permission from Cilag Limited.

Diaphragms come in many sizes and in three major designs:

1. *Flat-spring diaphragm*. This has a firm or watch spring and is easily fitted, remaining in a horizontal plane on compression. It is suitable for most normal vaginas and is often tried first.

2. *Coil-spring diaphragm*. This has a spiral coiled spring which makes it softer than the flat spring but it may be more difficult for the woman to control during insertion.

3. *Arcing 'all-flex' diaphragm*. This combines features of both the above and consists of a rubber dome with a firm double metal spring. This combination of flat and coil spring produces an arc (see Fig. 22.1) when viewed from the side as the diaphragm is compressed. This makes it useful when the woman has difficulty getting the device to cover the cervix. This diaphragm is particularly suitable for women who tend to insert the device into the anterior fornix, like some with a retroverted uterus.

Generally diaphragms lie diagonally across the cervix, the vaginal vault and much of the anterior vaginal wall. They are available in 5 mm incremental sizes from 55–100 mm.

Since 'ballooning' of the upper two-thirds of the vagina is known to occur during intercourse (Johnson et al 1974) it is not possible to establish a sperm-tight fit between the diaphragm and the vaginal wall. Therefore on a theoretical basis, the main functions of the diaphragm are:

1. To act as a retainer of spermicide at the most important site namely the external cervical os (i.e. preventing its dissemination elsewhere during the movements of intercourse);

2. To keep sperm away from the receptive alkaline cervical mucus, long enough for them to die in the acid vagina;

3. Preventing this mucus from reaching the acid vagina and thereby tending to make it less spermicidal and providing a protective film for the sperm in which they could reach the external os;

4. Preventing physical aspiration of the sperm into the cervix and uterus.

Use of this very practical method requires careful training of the clinicians (often nurses) who must fit the correct size, assess the retropubic ledge, and the ease with which the cervix can safely be covered, and above all, of the women themselves. For a full account see Chapter 3 in Guillebaud (1985) and the instruction leaflet of the Family Planning Association. There is, however, no substitute for 'apprenticeship' training in by an experienced teacher in a clinic. The current Family Planning Association guidelines are that vaginal occlusive methods be used in conjunction with spermicides. Moreover it is believed, without any scientific basis, that spermicides add significantly to the effectiveness of caps and diaphragms.

Typical instructions, such as those of the FPA and those included in diaphragm packages (Fig. 22.2), state that:

1. A diaphragm may be inserted up to 3 hours before intercourse. If the delay will be longer, an extra dose of spermicide is advised (e.g. by pessary).

2. It should be used with two 2–3 inch strips of spermicide placed on each side of the diaphragm and some spread around the leading edge.

3. It must be left in place for at least 6 hours and, ideally, be removed no more than 24 hours after intercourse.

4. In the event of repeated intercourse, an additional applicator-full of spermicide or a pessary must be placed within the vagina.

Many of these assumptions have never been tested in proper controlled trials. Recently, some Family Planning practitioners have questioned the importance of spermicides (Craig & Hepburn 1982, Serlin 1981). The Australian Family Association, for example, leaves use of spermicide to the patients' choice. Pending more data most authorities feel that spermicides should continue to be used. Few researchers and women are willing to test the effectiveness of a diaphragm used without a spermicide. Such a study is currently in progress at the Margaret Pyke Centre, London. The pharmaceutical industry is attempting to make spermicides more acceptable by making them less 'messy', improving or eliminating the smell and taste thereby reducing the problems of non-compliance with which they are associated.

Effectiveness

When used properly at every episode of intercourse, a diaphragm plus spermicide can be highly effective with failure rates varying from 2–15 per 100 woman years (see Table 22.1). Lower failure rates tend to occur in older women, in highly motivated women and in those who have already been using the method for more than 5 months. All these special factors applied in the Oxford/FPA study into which such highly selected women were recruited (Vessey et al 1982). In the second study giving atypically

Table 22.2 Effectiveness of the diaphragm. Failure rater per 100 women years

Author	Number of women	Age & status	Pregnancy rate
Bounds et al 1984	123	90% 20–34 yrs 90% married/ consensual union	10.5
Edelman et al 1984	721	47% < 25 yrs 49% unmarried	12.5
Lane et al 1976	2168	61% 21–34 yrs 71% unmarried	1.9–2.2
Vessey et al 1982	4217	25–39 yrs all married	1.9

good results (Lane et al 1976) there is some doubt as to exposure, i.e. frequency and regularity of intercourse in some of the recruited population. The results of these two studies are not therefore applicable to many young women especially those setting out to use this method for the first time. Better estimates for such women of about 10–12.5 per 100 woman years come from the studies by Edelman (1984) and Bounds et al (1983). Results of selected studies are listed in Table 22.1. This method of contraception is therefore ideal for those in whom a pregnancy will not be totally unwanted and older, highly motivated women who will use the method with care and at all times. It also provides useful protection against sexually transmitted diseases (STDs) (see below).

Protection against cervical carcinoma

There is clear evidence that the use of a barrier method of contraception may reduce the risk of cervical carcinoma. In the Oxford/FPA study the incidence rate among diaphragm-users was 0.17 per 1000 woman years as compared to 0.95 in oral contraceptive pill-users and 0.87 in those using an intrauterine contraceptive device (Vessey et al 1976).

Protection against STD

Diaphragms protect against STD partly because they are usually used with a spermicide and partly because they act as a mechanical barrier to sperm and ascending infections. Diaphragms are not protective against the spread of HIV by sexual intercourse because of:

1. The contact between vaginal secretions and the male partner;
2. Loss of contact between the vagina and the diaphragm due to ballooning of the upper vagina;
3. Contact between semen and the vagina.

The diaphragm is not suitable for women with:

1. An anatomical abnormality of the vagina, cervix or uterus (e.g. fibroids grossly distorting pelvic anatomy);
2. A large cystocele, rectocele or uterine prolapse;
3. Repeated urinary tract infections which may be aggravated by diaphragm use;
4. Allergy to latex rubber or spermicide;
5. Aversion to touching the genital area.

The first three may not contraindicate the other caps, to be described.

Cervical/vault caps

Casanova (1725–1798) was perhaps the most famous advocate of cervical caps when, in the mid-eighteenth century he recommended the use of a squeezed out half-lemon inserted over the cervix. This is an early example of the use of cap and spermicide as the critic acid acted as the latter (Guttmacher 1973). Earlier than this women of Sumatra moulded opium into a cup-like shape and inserted it high into the vagina covering the cervix. Chinese and Japanese women covered the cervix with oiled silk paper (misugami). Cervical caps made from beeswax melted and moulded into 5–10 mm shapes were made by Hungarian women.

Friederick Adolphe Wilde, a German gynaecologist, made the first cervical caps from wax impressions of the cervix in 1838 (Himes 1970). In the UK, Allbut in *The Wife's Handbook* was the first to describe use of the cap. Marie Stopes recommended the cap in preference to the diaphragm as she felt that the latter produced uncomfortable distension of the vagina.

The present day cervical caps are small, firm cup-shaped structures which are placed over the cervix. Three types of caps are currently in use:

1. The *cervical cap* is a thimble-shaped cap that fits snugly over the cervix. The most commonly used type is the cavity rim cap with an integral thickened rim incorporating a small groove. The available internal diameters of the upper rim are 22, 25, 28 and 31 mm.

2. The *Dumas* or *vault cap* is a relatively shallow, bowl-shaped rubber cap with a thinner dome through which the cervix can be felt. It covers without fitting so closely to the cervix as the cervical cap. Five sizes ranging from 55–75 mm in 5 mm steps are available.

3. The *Vimule* has features of both the vault and cervical cap. It is available in three sizes, 45, 48 and 51 mm.

Cervical/vault caps function by occluding the cervix and impeding sperm entry into the endocervical canal. It is recommended that spermicides be used in conjunction with these devices. The bowl should be one-third filled with spermicide. However, the same doubts exist over the absolute necessity for this, as with diaphragm use. Unlike the latter, which is maintained in place by spring action, cervical/vault caps are held in place by suction. The comments above about the vital importance of training of clinicians and of good teaching of all new users apply here as much as to the diaphragm.

Caps have the following advantages over the diaphragm:

1. They can be used in women with uterovaginal prolapse, poor muscle tone or absence of a good retropubic ledge;

2. They have no rim, a feature sometimes felt by the male partner;

3. They are less likely to produce any urinary symptoms, making them particularly useful for a woman with recurrent cystitis;

4. Fitting is unaffected by changes in the size of the vagina, either during intercourse or as a result of changes in body weight.

Despite all this, the method still remains very underused and has declined in popularity over the years. Koch (1982) of America estimated that 50% of women motivated to use the cap are unable to do so because of difficulty in obtaining a good fit or dislodgment during intercourse. Family planning practitioners are also to blame as many are not trained or even motivated to offer this as a method. Renewed interest has been shown particularly in America probably as a result of the withdrawl of intrauterine devices, further limiting their choice of contraception.

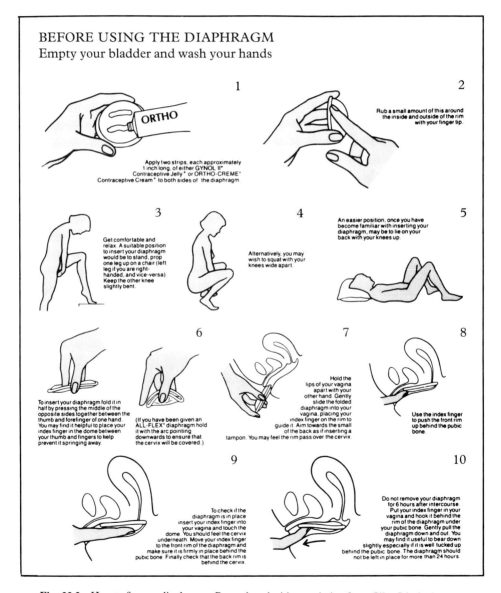

Fig. 22.2   How to fit your diaphragm. Reproduced with permission from Cilag Limited.

Effectiveness

Data until the late 1970s came from studies on the use of firm cervical devices made from plastic, metal and ivory. Failure rates ranged from 5–10% (Lehfeldt 1949). There have only been a few studies on the current cervical devices: Tietze et al (1953) estimated the failure rate to be 7.6 per 100 women years. More recently, efficacy ranges from 8.4 pregnancies per 100 women years (one-year cumulative life-table rate) (Koch 1982) to 19.6 per 100 women years (Boehm 1983) have been reported. The results of studies performed in the 40s and 50s found that cervical erosions associated with cervical caps were not the result of cap use but were present beforehand. Moreover, Koch (1982) found that of 31 women with cervical erosions who used the cap, 23 showed an improvement after cap use.

No serious side-effects appear to be associated with the use of the cap. Some women have reported irritation and this could be related to use of either the spermicide or a reaction to rubber. The cavity rim cap or vimule has, because of its design, been known to cause suction rings around the cervix, lesions of the portio vaginalis ranging from erythematous impressions to abrasions and lacerations. Bernstein (1982) reported these findings amongst women who wore the cap for up to 7 days in some cases. Both ulcers and other vaginal trauma from the rim of the diaphragm can also rarely occur. Three diaphragm cases in 10 years, have been observed at the Margaret Pyke Centre, where approximately 3000 women are supervised using caps, mainly the diaphragm, each year (Guillebaud, personal communication).

Other (personal) problems associated with cervical cap (and also in some couples, with diaphragm) use are:

1. Odour from vaginal secretions especially if the cap has been in place for several days;
2. Difficulty in insertion and removal of the cap;
3. Discomfort during intercourse to either partner;
4. Fear of dislodgement by some couples.

Although these are not serious problems they may affect acceptibility and use-effectiveness.

Sponge

Although now available as a marketed contraceptive, the practice of inserting a moistened sponge into the vagina before intercourse has been advocated since early biblical times. A section of the Talmud from the 2nd century AD recommended the insertion into the vagina of a sponge called a 'Mukh' to prevent conception (Preuss 1978). The first mention of use of a sponge moistened with a spermicidal substance was in Europe in 1732 (Himes 1970). The first of the present day sponges exposed to proper clinical trials did not contain a spermicide but was made of collagen of animal origin and, unlike the Today® sponge, was intended to be reusable. Apart from its role in covering the cervix it was supposed to absorb the ejaculate. However there were high pregnancy rates and problems with acceptability. Some couples noted vaginal dryness and discomfort during intercourse, and in addition, a fear of infection restricted its use (Chavpil 1979). Researchers found motile sperm within the endocervical canal. This encouraged research into developing a spermicide-impregnated sponge which resulted in the Today® sponge, a polyurethane sponge containing nonoxynol-9.

This is a mushroom-shaped sponge containing 1 g of nonoxynol-9. It has a dimple on the upper surface designed to fit snugly over the cervix and a loop to facilitate removal. The sponge is intended to have three types of contraceptive action:

1. To release spermicide during intercourse,
2. To absorb ejaculate,
3. To block access of sperm to the cervix.

It requires no medical supervision and can be purchased over the counter. The woman simply moistens it with tap water and inserts it into the vagina so that it covers the cervix. Use-effectiveness appears to be in the range of 9–25 per 1000 women years. Results from multicentre clinical trials have been variable. A USA study (Edelman et al 1984) yielded failure rates of about 17 per 100 women years for the sponge and 12.5 for the diaphragm, a significant difference. Unfortunately, about 20% of the women were lost to follow-up.

In the Margaret Pyke study, 251 women were recruited and were randomly allocated to the sponge and the diaphragm (Bounds & Guillebaud 1984). The observed failure rates, with 99% follow-up, were 25 for the sponge and 11 for the diaphragm (1-year cumulative life-table rates).

Since the USA and UK studies indicated high method-failure rates despite optimal teaching, it would appear that this method should only be recommended for those women who have a relatively reduced innate fertility or those women for whom another pregnancy would not be totally unwelcome. Those most suitable for this method are (Guillebaud, 1985):

1. Older women. Fertility declines most steeply after the age of 45. The sponge may be appropriate from the age of 45 through until one year after the menopause.

2. Lactating women. The method could be used until uterine bleeding begins to return at weaning.

3. Spacers. Those women who are spacing their family and do not want the most effective contraception.

4. Women experiencing secondary amenorrhoea before its spontaneous resolution.

5. Those using another form of contraceptive. The cap can be used as an adjunct to other methods such as the IUCD.

It should not normally be recommended for young and highly fertile women who are not ready for a pregnancy. The high failure rate, more than 20 times that of the combined oral contraceptive pill, must clearly be pointed out to this group of young women.

Condom

This oldest reliable method of contraception has long been stigmatized by its association with clandestine sex, prostitution and venereal disease. Even today as he purchases his sheaths a married man may sense that the retailer assumes they are probably not for intercourse with his wife. Today condoms are receiving new attention from health personnel, government campaigns and family planning clinics concerned with the increasing incidence of sexually transmitted diseases and HIV infections. An estimated 40 million couples use the condom worldwide, but with striking geographical differences. Japan accounts for more than a quarter of all condom users in the world, and 75% of couples who use any contraceptive in that country use this method. The idea of the condom as a way of reducing the risk of sexually transmitted diseases is certainly not a new one. In the 17th century when Mme de Sevigne warned her daughter she recommended condoms as 'armour against love, gossamer against infection'. Little did she realize how prophetic her comments would be. Casanova mentioned its use in his memoirs both as a contraceptive and as prophylaxis against sexually transmitted diseases.

The earliest recorded use of condoms is in Egyptian art depicting men wearing sheaths. Romans were reputed to have worn sheaths made from animal bladders to prevent sexually transmitted diseases. In 1564 the Italian anatomist Fallopio provided the first written description of the condom when he claimed that a linen sheath worn over the penis during intercourse prevented the spread of disease. In folklore the invention was much later, by Dr Condom, reputedly a physician in the court of Charles II. The origin of the word condom is uncertain; one possibility is that it is derived from the Latin word 'condus', which means receptacle. The Persian word 'kondu' meaning a long storage vessel is another possibility.

Early commercially available condoms were made from animal intestinal membranes mainly prepared from the caecum of sheep, claves and goats and had an average thickness of 0.6 mm. They are still produced in limited numbers, are expensive and therefore beyond the reach of most couples. They do not shrink or stretch and are heavily lubricated. Some men still prefer them to those made of vulcanized rubber as they feel that they transmit sensation better than rubber. The process of vulcanization of rubber, developed by Hancock and Goodyear in 1839, made it possible to produce condoms in large quantities and at cheaper prices. However, most rubber condoms produced in the early 1900s were not only defective but had a limited shelf life of only 3 months (Shenfelt 1981). The latex process introduced in the 30s eliminated most of these problems and improved both the quality and the efficacy of condoms.

Effectiveness

Rates vary from 0.5–2.0 per 100 couple years (Tatum & Connell Tatum 1981) and 4 per 100 couple years (Glass 1974) to a higher level of 15, depending on motivation (Guillebaud 1985). Theoretical failure rates can be as low as 0.4 per 100 couple years in cases where there has been no sexual contact whatever without rubber intervening and the only failure is by condom rupture (Guillebaud 1985). Pregnancy rates are highest in the young and inexperienced and among couples who wish to delay rather than avoid pregnancy (Vessey et al 1982). Older couples have lower failure rates possibly due to greater motivation, reduced natural fertility and lower frequency of sexual intercourse. In the Oxford/FPA study of a highly motivated group of couples, the pregnancy rate varied between 0.7% and 6% depending on age and past experience of condom use (Glass 1974).

Protection against STD

There is little doubt that the condom reduces the incidence of ascending vaginal infections associated with sexual intercourse. Siboulet (1972) looked at the sexual partners of 700 women with gonorrhoea. He found that less than 1% of the 302 men who used condoms contracted gonorrhoea whereas 97% of those who did not use a condom contracted the disease. Barlow (1977) and Pemberton et al (1972) demonstrated that amongst men attending a STD clinic the risk of contracting gonorrhoea and syphilis in condom users was lower than in non-users. The relative risk among users compared to non-users was 0.4.

Condoms are being promoted as a protection against the transmission of HIV. However, they only prevent the transfer of semen between partners. HIV has been isolated from saliva, vaginal secretions and blood. Because there is an exchange of other body fluids such as saliva, and occasionally blood from the gums in 'French kissing' and with orogenital contact as part of intercourse, the virus can still be passed to a partner (Goedert et al 1985). In vitro tests have shown that the HIV does not pass across an intact condom (Conant et al 1986). Although up to 5 per 1000 condoms (0.5%) may have faults, this is currently acceptable to the British Standards Institute (Self Health 1987).

In reality it is difficult to gauge how well condoms protect against STD as most studies have relied on retrospective interviews with patients attending STD clinics. However, what is clear is that consistent use of condoms does significantly reduce the incidence of STD (Barlow 1977).

Protection against cervical cell abnormalities

Two studies have shown that the use of condoms may be protective against cervical cell abnormalities. In a UK case-controlled study the relative risk

of developing severe cervical dysplasia decreased with condom and diaphragm use while it increases with Pill use (Wright et al 1978). After 10
years the relative risk for women using any barrier method was 0.2
compared to 4.0 for Pill-users. In an American study 136 out of 139 women
with cervical cell abnormalities who received no treatment apart from their
partners using a condom showed complete reversal of the condition.
(Richardson & Lyon 1981). Unfortunately there was no control group in
this study.

Spermicides

These are a wide range of substances which chemically immobilize or
destroy sperm. Spermicides are among the oldest and simplest forms of
fertility control and make a useful contribution to increasing the efficacy of
other barrier methods. They comprise two main components: a relatively
inert base material, and an active spermicidal agent. Hence they operate
both physically and biochemically, forming a partial barrier and also
immobilizing sperm. The active ingredients are of five possible types:

1. Surface acting agents, of which the most widely used are nonoxynol-9,
10 and 11, octoxinol-9, benzalkonium chloride and memfegol;

2. Enzyme inhibitors, which are compounds small enough to enter
the seminal coagulum. They interfere with enzymes of the acrosome,
hyalouronidase and proacrosin which are necessary for fertilization.
Gossypol, a cotton seed extract, is an example of such an agent. It has been
used successfully as an antispermatogenic agent vaginally. It also disrupts
spermatogenesis when given orally to men (Anonymous 1978). However,
toxicity considerations have limited its use;

3. Bactericides such as quinine sulphate and phenylmercuric acetate
(PMA), none of which are in current use.

4. Acids such as lactic acid, boric acid;

5. Local anaesthetics and other membrane-active agents, e.g.
propranolol.

Among the first commercially available spermicides were pessaries
containing soluble cocoa butter and quinine sulphate. They were developed
in 1885 by Walter Rendell, an English pharmacist. In most of the early
chemical spermicides, quinine sulphate was the active ingredient. However
chinosol, lactic acid and boric acid were also used. Phenylmercuric
acetate (PMA) was introduced in 1937 and was a more effective
spermicide than quinine sulphate. It is no longer available because of
toxicity after vaginal absorption. The next important breakthrough in
spermicide research occurred in the 1950s with the advent of surfactants
or surface acting agents. These are now the principal active agents in
spermicidal agents worldwide. They act primarily by disrupting the sperm
membrane (Bernstein 1971) by interference with oxygen-uptake and

fructolysis. Spermicides come in various forms, e.g. creams, jellies, pessaries, aerosol foams, water-soluble film, foaming tablets and foaming pessaries. To be effective the products should disperse quickly yet remain in sufficient concentration at the cervix to exert an effect at ejaculation after intercourse. Bactericides and acids are used in some preparations in place of or in addition to surfactants.

Effectiveness

Measuring the effectiveness of spermicides is a complex and difficult process depending on a variety of factors such as the type and concentration of the active ingredients, the type of base material used and its ability to dissolve, quick and even dispersal in the vagina, and above all the motivation of the woman to use the product. Failure rates based on use effectiveness studies range erroneously from about 0.3 to 40 pregnancies per 100 women-years (Coleman & Piotrow 1979). These results involved different study populations ranging from highly motivated and intelligent patients to poor, socially deprived women from developing countries. There were also different spermicidal preparations, and different study procedures and follow-up, so it is difficult to make direct comparisons between the products involved. In order to achieve maximal efficiency, spermicides need to be placed high up in the vagina before intercourse.

Pessaries require a period of 10 minutes between insertion and the moment of ejaculation for dispersion to occur and a further pessary is recommended before each new episode of intercourse. Spermicides are more effective in vitro than they ever prove to be in vivo. The general teaching is therefore that spermicides are not effective enough to be used alone. They are recommended as an adjunct to other methods, although exceptions are made if a women considers spermicides as the only acceptable method of contraception. The foams appear more acceptable and effective in most studies when used as the sole method.

Protection against infection

Tests show that spermicides offer useful protection against *Neisseria gonorrhoea, Treponema pallidum, Chlamydia, Trichomonas vaginalis,* and *Candida albicans* (Cutler et al 1977, Jick et al 1982). Laboratory studies have shown that nonoxynol-9 and various commercially available spermicidal products inactivate the AIDS virus (Feldblum et al 1986, Hicks 1985). In one study HIV inactivation occurred within 60 seconds of exposure to a nonoxynol-9 concentration of 0.05% or greater. This concentration was also toxic to lymphocytes infected by HIV (Hicks et al 1985). Commercial spermicidal preparations contain at least 1% of nonoxynol-9 or equivalent. In vivo studies on the effects of spermicides on STD organisms have mostly been small and uncontrolled. But two British

Table 22.2 Failure rates of barrier methods with age and duration of use

Method	25–34 years of age Duration of use (months)			> 35 years of age Duration of use (months)		
	24	25–48	49+	24	25–48	49+
Condom	6.0	4.0	3.6	2.9	1.3	0.7
Diaphragm	5.5	4.0	2.3	2.8	1.7	0.8

case-controlled studies found cervical dysplasia and neoplasia (thought to be associated with human papilloma virus) less common among diaphragm users than among other women (Harris et al 1980, Wright et al 1978).

Safety

It is now recognized that most substances inserted into the vagina are absorbed into the systemic circulation and hence it is impossible to say that spermicides are entirely free of potential harmful effects. To date, no serious side-effects have been reported with use of the currently available products. In 1979 it was suggested from animal studies that nonoxynol-9 might have hepatotoxic effects and affect serum lipids. Only one human study has been reported in a small group involving four women who were noted to have a reduction in their serum cholesterol levels after using nonoxynol-9 for 1–14 days (Chapvil 1984). Concern about the possible teratogenic effects of nonoxynol-9 followed a report by Jick et al (1981) who found a two-fold increase in congenital abnormalities in babies born to mothers who were thought to have used spermicides at around the time of conception, compared to controls. This study was criticized on methodological grounds, particularly the fact that the researchers were unable to confirm that the patients had actually used the spermicide specifically at the time of conception. Subsequent studies failed to demonstrate an association between spermicide use and birth defects (Shapiro et al 1982). The study was not standardized for other variables associated with teratogenic effects such as drug-taking and cigarette smoking.

NEW DEVELOPMENTS

Female condom (Femshield®)

This a loose-fitting, soft thermoplastic polyether polyurethane sheath made to cover the vagina and the external genitalia. It is 15 cm in length and has a polyurethane ring on either end. The inner ring, measuring 65 mm, is used as an introducer and as a means of anchoring the device in

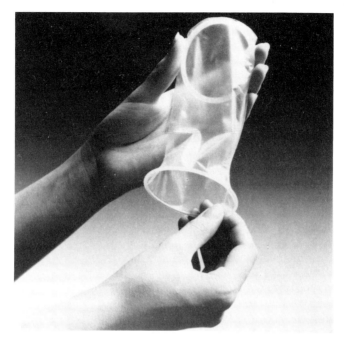

Fig. 22.3 Femshield (female condom). Reproduced with permission from Medicor International Limited.

the vagina. The outer ring, measuring 70 mm, lies against the external genitalia covering it and the base of the penis during intercourse (see Fig. 22.3). This idea was developed as a variant of the condom with the aim of overcoming most of the drawbacks associated with use of that method. The advantages apart from contraceptive would be that it would also reduce the incidence of STDs and particularly the transmission of HIV during vaginal intercourse. The results of the Margaret Pyke Centre study, using volunteers who were otherwise protected against pregnancy (79% using contraception and 21% previously sterilized) show that 50% of women and 54% of men considered the method acceptable (Bounds et al 1988). Moreover, 63% of the men and 79% of the women found the effects on sexual pleasure to be either unchanged or better when compared with the condom.

Since around 50% of couples in that study found the method acceptable according to the questions asked, the likely advantages are:

1. It can be purchased over the counter, with no 'fitting', few rules, and no clinic attendance;
2. It is under the woman's control therefore it can be fitted well in advance;
3. It offers protection against pregnancy as well as STD;

4. It is said to be stronger than the latex condom and hence less likely to rupture;
5. It is likely to be more effective than the condom (unproven as yet) because:
   a. it can be used before full erection
   b. 'slipping' means slipping out of the vagina and not off into the vagina as with the condom;
6. It permits continued intimacy during the resolution phase after intercourse;
7. Men prefer the lack of rubber membrane closely applied to the penis, i.e. 'freedom' to move in a secondary lubricated vagina;
8. It can be used for selected gynaecological indications including:
   a. menstruation
   b. vaginal discharge or during treatment with vaginal pessaries
   c. superficial dyspareunia
   d. in the puerperium.

In vitro studies show that the cytomegalovirus and HIV do not penetrate the Femshield® membrane (Bounds et al 1988). This device may become nationally available in the near future.

Disposable spermicide-coated diaphragms

These are made of sponge-like materials and are currently under study. They have been designed to overcome the perceived 'messiness' associated with the current spermicides.

New cervical caps

There has been great interest in the concept of a custom-fitted cervical cap which is made from a mould of the user's cervix. The idea of a non-spermicidal custom-fitted cervical cap designed to be left in place for 3 months at a time, with a one-way valve to allow the passage of cervical secretions and menstrual loss was most attractive. However in practice the failure rate was shown to be unacceptably high, with 9 accidental pregnancies among 29 women who used the Contracap® as their method of contraception for a total of only 72 women-months (Bounds et al 1986).

Intracervical devices

Both medicated and non-medicated devices with some kind of flange or protruding wings to anchor them in the endocervical canal are being investigated. Some are designed to block the cervical canal mechanically while still providing a valve mechanism to allow menstrual fluid and secretions to pass through. The medicated devices under investigation have a silastic rod containing either a progestogen or a spermicide.

Vaginal rings containing nonoxynol-9

The WHO has been testing a silicone ring that releases nonoxynol-9 at a constant rate over 30 days. There are as yet no data on efficacy.

Vaginal rings containing hormones

WHO-sponsored research into two types of rings, one releasing levonorgestrel and the other containing progesterone, is well under way in a number of centres. The levonorgestrel ring with an overall diameter of 55.6 mm, is designed to stay in the vagina for 3 months and releases 20 µg of levonorgestrel per day. In a multicentre trial involving 1000 women the pregnancy rate was calculated to be 3.5 per 100 woman years (WHO Report 1985). The problems encountered were similar to those associated with use of other progestogen-only methods, e.g. irregular vaginal bleeding, which accounted for most of the discontinuations. There was a 4% expulsion rate and 8% of women stopped using the method because of a vaginal discharge. The progesterone ring contains the natural hormone and was designed especially for breast-feeding women. It can remain in the vagina for 3 months and no results are as yet available.

New spermicides

An organic compound (RS 37367) developed by Syntex Research is reported to be 50 times more potent than nonoxynol-9. Drugs that inhibit the sperm's own enzymes, principally acrosin, show promise. Propranolol, a beta-blocker, used for hypertensive disorders among other indications, has also been shown to exhibit spermicidal properties (Zipper et al 1983). Used vaginally in its weak, beta-blocking form (D-propranolol) it was found to be as potent a spermicide as nonoxynol-9 (Tayob 1986).

REFERENCES

Anonymous 1978 Gossypol—a new antifertility agent for males. Chinese Medical Journal 4: 417
Barlow D 1977 Condoms and gonorrhoea. Lancet ii: 811–812
Bernstein G S 1971 Clinical effectiveness of an aerosol contraceptive foam. Contraception 3(1): 37–43
Bernstein G S, Kilzer L H, Coulson A H et al 1982 Studies of cervical caps: 1. Vaginal lesions associated with use of the Vimule cap. Contraception 26(5): 443–456
Boehm D 1983 The cervical cap: effectiveness as a contraceptive. Journal of Nurse Midwifery 28(1): 3–6
Bounds W, Guillebaud J 1984 Randomised comparison of the use-effectiveness and patient acceptability of the colltex (Today®) contraceptive sponge and the diaphragm. British Journal of Family Planning 10: 69–75
Bounds W, Kubba A, Tayob Y, Mills A, Guillebaud J 1986 Clinical trial of a spermicide-free, custom-fitted, valved cervical cap (Contracap®). British Journal of Family Planning 11: 125–131

Bounds W, Guillebaud J, Stewart L, Steele S J 1988 A female condom (Femshield®): a study of its user-acceptability. British Journal of Family Planning 14: 83–87

Casanova, J 1922 Memoires de Jacques Casanova de Seingalt. J. Rosez, Brussels, p 552

Chavpil M, Eskelson C D, Droegmueller W 1979 New data on the pharmokinetics of nonoxynol-9. In: Zatuchni G I et al (eds) Vaginal contraception: new developments. Harper & Row, Hagerstown, pp 110–115, 165–174

Coleman S, Piotrow P T 1979 Barrier methods: spermicides—simplicity and safety are major aspects. Population Reports Series H 5

Conant M, Hardy D, Sernatinger J, Spicer D, Levy J A 1986 Condoms prevent transmission of AIDS-associated retroviruses. Journal of the American Medical Association 255: 1706

Craig, S, Hepburn S 1982 The effectiveness of barrier methods of contraception with and without spermicides. Contraception 26: 347–359

Cutler J C, Singh B, Carpenter U et al 1977 Vaginal contraceptives as prophylaxis against gonorrhoea and other sexually transmissable diseases. Advances in Planned Parenthood 12(1): 45–56

Edelman, D A, McIntyre S L, Harper J 1984 Comparative trial of the Today® contraceptive sponge and diaphragm. American Journal of Obstetrics and Gynecology 150: 869–876

Feldblum P J, Rosenberg M J 1986 Spermicides and sexually transmitted diseases: new perspectives. North Carolina Medical Journal 47: 569–572

Fischl M A, Dickinson G M, Scott G B, Klimas N, Fletcher M A, Parks W 1987 Evaluation of heterosexual partners, children and household contacts of adults with AIDS. Journal of the American Medical Association 257: 640

Free M J, Alexander A J 1976 Male contraception without prescription. Public Health Reports 91(5): 437–445

Goedert J J, Biggar R J, Winn D M et al 1985 Decreased helper T-lymphocytes in homosexual men: sexual practices. American Journal of Epidemiology 122: 637–644

Glass R, Vessey M, Wiggins P 1974 Use-effectiveness of the condom in a selected family planning clinic population in the United Kingdom. Contraception 10: 591–598

Guillebaud J 1985 Contraception: your questions answered. Pitman Publishing, London

Guttmacher, A F 1973 Pregnancy, birth and family planning. Viking, New York, pp 287–289

Harris R W C, Brinton L A, Cowdell R H et al 1980 Characteristics of women with dysplasia or carcinoma in situ of the cervix uteri. British Journal of Cancer 42(3): 359–369

Hicks D R, Martin L S, Getchell J P et al 1985 Inactivation of HTLV-III/LAV-infected cultures of normal human lymphocytes by nonoxynol-9 in vitro. Lancet ii: 1422

Himes N E 1970 Medical history of contraception. Schocken Books, New York

Jick H, Walker A M, Rothman K J et al 1981 Vaginal spermicides and congenital disorders. Journal of the American Medical Association 245(13): 1329–1332

Jick H, Hannan M T, Stergachis A, Heidrich F, Perera D R, Rothman K J 1982 Vaginal spermicides and gonorrhoea. Journal of the American Medical Association 248(13): 1619–1621

Johnson V, Masters M, Cramer Lewis K 1974 In: Calderone M L (ed) Manual of family planning and contraceptive practice. Williams and Watkins, Baltimore, pp 237–238

Koch J P 1982 The Prentif contraceptive cervical cap: acceptability aspects and their implications for future cap design. Contraception 25(2): 161–163

Lane M E, Areco R, Sobrero A J 1976 Successful use of the diaphragm and jelly by a young population. Family Planning Perspectives 8: 81–86

Lefheldt H 1949 The firm cervical cap: 156 case records. Journal of Sex Education 1(4): 132–143

Mills A 1988 AIDS and barriers. In: Hudson C N, Sharp F (eds) AIDS and obstetrics and gynaecology. Proceedings of the 19th Study Group of the Royal College of Obstetrics and Gynaecology, London, March 1988

Pemberton J, McCann J S, Mahony J P H 1972 Sociomedical characteristics of patients attending a VD clinic and the circumstances of infection. British Journal of Venereal Disease 48(5): 391–396

Preuss J 1978 Biblical and talmudic medicine. Hebrew Publishing Company, New York

Richardson A C, Lyon A B 1981 The effect of condom use on squamous cell cervical intraepithelial neoplasia. American Journal of Obstetrics and Gynecology 140(8): 909–913

Self Health 1987 London Rubber Company, London, p 12

Serlin R 1981 Contraceptives: back to the barriers. 91(1264): 281–284

Shapiro S, Slone D, Heinonen O P et al 1982 Birth defects and vaginal spermicides. Journal of the American Medical Association 247: 2381–2384

Shenefelt P D 1981 The condom as a contraceptive and prophylactic—an appraisal. Wisconsin Medical Journal 80(9): 19–20

Siboulet A 1972 Maladies sexuelles transmissibles: interet des traitements prophylactiques. Prophylaxie Sanitaire et Morale 44(5): 155–159

Stewart G J, Tyler J P P, Cunningham A L et al 1985 Transmission of human T-cell lymphotropic virus type III (HTLV-III) by artificial insemination by donor. Lancet *ii*: 581–585

Tatum H J, Connell Tatum E B 1981 Barrier contraception: a comprehensive overview. Fertility and Sterility 36(1): 1–12

Tayob Y, Bounds W, Pearce R, Guillebaud J 1986 Propanolol: a novel effective spermicide compared with nonoxynol-9 and placebo. Abstracts of the 12th World Congress in Fertility and Sterility, Singapore, October 1986

Tietze C, Lefheldt H, Liebmann H G 1953 The effectiveness of the cervical cap as a contraceptive method. American Journal of Obstetrics and Gynecology 66(4): 904–908

Toth A, Lesser M, Labriola D 1984 Development of infections of the genito-urinary tract in wives of infertile males and possible role of spermatozoa in development of salpingitis. Surgical Gynaecology and Obstetrics 159: 565–569

Vessey M, Lawless M, Yeates D 1982 Efficiency of different contraceptive methods. Lancet *i*: 841–842

Vessey M, Doll E, Peto R, Johnson B, Wiggins P 1976 A long-term follow-up study of women using different methods of contraception—an interim report. Journal of Biosocial Science 8: 375–427

Westerom L 1980 Incidence, prevalence and trends of pelvic inflammatory disease and its consequences in industrialized countries. American Journal of Obstetrics and Gynecology 139: 880

World Health Organization 1985 Special programme of research, development and research training in human reproduction: 4th Annual Report. WHO, Geneva, pp 152

Wright N H, Vessey M P, Kenward B, McPherson K, Doll R 1978 Neoplasia and dysplasia of the cervix uteri and contraception: a possible protective effect of the diaphragm. British Journal of Cancer 38: 273–279

Zagury D, Bernard J, Liebowitch J 1985 HTLV-III in cells cultured from semen of two patients with AIDS. Science 226: 449–456

Zipper J, Wheeler R G, Potts D M, Rivera M 1983 Propranolol as a novel, effective spermicide: preliminary findings. British Medical Journal 287: 1245–1246

Index